Essentials of Dental Hygiene
Preclinical Skills

Mary D. Cooper, RDH, MSEd
Professor in Dental Hygiene
Indiana University Purdue University Fort Wayne
Fort Wayne, Indiana

Lauri Wiechmann, RDH, MPA
Coordinator, Dental Hygiene Program
Carl Sandburg College
Galesburg, Illinois

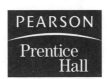

PEARSON
Prentice
Hall

Upper Saddle River, New Jersey 07458

Library of Congress Cataloging-in-Publication Data

Cooper, Mary Danusis.
  Essentials of dental hygiene: preclinical skills / Mary Danusis
Cooper & Lauri Wiechmann. — 1st ed.
    p. cm.
  ISBN 0-13-094104-2
1. Dental hygiene.   I. Wiechmann, Lauri.   II. Title.
  RK60.5.C667 2004
  617.6'01—dc22

                                              2003023259

Publisher: Julie Levin Alexander
Assistant to Publisher: Regina Bruno
Acquisitions Editor: Mark Cohen
Associate Editor: Melissa Kerian
Editorial Assistants: Mary Ellen Ruitenberg and Jaquay Felix
Channel Marketing Manager: Rachele Strober
Director of Production and Manufacturing: Bruce Johnson
Managing Production Editor: Patrick Walsh
Production Liaison: Danielle Newhouse
Production Editor: Marianne Hutchinson, Pine Tree Composition

Manufacturing Manager: Ilene Sanford
Manufacturing Buyer: Pat Brown
Design Director: Cheryl Asherman
Design Coordinator: Maria Guglielmo Walsh
Cover Designer: Kevin Kall
Cover Image: Getty Images/Brand X
Composition: Pine Tree Composition, Inc.
Manager of Media Production: Amy Peltier
New Media Project Manager: Stephen Hartner
Printing and Binding: Banta Book Group
Cover Printer: Phoenix Color Corp.

Pearson Education, Ltd., *London*
Pearson Education Australia Pty. Limited, *Sydney*
Pearson Education Singapore Pte. Ltd.
Pearson Education North Asia Ltd., *Hong Kong*
Pearson Education Canada, Ltd., *Toronto*
Pearson Educación de Mexico, S.A. de C.V.
Pearson Education—Japan, *Tokyo*
Pearson Education Malaysia, Pte. Ltd.
Pearson Education, Upper Saddle River, New Jersey

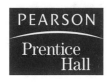

10 9 8 7 6 5 4 3 2 1
ISBN 0-13-094104-2

To my husband, George, and our son, George IV—you have brought me more joy than you will ever know. Some people wait a lifetime to have what I have with both of you. Thank you for your love and support and for being the rocks in my life. You are a blessing.

To my parents, Afrodhiti and the late Dimitrios Danusis—thank you for coming to this country to give your children an opportunity for a better life—for this sacrifice alone, I am forever indebted to you. I also want to thank you for instilling upon us a strong work ethic—you always taught us that anything is possible. Because of your support, I have made achievements I thought were not possible to reach.

To Lauri Wiechmann—thank you for your trust in me, for your dedication to dental hygiene, and for making this project most enjoyable.

To my students—your encouragement and support are the reasons I continue to enjoy teaching. I feel blessed to have each of you as a part in my life.

—Mary Danusis Cooper

To my husband, Jay, and our daughters, Kendra and Colleen—thank you for your patience, love, and support. You are the beacon of light in my life! There are few things in life that we are blessed with—I thank the Lord daily for each of you!

To my parents and family—thank you for the guidance and words of wisdom over the years. The path that led me here is marked with remembrances of your love.

To Mary Cooper—you are a wonderful mentor. Thank you for helping me follow my dreams. This has been a great trip with you!

To my present and former students—it is because of you that I continue to achieve professionally. I always wish the best for you!

—Lauri Wiechmann

Contents

Preface

Essentials of Dental Hygiene is written for the first-year, first semester of the dental hygiene curriculum. The purpose of this book is to develop basic introductory skills that will be utilized while providing dental hygiene care in the clinical setting. The challenge for us was to design the book focusing solely on the skills necessary to provide initial treatment for the dental hygiene patient. We recognize there are more skills and services involved in the comprehensive care of the patient—those additional skills and services will be covered in a follow up textbook.

The ten chapters are introduced in the order the dental hygienist provides treatment for the patient. Each chapter is written in an outline format, which offers the student a comfortable style for reading the material, while providing basic, fundamental information. Each chapter provides the first-year dental hygiene student the opportunity to learn about an individual process or skill in a step-by-step sequence. Not only are the skills provided—the hows—but also the reasons—the whys.

Objectives are listed at the beginning of each chapter. This provides the student with fundamental concepts contained within the chapter. Key terms are also provided at the beginning of each chapter as a quick, easy glossary reference. Contained within each chapter are text boxes containing interesting information the dental hygiene student will find useful.

References to current literature are made throughout the book. They reflect current research results and support the philosophy of life-long learning. At the end of the chapter are review questions, which serve as a self-evaluation for the student. Students can review the text, answer the questions, and reflect back to the material to reinforce the information. In addition, a companion CD-ROM supplements the procedures presented in the written text through video clips and additional photographs.

Each chapter presents the following information:

Chapter 1, "Infection Control," focuses on the basic clinical applications of infection control necessary to provide dental care.

Chapter 2, "Medical/Dental Histories," introduces common conditions patients present with and how to address these conditions in a thorough and professional manner.

Chapter 3, "Vital Signs," stresses the need for baseline readings such as blood pressure, temperature, pulse, and respiration and for determining contraindications for treatment based on the findings.

Chapter 4, "Extraoral and Intraoral Examinations," addresses techniques used and structures examined when providing an examination of the head and neck.

Chapter 5, "Examination and Charting of the Hard and Soft Tissues," discusses how to examine the dentition and to record findings on the dentition and periodontal charts respectively.

Chapter 6, "Preventive Dentistry," provides information used during oral hygiene instructions from plaque development to methods of plaque removal.

Chapter 7, "Ergonomics," stresses the importance of maintaining neutral body positions to protect the body from injury while providing dental hygiene care. Exercises are included that can be performed during the workday.

Chapter 8, "Instrumentation," introduces basic instrument setup used to provide dental hygiene care for the patient with minimal calculus and disease, since these are the patients most first-year students will perform on during their initial clinical exposure. Focus is on foundational skills and instrumentation principles.

Chapter 9, "Polishing," focuses on the theory of stain removal and explains the agents and techniques used to remove stain.

Chapter 10, "Fluorides," presents information needed to make an educated decision regarding the most appropriate and effective fluoride therapy for the patient.

Acknowledgments

We would like to convey our sincere appreciation to the contributors who dedicated many hours to developing this quality textbook. Each has made a personal contribution and commitment to helping dental hygiene students attain the knowledge and skills needed to provide direct care for patients.

We also acknowledge the support of individuals who helped us with photographs, videotape for the CD-ROM, typing, and mailing: Kim Norris, Stephanie Burkhardt, and Fritz Archer from Carl Sandburg College. Thank you to Harold Henson, from the University of Texas at Houston Dental Branch, School of Dental Hygiene, for providing some of the photographs for the Ergonomics chapter. Also, a special thank you to Elmer Denman from the Learning Resource Center at Indiana University Purdue University Fort Wayne, for his talent in taking several of the photographs.

Reviewers

Marsha E. Bower, RDH, MA, CDA
Assistant Professor
Monroe Community College
Rochester, New York

Pamela Brilowski, MS
Dental Hygiene Coordinator
Waukesha County Technical College
Pewaukee, Wisconsin

Suzanne M. Edenfield, EdD, RDH
Associate Professor
Armstrong Atlantic State University
Savannah, Georgia

Paula J. Fitch, RDH, MSEd
Associate Professor, Dental Hygiene
    Clinic Coordinator
Broome Community College
Binghamton, New York

Judith A. Hall, RDH, BS
Department Chair, Dental Hygiene
Delaware Technical and Community College
Wilmington, Delaware

Marilyn Kalal, RDH, MS
Professor of Dental Hygiene
Quinsigamond College
Worcester, Massachusetts

Contributors

Mary D. Cooper, RDH, MSEd
Professor in Dental Hygiene
Indiana University Purdue University Fort Wayne
Fort Wayne, Indiana

Nancy Cuttic, BSDH, MEd
Associate Professor
Harcum College
Bryn Mawr, Pennsylvania

Anne N. Guignon, RDH, MPH
Private Practice
Houston, Texas

William A. Johnson, DMD, MPH
Director, Dental Auxiliary Programs
Chattanooga State Technical
Community College
Chattanooga, Tennessee

Nancy K. Mann, RDH, MSEd
Clinical Assistant Professor in Dental Hygiene
Indiana University Purdue University Fort Wayne
Fort Wayne, Indiana

Mary Kaye Scaramucci, RDH, MS
Associate Professor in Dental Hygiene
University of Cincinnati, Raymond and Walters
   College
Cincinnati, Ohio

Lauri Wiechmann, RDH, MPA
Coordinator, Dental Hygiene Program
Carl Sandburg College
Galesburg, Illinois

Chapter 1

Infection Control

Mary Kaye Scaramucci, RDH, MS

MediaLink

A companion CD-ROM, included free with each new copy of this book, supplements the procedures presented in each chapter. Insert the CD-ROM to watch video clips and view a large collection of color images that is also included. This multimedia library is designed to help you add a new dimension to your learning.

KEY TERMS

aerosols. Creation of airborne microorganisms.

antimicrobial. A substance or drug that inhibits or controls the growth of microorganisms.

aseptic. Techniques and methods used to reduce and/or eliminate the likelihood of spreading disease microorganisms.

bioburden. Microbial or organic material on a surface, instrument, or object.

biofilm. Microorganisms that accumulate in moist environments, increasing patients' susceptibility to a communicable disease.

carrier. An individual who has been exposed to and harbors an infectious agent, displays no clinical signs or symptoms of disease, yet serves as a source of infection.

communicable disease. An infectious disease that can be transferred by direct or indirect contact.

contamination. A surface, instrument, or object that has been infected with pathogenic microorganisms.

cross-contamination. The process of spreading infection from one person to another by way of contact with an infected surface, object, or instrument.

direct contamination. Transfer of a communicable disease from the host (person infected with the disease) to another person.

disinfection. The process of killing or reducing pathogenic microorganisms; does not include the destruction of bacterial spores.

endemic. Native to a particular country, nation, or region; generally refers to a disease that is under control.

immunization. To give immunity to a person by inoculation.

incinerate. To burn to ashes.

incubation. The period of time from exposure to a pathogenic microorganism and the appearance of signs or symptoms of the disease.

indirect contamination. Transfer of a communicable disease from the host to an inanimate object (i.e., contaminated instrument) to another person.

latency period. The time in which a communicable disease appears to be dormant, showing no signs or symptoms of that disease yet having the potential for recurrent infection.

microbe. A disease-causing organism that can be seen only with a microscope, not with the naked eye.

opportunistic infection. Infections with any organism (especially fungi and bacteria) that occur due to the opportunity allowed by the altered state of the host.

OSHA. Occupational Safety and Health Administration; a division of the U.S. Department of Labor whose purpose is to ensure the safety and protection of employees.

pathogenic. Disease-causing microorganisms.

perinatal. Involving or occurring during the period closest to birth.

personal protective equipment (PPE). Consists of surface barriers for equipment and clothing for the operator and patient.

residual bacteria. Species of microorganisms that are always present in or on the body.

sanitation. The process of cleaning to remove dust, dirt, and gross debris, and not necessarily destroying pathogenic microorganisms but reducing them to a safe level.

seroconversion. The time at which an individual, once inoculated, has developed immunity to a pathogenic disease.

spatter. Large particles of moisture that may carry infectious agents.

spores. A resistant form of bacteria that does not have the capabilities of reproduction.

spray. Small particles of moisture that may carry infectious agents.

sputum. Saliva mixed with mucus from the respiratory tract that is ejected from the mouth.

sterilization. The process used to destroy, by physical or chemical means, all pathogenic microorganisms, including bacterial spores.

transient bacteria. Microorganisms that are *not* always present in or on the body.

universal precautions. Procedures designed to ensure treatment is rendered in a safe manner regardless of the health of the patient.

LEARNING OBJECTIVES

After reading this chapter, the student should be able to:

- apply the clinical aseptic practices that protect the patient, community, and dental team from disease and cross-contamination;
- describe the mechanisms for the transfer of infectious diseases;
- discuss the disease process, transmission, and clinical management of infectious diseases;
- compare and contrast sanitation, disinfection, and sterilization;
- list and discuss three methods of sterilization;
- describe the method for disinfecting surfaces in the operatory;
- identify five chemical solutions approved for surface disinfection;
- determine which immunizations and vaccines provide personal protection for the dental team;

- compare and contrast the use of barriers versus disinfection for surface decontamination to prevent disease transmission;
- demonstrate the short scrub and handwashing technique and determine when each should be implemented;
- demonstrate the decontamination of the operatory before and between patient care;
- describe the process in preparing contaminated instruments for sterilization;
- explain the purpose and use of the material safety data sheets (MSDS) in the dental office;
- identify the components of the MSDS;
- recognize the hazard symbols as they relate to products used in dentistry;
- recognize asepsis as a valuable component of the dental hygiene care plan;
- describe the responsibility for protecting patients, colleagues, and personnel from disease transmission.

I. Introduction

The oral cavity maintains one of the most concentrated microbial populations of the entire body. Dental personnel are in contact with potentially pathogenic microorganisms every working day. Proper handling and preparation of equipment should ensure that all instruments and equipment are completely free of viable bacteria, viruses, and spores, and that their usefulness is maintained. Goals for universal precautions include the following:

A. Reduce or eliminate the number of available pathogenic microorganisms

B. Break the cycle of infection and eliminate cross-contamination

C. Treat every patient and instrument as a vehicle for transmission of an infectious disease

D. Protect patients and personnel from infections, and protect all dental personnel from the threat of malpractice[1]

II. Communicable Diseases (Table 1–1)

A variety of diseases can be transmitted by blood, blood products, secretions, and saliva. Maintaining aseptic practices is of utmost importance to protect the dental team from contamination and subsequently protect patients from cross-contamination. The following are common diseases that have the potential to be transmitted during dental hygiene care.

A. Hepatitis: A highly infectious viral disease that causes inflammation of the liver and is transmitted by means of body secretions, blood, and blood products

    1. Five forms of hepatitis

        a. Hepatitis A (HAV): Formerly known as infectious hepatitis; the least serious form

            (1) Epidemiology: Approximately 100,000 infected cases reported in the United States each year

            (2) Incubation and symptoms

                (a) Incubation period: 15 to 50 days

Table 1–1   Communicable Diseases Chart

Disease	Incubation	Symptoms	Transmission	Precautions	Vaccine
HAV	15–50 days	Flu-like	Fecal contamination	Handwashing and sanitary waste disposal	Yes. HAVRIX and VAQTA (recalled)
HBV	45–160 days	Fever, extreme fatigue, joint pain, jaundice, rash	Blood, saliva, semen, vaginal fluids	Immunization, barriers/disposables, disinfection, sterilization	Yes Recombivax HB & Enerix B
HCV	2–20 weeks	None or those similar to HBV	Percutaneous exposure to blood or plasma	Barriers/disposables, disinfection, sterilization	No
HDV	Abrupt	Resemble HBV	Same as HBV	Same as HBV	Yes. Same as HBV
HE/GV	15–50 days	Same as HAV	Contaminated water, feces, saliva	Same as HAV	No
Herpes	Varies after initial exposure	Usually a vesicular lesion	Depending on virus form: fluid in vesicles, saliva, urine, cervical secretions, breast milk, semen	Postpone treatment when symptoms are present, barriers/disposables, disinfection, sterilization	No
HIV	Varies depending on stage of disease	Flu-like to debilitation depending on stage	Evident in blood, vaginal secretions, breast milk, and semen	Barriers/disposables, disinfection, sterilization	No. 40 experimental vaccines in clinical trials
Syphilis	Primary: 3 weeks Secondary: 6 months Tertiary: 10+ years	Chancre, body rash, fever, weight loss	Direct contact with the lesion or sexual contact; infected mothers can pass on to unborn children	Transmission is low; barriers/disposables, disinfection, sterilization	No
Gonorrhea	2–7 days	Lesion at site of infection with possible inflammation of throat and oral cavity	Direct contact with the lesion or sexual contact	Same as syphilis	No
Tuberculosis	12 weeks	Fever, weight loss, night sweats, cough with sputum	Inhalation of infectious droplet (sputum)	Barriers/disposables, disinfection, sterilization	No

Courtesy of Mary Kaye Scaramucci, RDH, MS. University of Cincinnati, Raymond Walters College, Dental Hygiene Program.

(b) Symptoms: None or flu-like[2, 3]

(3) Mode of transmission

   (a) Person-to-person contact, generally through fecal or oral route contamination facilitated by poor hygiene or sanitation and intimate contact; also waterborne and through food

   (b) Those at risk include
- Childcare providers
- International travelers
- Healthcare workers[4, 5]

   (c) Once exposed to HAV, immunity to reinfection following recovery[5]

   (d) Rarely enters the carrier state[3, 4]

(4) Precautions: Prevention includes

   (a) Meticulous handwashing by all individuals who come in direct contact with the infected person

   (b) Sterilizing instruments

   (c) Using disposable items

   (d) Using universal precautions

   (e) Obtaining vaccinations

   (f) Drinking bottled water when traveling abroad

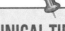

PRECLINICAL TIP

Cleansing Your Knowledge: Incubation period is the interval between exposure to an infection and the first visible signs and symptoms of the infection. The individual is unaware of the presence of the disease, but may be contagious.

b. Hepatitis B (HBV): A potentially fatal bloodborne disease
   (1) Epidemiology: Approximately 1 million cases reported in the United States, with 300,000 new cases each year[3, 5]
   (2) Incubation and symptoms
       (a) Incubation period: 45 to 160 days[2, 5]
       (b) Symptoms: Fever, malaise, extreme fatigue, skin rash, joint pain, and jaundice
   (3) Mode of transmission
       (a) Direct contact with infected body fluids; while all body fluids carry the virus, only blood, saliva, semen, and vaginal fluids are infected[3, 5]
       (b) Those at risk include
           • Healthcare workers
           • Parenteral drug users
           • Infants born to HIV-infected mothers
           • Homosexuals/heterosexuals with many partners not practicing safe sex
           • Travelers to areas where HBV is endemic[6]
           • Those who have body piercing(s)
           • Those who use infected toothbrushes, razors, or similar hygiene aids
       (c) Five to 10 percent of all HBV develops into the carrier state, while approximately 15,000 cases become chronic disease carriers;[3, 5] both types of carriers are extremely contagious
   (4) Precautions: Prevention includes
       (a) Obtaining vaccination; vaccines for active immunization are also available in the form of anti-HBs immune globulin[7]—globulins derived from blood plasma of human donors who have high titers of antibodies against hepatitis B surface antigen
       (b) Practicing universal precautions
       (c) Using disposable equipment and barriers
       (d) Decreasing aerosol production; for example, avoiding use of ultrasonic scalers or air polishers and performing minimal polishing
c. Hepatitis C (HCV): Formerly known as non-A/non-B hepatitis; most commonly associated with blood transfusions
   (1) Incubation and symptoms
       (a) Incubation period: 2 to 20 weeks[5, 8]
       (b) Onset possibly insidious with no clinical symptoms, or symptoms can be same as HBV
       (c) Chronic liver disease is common
   (2) Mode of transmission
       (a) Percutaneous exposure to contaminated blood or plasma through needles, syringes, transfusions, accidental needle stick injuries, and IV drug use
       (b) Kidney dialysis patients
       (c) Intimate sexual contact or perinatal exposure[5, 8]
       (d) Body piercings
       (e) Use of infected toothbrush, razor, or similar hygiene aids

📌

PRECLINICAL TIP

Cleansing Your Knowledge: Prior to 1992, there was an increased risk of contracting HCV through blood transfusions and organ transplants because there was no testing for the presence of HCV. Today's tests identify those who are infected with the virus and provide a screening for potential blood donors.

(3) Precautions: Prevention includes following all measures recommended for HBV

(4) No vaccine presently available for pre- or post-exposure prophylaxis[5]

   d. Hepatitis D (HDV): Also known as delta hepatitis, causes infection only in the presence of HBV

     (1) Incubation and symptoms

       (a) Abrupt onset

       (b) Signs and symptoms resemble HBV

       (c) Infection occurs simultaneously with HBV or attaches to an HBV carrier or chronic carrier; in addition, a delta carrier state may develop[3, 5]

     (2) Mode of transmission

       (a) Same as HBV

       (b) Occurs primarily in individuals who have had HBV

     (3) Precautions: Since HDV is dependent upon HBV, prevention includes the same measures used to prevent HBV, such as HBV vaccination and decreasing aerosol production by healthcare worker

   e. Hepatitis E and G are predominantly found in third-world countries where water supplies are unsanitary

     (1) Incubation and symptoms: Onset and symptoms are the same as HAV

     (2) Mode of transmission

       (a) Water contamination

       (b) Person-to-person by fecal or oral route

     (3) Precautions: Prevention includes

       (a) Meticulous handwashing, especially prior to handling food

       (b) Sanitary waste disposal

       (c) Drinking bottled water

B. Herpes virus

1. Consists of a variety of disease entities

   a. Herpes simplex 1 (HSV-1): Associated with lesions of the oral/facial region

   b. HSV-2: Associated with genital lesions and proctitis—sexually transmitted

   c. Epstein-Barr virus (EBV): Responsible for infectious mononucleosis

   d. Varicella-zoster virus (VZV): Results in chicken pox in children and shingles in adults

   e. Cytomegalovirus (HMCV): Responsible for the fetal or adult infection called cytomegalovirus disease

2. Viral latency

   a. All forms of the herpes virus have a latency period and will lie dormant among neural ganglia until triggered by a stimulus such as sunlight, stress, or illness

   b. After initial exposure, the virus will lay dormant in specific nerve ganglia: HSV remains dormant in the trigeminal ganglia, EBV is dormant in the throat and B-lymphocytes, and VZV migrates to the dorsal root and sensory ganglia

PRECLINICAL TIP

Cleansing Your Knowledge: Chicken pox and shingles are the result of the varicella-zoster virus. Mononucleosis is the result of the Epstein-Barr virus. Cytomegalovirus disease is caused by the cytomegalovirus. Oral and genital herpes is the result of herpes simplex 1 and 2 respectively.

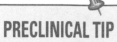

PRECLINICAL TIP

Cleansing Your Knowledge: Note when *not* to treat a patient with herpes. Do not treat if lesion is open and weeping. While the virus is not present when the lesion is crusted and dried, there is the potential to break open a dried lesion to cause bleeding and prolong the healing process. Ideally, it is best to treat when the lesion is completely healed. However, applying a nonpetroleum-based lubricant to a dried lesion can prevent reinjury.

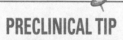

PRECLINICAL TIP

Cleansing Your Knowledge: While HIV has been found in many fluids, there is no specific evidence linking any fluids other than blood, semen, vaginal secretions, and breast milk in the transmission. Studies suggest that the reasons are poor routes of transmission, susceptibility of the host, virulence of the HIV strain, and dose of virus and inoculum size. In particular, research has shown that saliva appears to inhibit HIV infection of target cells, thus *not* serving as a mode of transmission.[3]

    c. Initial exposure occurs by direct or indirect contact with the fluid from the vesicles or respiratory droplet, depending on the virus form

    d. Recurrent lesions are precipitated by sunlight, stress, illness, or trauma, and usually reappear in the proximity of the primary site of infection

3. Mode of transmission

    a. Herpes simplex 1 and 2 shed virus in the fluid from the vesicle; can spread from person to person and to other areas of the infected person;[9] some research indicates a relationship between herpes simplex 1 and Bell's palsy

    b. Epstein-Barr virus is found in the saliva of infected individuals; virus is excreted even when the individual has no symptoms of the disease[3]

    c. Varicella-zoster is discharged from ruptured vesicles on the skin and via the respiratory tract (coughing, breathing)[3]

    d. Cytomegalovirus is found in urine, saliva, cervical secretions, breast milk, and semen[3]

4. Precautions and treatment

    a. Postpone treatment when signs and symptoms of the disease are present; avoid contact with weeping lesions because contact can spread the virus from person to person or to other areas on the infected person

    b. Adhere to strict universal precautions

    c. No approved vaccines are currently available; however, two vaccines are in clinical trials[10]

C. Human immunodeficiency virus (HIV) infection and acquired immune deficiency syndrome (AIDS) are in epidemic proportions around the world

1. HIV: Compromises infected person's immune system, rendering him or her unable to fight off opportunistic infections

2. AIDS: Last stage of the infectious process, resulting in death

3. Mode of transmission

    a. Transmission of the virus is by way of blood, vaginal secretions, breast milk, and semen;[3] HIV has been found in blood, saliva, tears, urine, spinal fluid, semen, vaginal secretions, breast milk, and amniotic fluid

    b. Vehicles for transmission of the virus include

        (1) Engaging in unprotected sex with an HIV-infected person

        (2) Using contaminated needles

        (3) Having direct contact with infected blood or blood products

        (4) Receiving a transplant from an HIV-infected body part

        (5) An infected mother giving birth via vaginal delivery[3]

4. Precautions and treatment

    a. Use proper universal precautions, with disinfection, sterilization, personal protection equipment (PPE), and barriers to prevent spreading the virus

    b. No vaccine is currently available; however, there are medications for those who are HIV positive to help delay seroconversion to AIDS[1]

D. Syphilis: A sexually transmitted disease caused by the *Treponema pallidum spirochete* bacterium; if left untreated, can lead to death

1. Incubation and symptoms
   a. Primary stage: Exhibits a single chancre lesion, which appears at the site of contact approximately three weeks after the initial exposure—this lesion can occur orally
   b. Secondary stage symptoms occur approximately six months after initial exposure
      (1) Symptoms include
         (a) Body rash
         (b) Fever
         (c) Weight loss
         (d) General flu-like ailments
      (2) If left untreated, syphilis will progress into the tertiary stage
   c. Tertiary stage: Bacterium attacks the body's organs, including the brain, nerves, heart, and liver; latent stage usually manifests 10 or more years after the initial infection[1, 3, 11]
2. Mode of transmission: Bacterium is transmitted via
   a. Oral, vaginal, and anal sex
   b. Direct contact with the lesion by kissing or touching
   c. Infected mothers to child in utero
3. Treatment of choice: Penicillin G for all stages, with tetracycline or doxycycline as alternatives
   a. These antibiotics will cure infection but do not serve as a vaccine
   b. Reinfection can occur upon re-exposure to the bacteria[1, 3, 11]
4. Precautions: Although chances of primary syphilis appearing in the oral cavity are relatively low, the operator should be aware of the potential for cross-infection
   a. Oral symptoms often occur before body symptoms
   b. Use appropriate universal precautions to prevent transmission

E. Gonorrhea: A sexually transmitted disease caused by the *Neisseria gonorrhoeae* bacterium; while oral lesions are infrequent, oral infections can occur
1. Incubation and symptoms
   a. Initial lesion: An infection of the mucous membrane of the genitalia with symptoms of pain—appears 2 to 7 days after exposure
   b. Infection can be spread to the oral cavity, resulting in inflammation of the throat and/or oral cavity with painful ulcerations throughout[11]
2. Mode of transmission: Bacterium transmitted through sexual or direct contact with the infected area
3. Treatment
   a. Penicillin
   b. Trimethoprim/sulfamethoxazole for penicillin-resistant strains
   c. Carrier state in some individuals is up to 6 months after treatment
4. Precautions: Use universal precautions to prevent transmission

F. Tuberculosis (TB): A chronic infectious disease caused by the *Mycobacterium tuberculosis,* which infects the lungs and results in tissue necrosis; lymph nodes, meninges, kidneys, bone, skin, and oral cavity can also become infected; TB has increased because it is becoming multidrug-resistant

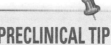

PRECLINICAL TIP

Cleansing Your Knowledge: Twenty percent of patients contracting gonorrhea present with some form of oral or oropharyngeal lesions. Since these lesions are nonspecific and resemble a multitude of common oral lesions, a diagnosis of gonorrhea can go undetected.[11] While the spread of gonorrhea from patient to dental healthcare worker has not been documented, there is concern of spreading oral lesions in aerosols generated during dental hygiene procedures if oral lesions are present.[1]

1. Incubation and symptoms: Signs and symptoms occur approximately 12 weeks after initial exposure to the bacterium
   a. Early symptoms include fever, weight loss, and slight cough with eventual sputum
   b. Later symptoms include night sweats, weakness, and a persistent cough[9]
2. Mode of transmission: Bacterium is transmitted via
   a. Inhalation of infectious droplet, particularly the sputum from persistent cough; utmost communicability usually occurs just prior to diagnosis of the disease[12]
   b. Ingestion or direct inoculation
3. Treatment: Infected individuals must be treated with anti-tuberculosis medications for 9 to 12 months
   a. With this regimen, most individuals will become noninfectious after 2 to 3 weeks
   b. Determine success of treatment by a skin test—most likely will show positive; therefore, a chest x-ray may be needed
4. Precautions: Major risk to healthcare workers is exposure to those individuals with unsuspected TB; therefore, follow universal precautions

III. **Elements (or Fundamentals) of Universal Precautions**

Infection control is a multifaceted discipline involving various procedures to prevent the spread of disease. A thorough universal precautions program includes sanitizing, personal protection, equipment asepsis, surface disinfection, and sterilization. Various governmental and nongovernmental agencies have developed recommendations and requirements for universal precautions in dental offices.

A. Agencies
1. Occupational Safety and Health Administration (OSHA): a government agency responsible for developing universal precaution protocols for the health and safety of employees
   a. In December 1991, the Occupational Exposure Bloodborne Pathogens: Final Rule was enacted
      (1) Consists of an extensive set of requirements the employer must have in place to protect the employee from contracting diseases transmitted by blood and other body fluids (Table 1–2)
      (2) Requires all healthcare workers to be immunized against hepatitis B or to sign a declination
   b. These standards cover issues relating to
      (1) Exposure control
      (2) Compliance methods
      (3) HIV
      (4) HBV
      (5) Vaccinations and postexposure evaluation
      (6) Hazard communication to employees
      (7) Record keeping
      (8) PPE
2. Centers for Disease Control (CDC): A government agency responsible for conducting research to determine how diseases are transmitted and to develop infection control recommendations;

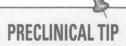

PRECLINICAL TIP

Cleansing Your Knowledge: Although the OSHA Bloodborne Pathogens Standard recognizes hepatitis B as an occupational risk, employees have the right to refuse inoculation. A mandatory declination statement provided by OSHA must be read and signed by the employee. However, the employee can be vaccinated at a later date if he/she requests it. (See Diagram 1–1 for example of form.)

Diagram 1–1   OSHA Bloodborne Pathogens Standard (29 CFR 1910.1030) Hepatitis Vaccine Declination

I understand that due to my occupational exposure to blood and other potential infectious materials I may be at risk of acquiring hepatitis B virus (HBV) infection. I have been given the opportunity to be vaccinated with hepatitis B vaccine, at no charge to myself. However, I decline hepatitis B vaccination at this time. I understand that by declining this vaccine, I continue to be at risk of acquiring hepatitis B, a serious disease. If in the future I continue to have occupational exposure to blood or other potentially infectious materials and I want to be vaccinated with hepatitis B vaccine, I can receive the vaccination series at no charge to me.

_____   _____
Employee Signature   Date

_____   _____
Witness Signature   Date

---

recommendations are designed to prevent contamination and cross-contamination, and include the following

a. Immunizations against various transmissible pathogens; many individuals receive vaccines at birth to develop immunity to various infectious diseases such as chicken pox, measles, and mumps

b. Hepatitis B vaccine (refer to Table 1–1)
   (1) Currently, two available vaccines are Recombivax HB and Enerix B,[2] both synthetic forms of hepatitis B virus
      (a) Recombivax has lower antigen level
      (b) Enerix has been shown to lose potency during storage[3]
   (2) Provides immunization against hepatitis B that in turn protects the individual from hepatitis D
   (3) Regimen consists of three 1.0 ml doses to provide the greatest immunogenicity
   (4) Injections given in the deltoid, as opposed to the gluteal muscle, have produced the best seroconversion rates[9]
   (5) Obtain an antibody titer to determine seroconversion within 6 months of the last injection; if seroconversion has not occurred, another series is recommended

c. Hepatitis A vaccine (refer to Table 1–1)
   (1) Two vaccines containing inactivated virus have been recently developed: HAVRIX and VAQTA
      (a) HAVRIX is formalin-inactivated vaccine
      (b) VAQTA is nonformalin-inactivated vaccine; recalled because of potency concerns[4, 5]
   (2) Administer in the deltoid muscle
   (3) Dosage differs according to the age of the individual receiving the vaccine—higher dosage for those older than 18
   (4) Follow a two- or three-dose schedule with a 0 to 6–12-month interval[4]

d. Immune globulin for HBV and HAV
   (1) Anti-HAV and anti-HBV antigens: Postexposure agents currently available[5]
   (2) Administer if the operator suspects exposure to HBV or HAV and has not been previously immunized

PRECLINICAL TIP

Cleansing Your Knowledge: Immune globulin is a sterile preparation of antibodies made from human plasma and provides protection against HBV and HAV through a passive transfer of antibodies.[4]

Table 1–2   Highlights of the OSHA Bloodborne Pathogens Standard

Exposure Determination
- List job classifications in which employees have occupational exposure.
- List tasks and procedures in which occupational exposure occurs.

Universal Precautions
- Gloves must be worn in the provided situations/circumstances and include the following:
  - Direct contact with potentially infectious body fluids
  - Examination of abraded or non-intact skin
  - Invasive procedures, instrumental examination of throat GI or GU tract
  - Presence of cuts/lesions on healthcare worker
  - Handling of contaminated instruments
  - Appropriate size, material and quality
  - Gloves cannot be washed or disinfected for reuse
  - Only general-purpose utility gloves can be reused if intact
  - Designed to minimize allergic reactions
- Masks must be worn when engaged in procedures likely to generate droplet of blood or other body fluids.
- Protective eyewear must have solid side-shields.
- Protective clothing must
  - Be worn when engaged in treatment that will generate spraying or spattering of blood or other body fluids
  - Be appropriate for the procedure being performed
  - *Not* permit blood or body fluids to pass through and reach undergarments or skin
  - Be removed prior to leaving the work area
- Surgical caps and shoe covers must be worn when engaged in procedures likely to involve gross contamination.
- Handwashing includes the following:
  - Wash as soon as possible if contaminated with blood or body fluids
  - Wash prior to donning gloves and immediately after removing gloves
  - If facilities to wash hands are not available, antiseptic hand cleaners or towelettes must be available; hands then need to be washed with soap and water as soon as possible
- Sharps precautions must include the following:
  - Needles are not to be purposely bent or broken by hand
  - Contaminated sharps are not to be recapped unless necessary for specific medical procedures; then recapping cannot be performed manually
  - Containers must be readily and easily accessible, puncture resistant, and leakproof
  - Container must not be overfilled
  - Container must be labeled or color-coded and closed immediately prior to replacement

Engineering and Work Practice Controls
- Resuscitation equipment must be kept in a strategic location and readily available to key personnel.
- General housekeeping and laundry practices must include the following:
  - All areas are clean, orderly, and in a sanitary condition
  - Housekeeping personnel have instruction in acceptable precautionary measures
  - Written schedule for cleaning and disinfecting equipment and surfaces must be implemented and maintained
  - Protective coverings for equipment and environmental surfaces must be removed and replaced as quickly as possible once contaminated
  - Soiled linen must be contained at the site of use, placed in leakproof bags, and sorted or rinsed in the area of use
  - Linens contaminated with blood or other infectious body fluids must be labeled or color-coded
- Infectious waste should be either incinerated or autoclaved prior to disposal in sanitary landfills.
  - Liquid infectious waste in most areas can be poured down a drain connected to a sanitary sewer
  - Waste containers must be closable, leakproof, labeled, tagged, or color-coded as infectious
  - If tags are not used, red bags or containers must be used
  - Reusable infectious waste containers must be cleaned and decontaminated on a regular basis

Hepatitis B Prophylaxis
- Employers must provide the HBV vaccination and postexposure followup.
- Pre-exposure vaccine must be offered free of charge.
- Exposure events must be documented in detail to include the source of the individual's blood to be tested, consent for testing, and evidence of HBV/HIV infection.
- Test results must be made available to exposed employee.
- Pre-exposure vaccine is offered within 10 days of initial employment or work assignment.

Table 1–2 (Continued)

- A prescreening program is not a prerequisite for the HBV vaccination.
- Employees refusing the vaccination must sign a declination statement as written in the standard.

Training and Education
- Programs must be provided upon initial employment and at least annually thereafter.
- Programs must be conducted during working hours at no cost to employee.
- Person providing the training must be knowledgeable in subject matter.
- Program content must include the following:
  - Precautionary measures, epidemiology, modes of transmission, symptoms, and prevention of HIV and HBV
  - Location and use of personal protective equipment
  - Explanation of universal precautions
  - Explanation of labeling and color-coding
  - Explanation of procedures to be followed pending occupational exposure
  - Access to a copy of the OSHA standard
  - Opportunity for a question and answer session

Record Keeping
- Document employee vaccination and postexposure followup.
- Maintain confidentiality through duration of employment and 30 years thereafter.
- Maintain training records for 3 years and include dates, content, and identification and job titles of attendees and facilitators.

Courtesy of the Occupational Safety & Health Administration Regulations (Standards-29CFR) Bloodborne Pathogens.-1910.1030

      (3) Administer injections in the deltoid or gluteal muscle immediately after exposure in a two-dose schedule, 4 weeks apart[4]

  e. HIV vaccine (refer to Table 1–1)

      (1) Approximately 40 experimental vaccines worldwide are in clinical trials[13]

      (2) AIDSvax vaccine, a synthetic portion of HIV virus,[13] shows the most promise

  f. Tuberculosis test (refer to Table 1–1)

      (1) Currently, there is no vaccine for tuberculosis because the risk for acquiring the infection is low for the U.S. population; however, researchers are testing the use of Bacillus of Calmette and Guerin (BCG) to minimize the risk of transmission and provide treatment for individuals who have active infectious TB when other strategies are not effective[13]

      (2) Test healthcare workers for possible exposure to the *M. tuberculosis* bacterium

         (a) Tuberculin skin testing consists of an injection of active material in the lower part of the arm

         (b) Chest x-ray or phlegm culture may also be needed to confirm the diagnosis

B. Personal protective equipment (PPE): Surface barriers for equipment and clothing for the operator and patient; use during preappointment (setup), patient care, and postappointment cleanup

  1. Masks: Must cover nose and mouth

    a. Designed to prevent dental personnel from inhaling pathogens and spatter (Figure 1–1)

    b. OSHA recommends wearing masks whenever splashes, sprays, spatter, or aerosol have the potential for nose and/or mouth contamination

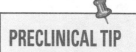

PRECLINICAL TIP

Cleansing Your Knowledge: Some states recommend testing healthcare providers for TB on a yearly basis.

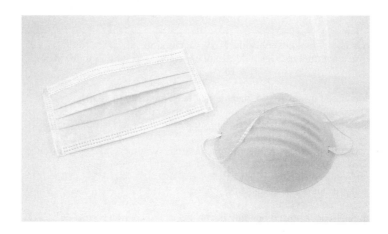

Figure 1–1   Masks.

    c. For most dental procedures, filtration is considered 95 percent efficient for particles 1 to 3 microns in diameter;[1] particle sizes smaller than 3 microns have been shown to be infectious pathogens and can penetrate to the alveoli of the lower respiratory tract, causing an increased infectivity[2]

    d. Change mask between patient treatment or during treatment if it becomes wet to minimize microorganisms passing from one person to another; research has shown wet masks may need to be replaced every 20 minutes to ensure high filterability[1]

2. Eyewear: Protective devices for the eye; also required whenever splashes, spatter, spray, or aerosols are generated (Figure 1–2)

    a. OSHA recommends safety goggles with side shields or a chin-length face mask

    b. When the operator wears a chin-length face shield, a mask is also required to prevent inhalation of aerosolized particles

    c. Eyewear should also be worn by all patients for protection; patients who wear prescriptive eyewear can leave their glasses on during treatment; however, wearing safety goggles will prevent spatter and/or damage to prescription glasses

3. Gloves

    a. Worn by the operator during patient treatment and decontamination of the treatment area (Figure 1–3)

    b. Made of latex and non-latex materials

Figure 1–2   Face shield and protective eyewear.

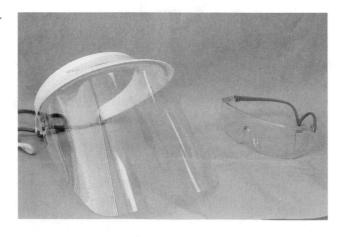

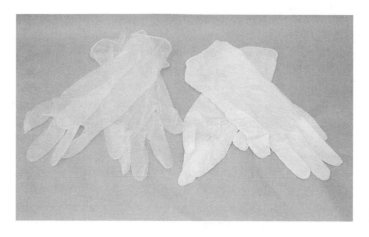

Figure 1–3   Gloves.

c. OSHA recommends a combination of disposable, single-use examination or surgical gloves and utility gloves; utility gloves are durable and designed for cleanup procedures, thus reducing the risk of puncture wounds

d. To prevent cross-contamination, change gloves between patients, when chain of asepsis is broken, or when their ability to function as a barrier is compromised

e. Types of gloves
   (1) Patient treatment gloves
       (a) Examination gloves: Nonsterile and usually sized as small, medium, or large; fitted to wear on either the right or left hand and manufactured in bulk; can also be right-left specific
       (b) Surgical gloves: Sterile and packaged in pairs; designed for a right and left hand and sized to be more form fitting
   (2) Utility gloves
       (a) Should be made of a durable, heavy-duty rubber (Figure 1–4); nitrile gloves also available for latex-free environments
       (b) Wear to decontaminate a treatment room and prepare instruments for sterilization
       (c) Wash and disinfect between use; sterilize if possible
       (d) Discard when punctured or torn

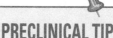

PRECLINICAL TIP

Cleansing Your Knowledge: Latex sensitivity appears as a nonspecific contact dermatitis along the confines of glove-to-skin contact. Insufficient hand rinsing or drying, a reaction to glove powder, or exposure to disinfectants can cause latex sensitivity. All result in direct physical or chemical injury to skin cells rather than an allergic response. A true latex allergy can also appear as a nonspecific contact dermatitis. Other symptoms include itching, hives, sneezing, swelling, and breathing difficulties. A qualified allergist should perform a definitive diagnosis for latex allergy.

Figure 1–4   Utility gloves.

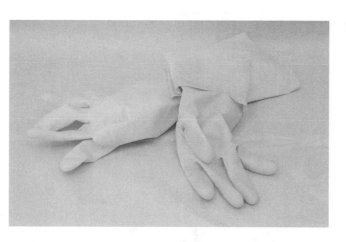

(e) Avoid cloth-lined utility gloves because the lining could become contaminated and difficult to disinfect; made of latex or latex-free material

(3) Over gloves (food-handler gloves)

(a) Used to cover contaminated gloves when providing indirect patient care, such as charting or writing notes

(b) May be contaminated during placement or removal and should not be worn to provide direct patient care

4. Clothing

a. Protects operator from occupational exposure by forming an effective barrier

b. OSHA recommends wearing an impervious material that serves as a barrier to cover exposed skin (Figure 1–5)

c. Appropriate clothing consists of lab coats, clinic jackets, and disposable gowns or garments that completely cover exposed skin, especially necklines and wrists

d. Remove clothing immediately once it is penetrated with blood or saliva

e. Provide separate bags for clean and contaminated clothing; follow protocol for caring for contaminated clothing

(1) Avoid handling with bare hands

(2) To ensure universal precautions, place contaminated clothing in a bag labeled *hazardous*

(3) Options required by OSHA when laundering contaminated clothing include

(a) Using disposable gowns made of an impervious, lightweight material

(b) Using an outside laundry service

(c) Using an onsite washer and dryer at facility

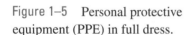

PRECLINICAL TIP

Cleansing Your Knowledge: PPE garments cover the articles of clothing the operator wears and are designed to be changed daily or when visibly soiled. PPE should *not* be worn outside the general treatment area or taken home.

Figure 1–5   Personal protective equipment (PPE) in full dress.

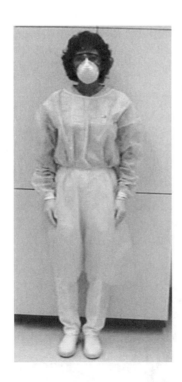

(d) Designating one employee to be responsible for washing the protective clothing in the office

5. Equipment barriers, if used properly, are considered more effective than disinfection to prevent the spread of pathogenic microbes; however, the OSHA Bloodborne Pathogens Standard does not require barriers (Figure 1–6a & 1–6b)

  a. Types of barriers to cover equipment that cannot be sterilized include

    (1) Plastic wrap

    (2) Aluminum foil

    (3) An imperviously backed absorbent paper

  b. Cover or wrap surfaces that cannot be sterilized, such as

    (1) Countertops

    (2) Handpiece and air/water syringe cords

    (3) Stools and chairs

    (4) Light handles

    (5) Writing utensils

    (6) Instrument trays

    (7) Any item that may become contaminated

  c. Change covers immediately after use; if properly used, the covered item will not need to be disinfected[14]

C. Handwashing: Critical component of the infection-control process

  1. Permits the removal of all transient bacteria and as many of the residential bacteria as possible

  2. Types of handwashing

    a. Short scrub

      (1) Purpose

        (a) Designed to clean nails, hands, and forearms with a germicidal soap and soft, sterile brush

        (b) Performed at the beginning and end of each day, although thorough washes should occur between patients

      (2) Techniques

        (a) Lather using multiple scrub and rinse cycles for approximately 2 minutes

        (b) Begin with fingertips, working down each finger and thumb while keeping the hands above elbow level to prevent contaminated water from running onto clean fingers

PRECLINICAL TIP

Cleansing Your Knowledge: Effective use of barriers can prevent the need to use a disinfectant between patients. However, the barrier must be carefully removed when contaminated so that the item being covered does not become contaminated. If the covered item becomes contaminated, then it must be disinfected prior to placing another barrier.

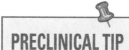

PRECLINICAL TIP

Cleansing Your Knowledge: Handwashing techniques may vary by dental hygiene programs. Regardless of which method is used, remove jewelry before handwashing.

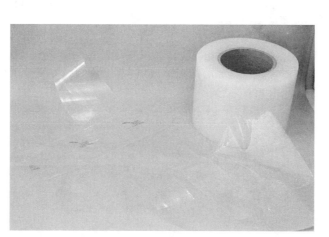

Figure 1–6a Types of barriers.

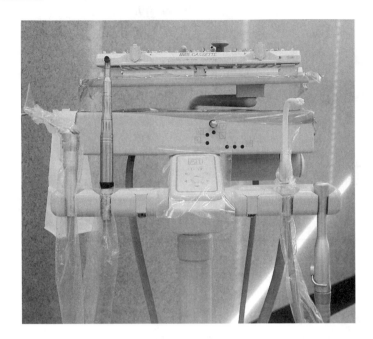

Figure 1–6b   Equipment covered
with barriers.

(c) Scrub hands and forearms

(d) Rinse hands, then forearms, permitting the runoff rinse water to drip from the elbows to prevent recontamination[15]

(e) Dry with sterile towels

b. Handwash

(1) Purpose

(a) Designed to clean hands and forearms using an antimicrobial hand soap—scrub brush not required

(b) Perform between patients or any time gloves are removed during patient treatment

(2) Technique

(a) A lather and rubbing cycle of 10 to 20 seconds is repeated two or more times[15]

(b) Begin at fingertips and work down each finger to include the thumb; wash palm of hands and forearms last

(c) Rinse and dry hands first to prevent recontamination, then rinse forearms

(d) Use paper towel to turn faucets off if not a hands-free system[15]

3. Issues

a. Hands should be well manicured, free of cuts, scrapes, chipped nail polish, and hangnails, since these areas are potential gateways for infectious bacteria

b. Keep nails short to prevent blood impaction and bacterial contamination underneath the nail; long nails also have the potential to puncture gloves and possibly traumatize the patient's tissue; fingernail polish has been shown to have an adverse reaction with chemicals in glove materials, compromising glove quality

c. Remove rings to prevent damage to gloves and microbial retention around and under them

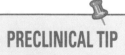

PRECLINICAL TIP

Cleansing Your Knowledge: To check proper length of nails, view the fingers from the palm side of the hand. The nails should *not* be showing above the fingertips.

       d. Pay particular attention to fingertips and thumbs, since these areas are easily overlooked and not washed thoroughly

       e. Use cool or lukewarm water instead of hot to protect hands; frequent handwashing and harsh detergents can create chapping and cracking

       f. Use hand creams and moisturizers sparingly between gloving

         (1) Avoid products that contain petroleum, mineral oil, or lanolin, since they can interfere with the integrity of latex gloves[15]

         (2) Glycerin-based hand creams have not been proven to interfere with the integrity of hand gloves

  4. Effective solutions

       a. Plain soap and water effectively removes dirt and some transient bacteria but does not inactivate pathogenic microbes; solutions containing an antimicrobial destroy most transient bacteria and reduce the number of pathogenic bacteria

       b. Effective solutions should possess the following properties

         (1) Broad-spectrum antimicrobial—effective against a wide variety of microorganisms

         (2) Fast acting—possesses rapid lethal action on all vegetative and spore forms

         (3) Substantivity level—remains on the hands to kill bacteria after hands are dry; unlike plain soaps, antibacterial agents used repeatedly throughout the day provide an antimicrobial barrier over time[15]

         (4) Few allergic or adverse reactions[15]

       c. Common antimicrobial agents include solutions containing chlorhexidine gluconate, triclosan, para-chloroxylenol, and iodophors[15]

D. Sanitization

  1. Purpose

       a. Sanitizing treatment area is a critical first step in the infection control process

       b. Designed to remove dust, dirt, and debris, yet does not necessarily remove any infectious agents

  2. Application

       a. Accomplished with a damp paper towel and antimicrobial soap and water

       b. Sanitize items in the treatment area that do *not* have direct contact with the patient's oral cavity; examples include

         (1) Dental light

         (2) Leather/vinyl parts of dental chair (back, seat, headrest, and armrests) and operator stool

         (3) Dental chair base

E. Disinfection

  1. Purpose

       a. Reduces the number of pathogenic microbes to a safe level by applying a disinfectant (chemical agent)—disinfectants destroy or inactivate most species of pathogenic microorganisms; attempt is to destroy most of the pathogenic bacteria, since all bacteria cannot be removed

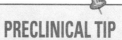

PRECLINICAL TIP

Cleansing Your Knowledge: Liquid soap is preferred to bar soap. Bar soaps *do not* provide residual antiseptic protection as do many liquid soaps. Because a single bar of soap is used by many individuals and usually sits in a pool of water at the sink, it serves as a reservoir for microorganisms.

2. Application
   a. Required for all surfaces, equipment, or instruments that have
      (1) Direct contact—actual contact with oral cavity, such as an air/water syringe tip
      (2) Indirect contact—touched by something that cannot withstand the rigors of sterilization and that has had direct contact with patient's oral cavity, such as a hand mirror picked up by the operator who was working in the patient's mouth
   b. Items that should be disinfected include
      (1) Countertops
      (2) Drawer handles
      (3) Unit switches
      (4) Unsterile supplies such as pens and pencils
      (5) Instrument trays
   c. Technique consists of
      (1) Spraying disinfecting solution directly into gauze
      (2) Wiping item to clean debris or bioburden (cleaning the surface)
      (3) Spraying solution directly into gauze again, wiping (disinfecting surface), and air drying for at least 10 minutes
3. Properties of a good disinfectant
   a. Registered with the Environmental Protection Agency (EPA) as an antimicrobial pesticide
   b. Employs rapid, broad-spectrum antimicrobial kill and is tuberculocidal, bactericidal, fungicidal, and virocidal
   c. Offers residual activity—agent continues killing microorganisms after it has dried
   d. Contains antimicrobial activity in the presence of bioburden so disinfection begins prior to cleaning
   e. Offers minimal toxicity and environmental compatibility
   f. Product is odorless, inexpensive, and easy to use[16, 17]
4. Types of disinfectants (Table 1–3)
   a. Chlorine agents such as sodium-hypochlorite and chlorine dioxide

---

PRECLINICAL TIP

Cleansing Your Knowledge: While the spray-wipe-spray technique is used for appropriate disinfection, the operator must use care when spraying a chemical disinfectant to prevent aerosolization of the disinfectant. Suggestions include spraying the disinfectant close to the item being cleaned to help contain the spray, using paper towel to absorb the spray, or spraying the disinfectant into a gauze square. It is also recommended to wear a mask, gloves, and protective eyewear when using a spray disinfectant.

Table 1–3   Types of Disinfectants

Agent	Effectiveness	Exposure Time	Cautions
Chlorines	Broad-spectrum antimicrobial	Germicidal in 3 minutes	Corrosive and caustic
Phenols	Broad-spectrum biocidal and tuberculocidal	Germicidal in 10 minutes	May leave residue or film
Iodophors	Broad-spectrum biocidal and tuberculocidal	Germicidal in 10 minutes	Use at room temperature; can discolor some surfaces
Gluteraldehydes	Broad-spectrum antimicrobial and tuberculocidal	Immersion sterilant for 10 or more hours	Highly toxic and corrosive
Quat-Alcohol Compounds	Broad-spectrum antimicrobial and tuberculocidal (high alcohol)	Germicidal in 5 (high alcohol) or 10 (low alcohol) minutes	High amounts may cause surface staining

Courtesy of Mary Kaye Scaramucci, RDH, MS. University of Cincinnati, Raymond Walters College Dental Hygiene Program.

        (1) Broad-spectrum antimicrobial
        (2) Prepared daily with an effective dilution in water of 1:10 or 1:100 that cannot be reused
        (3) Germicidal in 3 minutes on a precleaned surface
        (4) May corrode metal and be extremely caustic to human tissue and harmful to equipment and materials; wear protective eye wear, gloves, and mask while using[16, 18]
    b. Complex phenols consisting of more than one phenolic agent that work together
        (1) Broad-spectrum biocidal and tuberculocidal activity
        (2) Effective cleaning ability limited to one day of use; most must be remixed daily
        (3) Germicidal in 10 minutes on precleaned surface
        (4) Compatible with such materials as metals, glass, plastic, and rubber
        (5) Possibly leaves a residue or film on treated surface[16, 18]
    c. Iodophors contain-iodine and water-soluble surfactants
        (1) Broad-spectrum biocidal and tuberculocidal activity
        (2) Germicidal in 10 minutes on precleaned surface
        (3) Effective cleaning ability with residual activity limited to one day of use; must be remixed daily
        (4) Use at room temperature; can be unstable at higher temperatures
        (5) Compatible with most materials, but can discolor some surfaces[16, 18]
    d. Gluteraldhydes in 2 percent solutions—not recommended as a spray disinfectant by OSHA, since they are highly toxic and corrosive;[16, 18] recommended as an immersion sterilant (see section on sterilization for a complete description of gluteraldhydes)
    e. Quat/alcohol compounds—quaternary ammonium chlorides in combination with isopropanol or ethanol, creating fifth-generation agents
        (1) Broad-spectrum antimicrobial
        (2) Available in two concentrations—those with less than 40 percent and those with more than 40 percent alcohol
            (a) Higher alcohol concentration is tuberculocidal
            (b) Lower alcohol concentrations are generally not tuberculocidal
        (3) Contact time is 5 minutes for high alcohol concentrations and 10 minutes for lower concentrations[16, 18]
        (4) Excessive amounts of the quat compound may cause surface staining[18]
F. Sterilization (Table 1–4)
    1. Purpose
        a. Destroys all pathogenic microorganisms including spores
        b. Provides the highest level of patient protection
    2. Protocol
        a. After use, sterilize instruments and equipment that have come into contact with blood and saliva
        b. If items cannot be sterilized after use, by heat or immersion, they should *not* be used but discarded

---

PRECLINICAL TIP

Cleansing Your Knowledge: Quaternary ammonium compounds have been around since the 1930s. They have evolved over time and are now in their fifth formulation—thus the reference to fifth-generation agent.

Table 1–4   Methods of Sterilization

Device	Conditions	Advantages	Disadvantages
Steam	250°–273° F, 15–30 lbs. pressure, 3–30 minutes	Quick process; accommodates wide variety of materials	Corrodes carbon-steel instruments; dulls cutting edges; unsuitable for rubber, oils, powders
Dry heat	320°–375°F, 1 hour	Appropriate for materials that cannot withstand steam; does not dull cutting edges; does not corrode carbon-steel instruments	Long exposure time
Chemical	270°F, 25 lbs. pressure, 20 minutes	Short exposure time; does not corrode carbon-steel instruments	Produces strong odor
Liquid	Uninterrupted immersion 6–10 hours	None	No assurance that spores are killed; long exposure time

Courtesy of Mary Kaye Scaramucci, RDH, MS. University of Cincinnati, Raymond Walters College Dental Hygiene Program.

3. Methods of sterilization
   a. Steam under pressure, also known as steam sterilizer or autoclave (Figure 1–7a and 1–7b)
      (1) Sterilization occurs by the action of steam under pressure in a metal chamber
         (a) Maintain an airtight chamber so water can be heated to create steam under pressure needed for sterilization
         (b) Offers a transfer of latent heat energy to the objects being sterilized
      (2) Ideal conditions: Sterilization can begin when the chamber reaches 250° Fahrenheit (standard cycle) or 273° Fahrenheit (flash cycle) at 15 to 30 lbs. per square inch (psi)
         (a) Processing time varies from 3 to 30 minutes depending on whether the objects are wrapped or unwrapped, and/or the type of wrap that is used

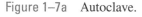

Figure 1–7a   Autoclave.

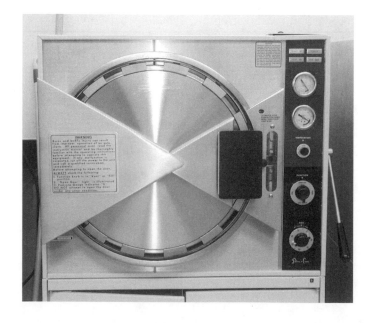

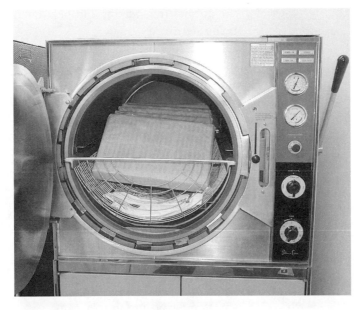

Figure 1–7b   Autoclave loaded with instruments.

    (b) Unwrapped instruments may be sterilized using a shorter exposure time; avoid routine use of flash method, since it lessens sterility assurance

    (c) Instrument wraps should be able to withstand steam heat;[3] available in paper, plastic, or cloth, and designed as pouches, bags, or sheets

  (3) Advantages: Provides a quick process that can sterilize a wide variety of materials

  (4) Disadvantages

    (a) Can corrode carbon-steel instruments as well as dull the cutting edges of scaling instruments

    (b) Unsuitable for rubber products, oils, and powders

b. Dry heat sterilization (Figure 1–8)

  (1) Process: Works much like an oven, except the heat is constant without a fluctuation in temperature; involves heating

Figure 1–8   Dry heat sterilizer.

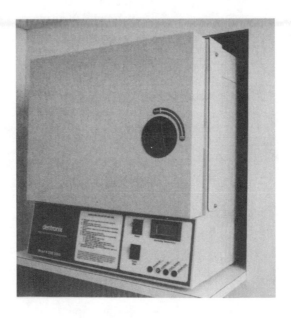

the air and transferring the heat energy to the instruments being sterilized

(2) Ideal conditions: Sterilization can begin once the chamber reaches 320° to 375° Fahrenheit

    (a) Processing time is one hour; however, a forced-air (rapid heat tranfer) dry-heat sterilizer can process instruments in 6 to 12 minutes for unwrapped and wrapped respectively

    (b) Instrument wraps should be able to withstand the high temperatures of dry heat and not burn or melt[3]

(3) Advantages

    (a) Useful for materials that cannot withstand steam under pressure, such as oils, powders, greases, and some handpieces

    (b) Does not dull the cutting edges of scaling instruments or corrode metal

(4) Disadvantages

    (a) Long exposure time

    (b) Destroys heat-sensitive materials, such as plastics and waxes

    (c) Unsuitable for all liquids

c. Chemical vapor sterilization (Figure 1–9)

(1) Process: Involves the heating of special chemicals, such as 0.23 percent formaldehyde, 72.38 percent ethanol and acetone, ketone, water, and other alcohols, to produce vapors that kill microorganisms[3]

(2) Ideal conditions: Sterilization begins once the chamber reaches 25 lbs. psi at a temperature of 270° Fahrenheit

    (a) Processing time is 20 minutes

    (b) Use instrument wraps and choose one based on manufacturer's recommendations; if wraps are *not* used, then instruments will *not* remain sterile after processing

(3) Advantages: Short exposure time; does *not* corrode metal instruments

(4) Disadvantage: Ventilation must be used, since the chemicals can produce a strong odor

Figure 1–9   Chemical vapor
sterilizer.

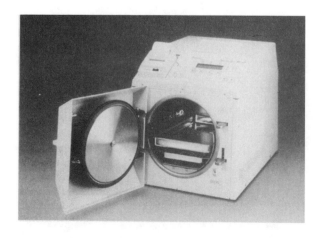

d. Liquid chemical solutions, also known as *cold sterilization*
   (1) Gluteraldhydes in 2 percent solutions (refer to Table 1–3)
       (a) Broad-spectrum antimicrobial and tuberculocidal activity
       (b) Immersion sterilant for 10 or more hours
       (c) Highly toxic to human tissue and corrosive to certain metals; wear protective eyewear, gloves, and mask
   (2) Process: Equipment is immersed in specific solutions designated as sterilants
   (3) Ideal conditions: Chemical solution is prepared and placed in a container that can hold equipment or instruments
       (a) Immerse items to be sterilized uninterrupted for 10 hours
       (b) After immersion, rinse items in sterile water
   (4) Advantages: None, since sterilization cannot be guaranteed
   (5) Disadvantages: No assurance that spores will be killed; requires a long exposure time

G. Quality assurance monitoring programs provide performance data to support and assure that sterilization occurs on a consistent basis. Biological, physical, and chemical indicators are the three major monitoring techniques available to the dental team. While OSHA does not regulate monitoring systems, many states require regular monitoring and ongoing data collection and documentation. A combination of all three techniques should be performed with each sterilization cycle.

1. Biological monitors (Figure 1–10)
   a. Designed to monitor autoclave, chemical vapor, dry heat, and ethylene oxide sterilizers
   b. ADA and CDC recommend weekly testing of sterilizers in the dental office[19]
   c. Consist of spore-impregnated strips or self-contained in vials
   d. Procedure for use
      (1) Label and place test strips or vials in the sterilizer and process with a normal load of instruments

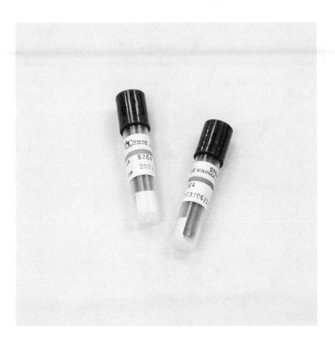

Figure 1–10   Biological monitors.

    (2) Label another strip or vial as the control and do *not* place in a sterilizer

    (3) After the sterilization process is complete, incubate strip or vial for a period of time based on manufacturer instructions; incubation period can range from 24 hours to 7 days

    (4) Presence of microbial growth is determined by a color in the test vial or strip; if there was no change from the original color in the test vials/strips, and the control vial/strip has changed color, then the sterilization cycle was a success[20]

2. Physical indicators (Figure 1–11)
    a. Consists of visual monitoring and documentation of the sterilizer gauges and readouts
    b. While correct readings cannot guarantee sterility, they can provide the first indication of equipment failure[20]

3. Chemical indicators (Figure 1–12)
    a. Consists of heat-sensitive compounds that change color when exposed to sterilizing temperatures; examples include autoclave tape and indicator labels on packages
    b. Serves to distinguish what has or has not been heat processed, but does *not* guarantee sterility[20]

H. Material Safety Data Sheets (MSDS) have been required since 1994 when the Hazard Communication Standard, issued by OSHA, was registered as a federal rule (Table 1–5). The purpose of these sheets is to provide the employee with information regarding the hazards of various chemicals used in the dental office and how to protect every member of the dental team from the dangers associated with the chemicals (Figure 1–13)

Figure 1–11   Sterilizer gauges.

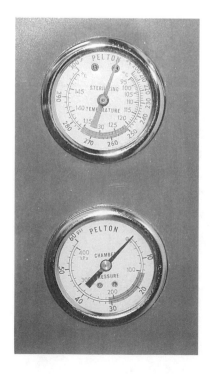

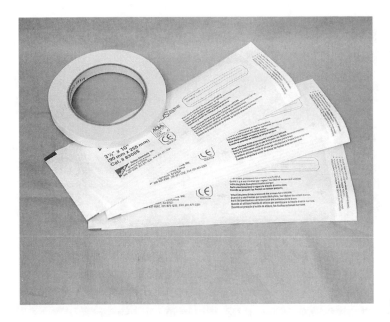

Figure 1–12   Autoclave tape and autoclave bags.

Table 1–5   Highlights of the OSHA Hazard Communication Standard

Responsible Parties
• Chemical manufacturers and importers determine hazards of their chemical product.
• Chemical manufacturers, importers, and distributors communicate the hazard and safety pre-
  cautions to the customers by supplying labels and MSDS.
• Employers identify, list, and label hazardous chemicals in the workplace and develop, imple-
  ment, and maintain a hazard communication program to include employee training.
Container Labeling
• Must be completed by the manufacturer, importer, or distributor prior to shipping.
• Must be written in English.
• Must include the identity of the hazardous chemical, appropriate warning, and the name and
  address of the manufacturer, importer, or distributor.
Hazardous Chemical Inventory
• Hazardous chemicals must be inventoried and cross-referenced with the MSDS.
Material Safety Data Sheets
• Must be written in English and reference the common name of the product as well as the spe-
  cific chemical name.
• Must be obtained for all hazardous chemicals.
• Must be placed in an accessible location.
• Must be reviewed by employees prior to working with a hazardous chemical.
Maintaining Inventory and MSDS
• Products should be inventoried for updated MSDS with each shipment.
• Outdated MSDS should be replaced with current sheets.
• The individual responsible for maintenance must be identified.
Employee Information and Training
• Training must be provided to all employees who may be exposed to hazardous chemicals.
• Training must be provided at the time of initial assignment, job reassignment, or when a new
  hazard is introduced into the workplace.
• Employees must have access to the following:
  • Hazard Communication Standard—must know existence and content
  • Components of the hazard communication program
  • Operating procedures in work areas where hazardous chemicals are present
  • Location of the MSDS and training manual
• Training information should include the following information:
  • How the program is implemented in the office
  • How to read and interpret MSDS
  • How employees can obtain and use the hazard information
  • Hazards of chemicals in the workplace
  • Specific procedures to provide protection
  • How to detect presence of hazardous chemical

Courtesy of the Occupational Safety & Health Administration Regulations (Standards - 29CFR) Hazard
Communication. - 1910.1200

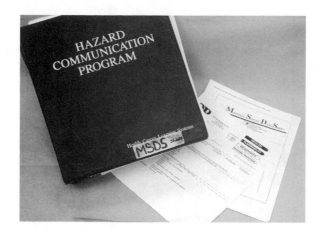

Figure 1–13   MSDS book and sheets.

1. MSDSs are supplied by the manufacturer of the chemical
   a. Criteria
      (1) There is no prescribed format for the form, but it must
         (a) Be written in English
         (b) Identify the common name of the product
         (c) Contain information regarding the specific chemical identity
2. MSDSs must include the following information
   a. Product label to identify product
   b. Chemical and common names for the active ingredient
   c. Chemical and common names and hazards of the chemicals contained within the mixture
   d. Carcinogenicity of the product
   e. Physical and chemical characteristics and hazards of the product (i.e., flash point, flammability, reactivity, explosivity)
   f. Health hazards, which include signs and symptoms of exposure, along with the primary route of entry
   g. Precautions and special protection required to safely handle the product
   h. Necessary procedures for cleaning up a spill or leak
   i. Name, address, and telephone number of the manufacturer or company preparing and distributing the MSDS sheets
3. MSDSs must be available to all employees by the employer; they must review the sheets before working with hazardous chemicals
   a. Maintain MSDSs in a binder in alphabetical order by product name
   b. Designate someone with proper training to be responsible for keeping the binder updated, although the dentist is responsible by federal law
4. Label containers of hazardous chemicals with hazard warning diamond to reference information from the MSDSs (Figure 1–14)
   a. Labels provide a quick method to identify the various hazards associated with a particular chemical
   b. Labels provide the identity of the hazardous chemical, appropriate hazard warning, and the required special protection for handling
   c. If the product is being transferred from the original container to a secondary container, a label is required for the secondary container; however, if the employee transfers the product to a sec-

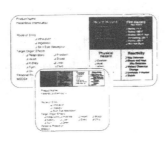
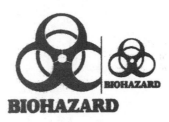
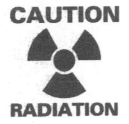
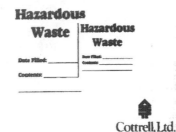

Figure 1–14   Labels for containers of hazardous chemicals.

ondary container for immediate use, a secondary label is *not* necessary[21]

5. Training: Employer is required to provide hazard communication training to all employees who may be exposed to chemicals

  a. Should occur with

    (1) New hires

    (2) Job reassignment resulting in exposure to new chemicals

    (3) Whenever new chemicals are introduced

  b. Under the OSHA Hazard Standard, the minimum content requirements for the training sessions include

    (1) How the hazard communication standard is implemented in the office

    (2) Reading and interpreting the MSDSs and how employees can obtain and use the hazard information

    (3) Hazards of the various chemicals used in the practice

    (4) How to prevent unnecessary exposure

    (5) Special protective equipment

    (6) How to detect the presence of hazardous chemicals

6. Keep a summary for three years of the training and names of those employees who participated in the training

IV. **Elements (or Fundamentals) of Universal Precautions**

  A. To decontaminate the treatment area, prepare and clean the operatory before and after patient treatment

    1. Preappointment procedures include sanitizing, disinfecting, placing barriers, flushing suction and water lines, and setting up equipment and unit dose supplies

      a. Sanitize clinical contact surfaces that neither the operator nor contaminated dental instruments contact—known as *splash, spatter, and droplet surfaces.*[22] Examples include, but are not limited to

        (1) Dental light and arm extension

        (2) Patient chair and base

        (3) Operator stool and mobile cart

        (4) Walls, floor, and cabinets

  b. Purge water supply at the beginning of each day by flushing water to reduce biofilm in water lines

  c. Disinfect or cover with appropriate barriers surfaces that are directly touched and contaminated during treatment, known as *touch surfaces,* and surfaces that are not directly touched but can come in contact with contaminated instruments, known as *transfer surfaces*[22]

   (1) Examples include, but are not limited to

    (a) Dental light handles

    (b) Hand-operated switches on the unit or chair

    (c) Instrument trays

    (d) Handpiece holders

    (e) Counter tops and writing utensils

   (2) Operator decides which items should be disinfected and covered

    (a) If items are covered, the cover must be intact throughout the treatment

    (b) If the barrier becomes compromised, the covered item must be cleaned and disinfected prior to the next patient

  d. Flushing

   (1) Flush air/water syringe and suction to prevent biofilm contamination[23, 24, 25]; use chemical flushing on a weekly basis[25]—only ADA approved product is Ultra[24]

   (2) Flush handpieces unless sterilized between uses

  e. Set up and protect equipment prior to treatment; supplies should be readily available as unit dose; examples include

   (1) If fluoride is in the realm of treatment, dispense in a dappen dish and cover rather than dispensing from the bottle during treatment to prevent contamination of the bottle; may also want to use one-use sealed packets

   (2) Dispense dental floss prior to treatment to prevent contamination of the dental floss dispenser

   (3) Set up and drape larger equipment, such as the ultrasonic scaler and the air polisher, with a barrier prior to its use

 2. Post-appointment procedures include disposing barriers, PPE, disinfecting equipment or touch/transfer surfaces that were *not* barrier protected, and preparing instruments or items for sterilization

  a. Properly dispose barriers, PPE, and waste in the regular waste

  b. Dispose any item that is soaked in blood or saliva (drips blood or saliva) in a biohazard waste container for incineration

  c. Disinfect equipment and surfaces that were not covered by barriers, using the spray-wipe-spray technique

  d. Flush water lines and evacuate tubing (HVE and/or saliva ejector) with detergent or water

  e. Disinfect water supply daily with an OSHA-acceptable disinfectant by adding the disinfectant to the water line on a weekly basis

B. Sterilize instruments or items containing blood or saliva after use

 1. Prior to sterilization, instruments should be free of bioburden

 2. Instruments should be cleaned in an ultrasonic cleaner, since this method of cleaning eliminates injury that could occur from manual

scrubbing; however, the autoclavable prophy angle should be cleaned by hand with gauze and a disinfectant because the gears can corrode when placed in an ultrasonic solution

3. Sterilize handpieces without oil; use sterile oil after or just before use; oil in handpiece during autoclaving "fries" the handpiece and shortens its life

4. Utilization of the cassette system affords the operator an easy and safe method for cleaning and sterilizing (Figure 1–15)

   a. Place instruments, metal air/water syringe tip, sharpening stone, test sticks, and prophylaxis paste grips in the cassette

   b. Close and lock the lid

   c. Place cassette in ultrasonic cleaner with a high-level disinfectant for approximately 12 minutes to remove bioburden (Figure 1–16)

      (1) If instruments are not in a cassette, place them loosely in the ultrasonic cleaner

      (2) *Do not* bind instruments, since this may prevent a thorough cleaning or can potentially nick or break working ends

   d. Remove cassette or instruments

   e. Rinse with water

   f. Ensure all bioburden has been removed; visually check all instruments; if debris remains, re-ultrasonic or carefully wipe with gauze

   g. Drip dry or place in instrument dryer

   h. Wrap cassette tightly in paper wrap, like a package

   i. Secure cassette wrap or other approved packaging material tape (Figure 1–17); place indicator tape on wrap cassette

      (1) Avoid writing directly on wrap because it creates microholes for recontamination after sterilization is complete; write on tape with pencil

      (2) Label package with contents and date prior to sterilizing

C. Other packaging materials: Available in plastic/paper pouches, nylon type clear plastic tubing, and paper bags; place loose instruments flat (*not* stacked) in packaging material and avoid puncturing the bag by wrapping sharp ends in gauze; wrap dental mirrors in gauze or bag alone to prevent scratching the mirror surface

   1. Plastic/paper pouches: Designed with clear plastic film on one side and heavy sterilization paper on the other side

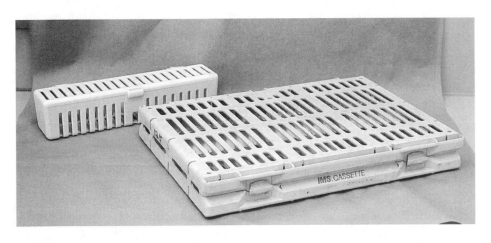

Figure 1–15   Types of cassettes for instruments.

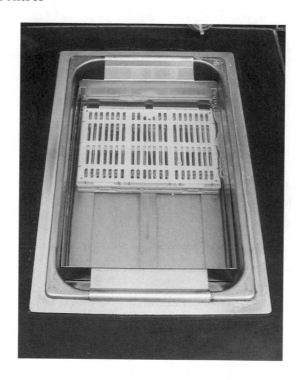

Figure 1–16   Ultrasonic cleaner.

      a. Available in many different sizes
      b. Self-sealing or tape sealable
      c. Easily opened after sterilization by peeling plastic away from paper
      d. Can be used in steam or unsaturated chemical vapor sterilizer
      e. Have chemical indicators printed on paper side of pouch
   2. Nylon type clear plastic tubing
      a. Available in different widths; comes on a roll and may be cut to varying lengths
      b. One type for use in steam and another for use in dry heat sterilizers
      c. Need to place indicator tape on bag
      d. Heat-sealed or tape sealable
      e. Easy open
   3. Paper bags
      a. Caution
         (1) Sharp and pointed instruments can easily puncture paper

Figure 1–17   Wrapped cassette and packaged autoclave bag.

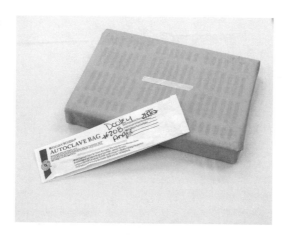

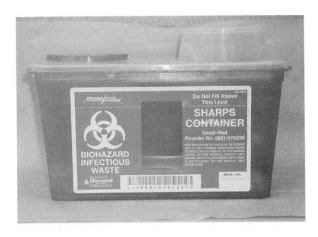

Figure 1–18   Sharps container.

(2) Paper gets wet during steam sterilization and can tear if handled before completely dried

D. Dispose most waste in regular trash; however, there are special circumstances when the regular trash is not appropriate

1. Place sharps, such as needles and irrigation canulas, in an official "sharps" container (Figure 1–18)
    a. Containers are usually red in color and display the universal contamination emblem
    b. Sterilize full containers prior to disposal or contact appropriate personnel for disposal

2. Dispose items that drip blood or saliva when held in the biohazard waste (Figure 1–19)
    a. Place in a red plastic bag with the universal contamination emblem
    b. Secure and incinerate bag

Figure 1–19   Biohazard waste bag.

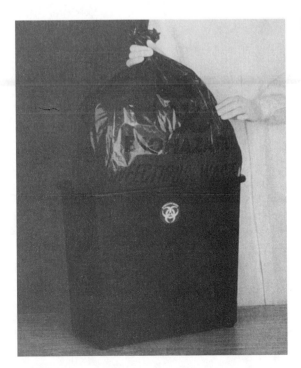

The dental hygienist has an ethical and profesional obligation to provide care to all patients in a safe manner. Therefore, it is vital to maintain the standards of universal precautions to prevent cross-contamination. By creating an organized system for exposure control, sound practices based on scientific evidence can protect the health of the dental team and their patients.

QUESTIONS

1. All of the following forms of hepatitis have the potential to result in a carrier state EXCEPT one. Which one is the EXCEPTION?
   a. HAV
   b. HBV
   c. HCV
   d. HDV

2. What is the primary concern with individuals who become carriers of specific forms of hepatitis?
   a. Carriers are just as contagious as those in the acute or chronic stage.
   b. The healthcare provider should have a titre test prior to treating a carrier.
   c. Carriers need to be immunized prior to receiving dental care.
   d. The healthcare provider should be immunized against HBV prior to treating carriers.
   e. Carriers cannot be seen for dental care.

3. Patients exhibiting oral signs and symptoms of the herpes virus should have treatment postponed because contact with weeping lesions can result in cross-contamination.
   a. The statement is correct, but the reason is not.
   b. The statement is incorrect, but the reason is correct.
   c. Both statement and reason are correct.
   d. Both statement and reason are incorrect.

4. The human immunodeficiency virus (HIV) has been found in many types of body fluids. Which of the following body fluids has *NOT* been related to transmission?
   a. Blood
   b. Saliva
   c. Breast milk
   d. Semen
   e. Vaginal secretions

5. Since the chance of spreading syphilis and gonorrhea from patient to dental healthcare provider is low, the dental hygienist should not worry about the use of appropriate procedures for universal precautions.
   a. Both statement and reason are correct.
   b. Both statement and reason are incorrect.
   c. The statement is correct, but the reason is incorrect.
   d. The statement is incorrect, but the reason is correct.

6. After which of the following timeframes will individuals diagnosed with tuberculosis and treated with antituberculosis medications for 9 to 12 months become noninfectious?
   a. 2 years
   b. 1 year
   c. 9 to 12 weeks
   d. 2 to 3 weeks
   e. 48 hours

7. All of the following denote a thorough universal precautions program EXCEPT one. Which one is the EXCEPTION?
   a. Sanitation
   b. Personal protection
   c. Sterilization
   d. Disinfection
   e. Antibiotic premedication

8. Against which of the following diseases does the OSHA Bloodborne Pathogens Standard require all healthcare workers to be immunized?
   a. HAV
   b. HIV
   c. TB
   d. HBV
   e. HCV

9. Disinfection of equipment and surfaces that have been protected by a plastic barrier is *not* necessary unless the barrier has become compromised.
   a. The statement is correct, but the reason is incorrect.
   b. Both statement and reason are correct.
   c. The statement is incorrect, but the reason is correct.
   d. Both statement and reason are incorrect.

10. All of the following are options for laundering contaminated clothing EXCEPT one. Which one is the EXCEPTION?
    a. All the dental healthcare workers can take the laundry home.
    b. Disposable gowns can be worn.
    c. An outside service can be used.
    d. The office can house an onsite washer and dryer.

11. All of the following are best times for the dental healthcare worker to wash his or her hands EXCEPT one. Which one is the EXCEPTION?
    a. Prior to donning gloves
    b. After glove removal
    c. At the beginning of the day
    d. At the end of the day
    e. When gloves are worn

12. Which products in hand creams does NOT interfere with the integrity of the gloves?
    a. Petroleum
    b. Mineral oil
    c. Lanolin
    d. Glycerin

13. Which of the following definitions is correct for disinfection?
    a. The application of a chemical agent to reduce the number of pathogenic microbes to a safe level
    b. The application of a chemical agent to kill all pathogenic microbes
    c. The application of a chemical agent to destroy spore-forming bacteria
    d. The application of a chemical agent to remove gross debris

14. To be MOST effective, how many minutes do most disinfectants need to air dry?
    a. 5
    b. 10
    c. 20
    d. 30

15. Which of the following conditions need to be met to achieve steam sterilization?
    a. 250° F, 15 psi, 30 minutes
    b. 350° F, 30 psi, 15 minutes
    c. 250° F, 25 psi, one hour
    d. 350° F, 15 psi, one hour

16. Which of the following conditions need to be present to achieve dry sterilization?
    a. 250° F for 30 minutes
    b. 250° F for one hour

c. 320° to 375° F for one hour
d. 320° to 375° F for 30 minutes

17. All of the following special chemicals achieve sterilization with chemical vapor sterilizers EXCEPT one. Which one is the EXCEPTION?
    a. Formaldehyde
    b. Ethanol
    c. Acetone
    d. Phenols

18. Which of the following conditions must be present to achieve chemical vapor sterilization?
    a. 250° F, 15 psi, 20 minutes
    b. 270° F, 25 psi, 20 minutes
    c. 320° F, 20 psi, 30 minutes
    d. 350° F, 20 psi, one hour

19. Which of the following immersion times do liquid chemical solutions, capable of sterilizing, require?
    a. 10 minutes
    b. 30 minutes
    c. 1 hour
    d. 10 hours

20. What does the color change on heat-sensitive compounds indicate on autoclave bags and tape?
    a. The contents have been exposed to sterilizing temperatures and are rendered sterile.
    b. The contents have been exposed to sterilizing temperatures, but sterility is not guaranteed.
    c. The contents have not been exposed to sterilizing temperatures, and sterility is not guaranteed.
    d. The contents have not been exposed to sterilizing temperatures, but sterility is guaranteed.

21. Material Safety Data Sheets (MSDSs) are required to provide the employee with all of the following information EXCEPT one. Which one is the EXCEPTION?
    a. Identify hazardous chemicals being used in the office.
    b. Provide associated protection from the dangers of the chemicals.
    c. Explain spill prevention and clean up.
    d. Recommend who uses the chemicals.

22. Splash, spatter, and droplet surfaces are clinical contact surfaces that are not touched by the operator or contaminated dental instruments. Therefore, these surfaces can be decontaminated by sanitizing.

a. The statement is correct, but the reason is incorrect.
b. The statement is incorrect, but the reason is correct.
c. Both statement and reason are correct.
d. Both statement and reason are incorrect.

23. Which of the following touch surfaces are directly touched and contaminated during treatment?
a. Dental light
b. Cabinets
c. Writing implements
d. Foot-activated pedals

24. Which of the following techniques can decontaminate touch surfaces?
a. Sanitizing
b. Disinfection
c. Sterilization
d. Antibiotics

25. The Bloodborne Pathogens Standard recommends dental healthcare workers use disposable examination or surgical gloves for patient treatment. It is recommended that utility gloves be used for decontamination of treatment area.
a. The first statement is TRUE. The second statement is FALSE.
b. The first statement is FALSE. The second statement is TRUE.
c. Both statements are TRUE.
d. Both statements are FALSE.

REFERENCES

1. Miller, C. H., & C. J. Palenik. *Infection Control and Management of Hazardous Material for the Dental Team,* 2nd ed. St. Louis: Mosby, 1998.

2. Wilkins, E. *Clinical Practice of the Dental Hygienist,* 8th ed. Philadelphia: Lippincott, Williams & Wilkins, 1999.

3. Cottone, J. A., G. T. Terezhalmy & J. A. Molinari. *Practical Infection Control in Dentistry,* 2nd ed. Philadelphia: Williams & Wilkins, 1996.

4. Centers for Disease Control. Prevention of hepatitis A through active or passive immunization: Recommendations of the advisory committee on immunization practices. Morbidity and Mortality Weekly Report, 45(RR15), December 1996.

5. Organization for Safety & Asepsis Procedures. Disease update: Viral hepatitis. *Monthly Focus,* 10, 2001.

6. Organization for Safety & Asepsis Procedures. Disease update: Hepatitis C. *Monthly Focus,* 8, 1998.

7. Organization for Safety & Asepsis Procedures. Health of the healthcare worker. *Monthly Focus,* 5, 2000.

8. Coates, E. A., L. Walsh, & R. Logan. The increasing problem of hepatitis C virus infection. *Australian Dental Journal,* 46(1), March 2001.

9. Dietz, E. *Safety Standards and Infection Control for Dental Assistants.* Albany: Delmar, 2002.

10. Roufos, A. Herpes: A vaccine to vanquish the beast? *Health,* 15(2), March 2001.

11. Siegal M. Syphilis and gonorrhea. *Dental Clinics of North America,* 40(2), April 1996.

12. Centers for Disease Control. The role of BCG vaccine in the prevention and control of tuberculosis in the United States: A joint statement by the advisory council for the elimination of tuberculosis and the advisory committee on immunization practices. Morbidity and Mortality Weekly Report, 45(RR-4), April 1996.

13. Organization for Safety & Asepsis Procedures, 1999 in review. *Monthly Focus,* 11, 1999.

14. Organization for Safety & Asepsis Procedures. Surface barriers. *Monthly Focus,* 4, 1999.

15. Organization for Safety & Asepsis Procedures. Hand asepsis. *Monthly Focus,* 3, 1998.

16. Organization for Safety & Asepsis Procedures. Environmental surface disinfection. *The Dental Assistant,* 69(4), November/December 2000.

17. Organization for Safety & Asepsis Procedures. Selecting safety & asepsis products. *Monthly Focus,* 1, 2001.

18. Smith, F. T. The germ fix. *RDH,* January 2000.

19. Miller, C. H. Use of spore tests for quality assurance in infection control. *American Journal of Dentistry,* 14(114), 2001.

20. Organization for Safety & Asepsis Procedures. Selecting & evaluating a sterilization monitoring service. *Monthly Focus,* 3, 2000.

21. Organization for Safety & Asepsis Procedures. MSDSs, chemical lists & other hazcom "musts." *Monthly Focus,* 2, 2000.

22. Organization for Safety & Asepsis Procedures. Environmental surface asepsis. *Monthly Focus,* 8, 2001.

23. Beierle, J. W. Biofilms: An introduction. *Journal of the California Dental Association,* 29(5), May 2001.

24. Lee, T. K., E. J. Waked, L. E. Wolinsky, R. S. Mito, & R. E. Danielson. Controlling biofilm and microbial contamination in dental unit waterlines. *Journal of the California Dental Association,* 29(9), September 2001.

25. Organization for Safety & Asepsis Procedures. Position paper: Dental unit waterlines. March 2000.

DECONTAMINATION OF TREATMENT AREA SKILL SHEET

Student _____

Date _____

Instructor _____

Re-evaluation
Instr: _____
Date _____

Instr: _____
Date _____

	S	U	Comments	S	U	Comments	S	U	Comments
Preappointment Sanitizing									
1. Dons eye protection, mask and utility gloves.									
2. Applies soap to damp paper towel.									
3. Sanitizes the following items:									
a. Dental light arm.									
b. Leather portions of patient chair and operator stool.									
c. Cabinets and wall, as appropriate.									
d. Operator stool legs.									
e. Patient chair base.									
f. Rheostat/foot controls.									
4. Washes utility gloves with antimicrobial soap.									
5. Flushes air/water syringe and suction for five minutes or disinfects with a chemical solution.									
Preappointment Disinfecting									
6. Uses the spray-wipe-spray technique with a disinfectant and paper towel/gauze and disinfects the following:									
a. Counter tops and drawer handles.									
b. Pens, pencils, clipboards.									
c. Hand mirror, patient eye protection.									
d. Air/water syringe and holder.									
e. Saliva ejector and holder.									
f. Handpiece holder.									
7. Removes utility gloves and washes hands.									
8. Applies barriers to the following items:									
a. Handles and switch on dental light.									
b. Master switch.									
c. Tubing.									
d. Patient chair.									
e. Operator stool.									
f. Countertop.									
g. Instrument tray.									
Post appointment									
9. Removes barriers with patient gloves ensuring surfaces have not been compromised.									
10. Properly disposes barriers and other trash.									
11. Removes patient gloves, washes hands, and dons utility gloves.									
12. Flushes air/water syringe and suction for several minutes.									
13. Cleans and disinfects items listed in #6 above using the spray-wipe-spray technique.									
14. Cleans and disinfects any compromised items in #8 listed above using the spray-wipe-spray technique.									
15. Disinfects utility gloves and washes hands.									
16. Leaves unit, at attention, with master switch in the off position.									

Courtesy of Mary Kaye Scaramucci, RDH, MS. University of Cincinnati, Raymond Walters College Dental Hygiene Program.

HANDWASHING SKILL SHEET

Student _____

Date _____

Instructor _____

Re-evaluation
Instr: _____
Date _____

Instr: _____
Date _____

	S	U	Comments	S	U	Comments	S	U	Comments
Short Scrub									
1. Removes all rings and watch.									
2. Uses cool or lukewarm water to rinse hands.									
3. Applies antimicrobial hand soap.									
4. Lathers soap and begins rubbing in the following manner:									
a. Starts at fingertips and works down each finger and thumb of each hand.									
b. Keeps hands above elbow level so water does not run down fingers.									
c. Moves to hands and forearms.									
5. Rinses hands, then forearms, permitting runoff rinse water to drip from the elbows.									
6. Repeats #4 and #5 for approximately five minutes.									
7. Dries hands first, then forearms, with paper towel.									
8. Turns faucets off with paper towel, if not using foot pedals.									
Handwash									
1. Removes all rings and watch.									
2. Uses cool or lukewarm water to rinse hands.									
3. Applies antimicrobial hand soap.									
4. Lathers and rubs for 10-20 seconds in the following manner:									
a. On each hand, starts at fingertips and works down each finger and thumb.									
b. Moves to palm of hands and forearms last.									
5. Rinses hands, then forearms, permitting runoff water to drip from the elbows.									
6. Repeats #4 and #5 above for a minimum of two times.									
7. Dries hands first, then forearms, with paper towel.									
8. Turns faucets off with paper towel, if not using foot pedals.									
Hand appearance; student's:									
1. Hands are well manicured and free of cuts, scrapes and hangnails.									
2. Nails are short and cannot be seen above fingertips.									
3. Rings and nail polish are removed.									

Courtesy of Mary Kaye Scaramucci, RDH, MS. University of Cincinnati, Raymond Walters College Dental Hygiene Program.

INSTRUMENT DECONTAMINATION AND STERILIZATON PREPARATON SKILL SHEET

Student _____

Date _____

Instructor _____

Re-evaluation
Instr: _____
Date _____

Instr: _____
Date _____

	S	U	Comments	S	U	Comments	S	U	Comments
1. Dons utility gloves.									
2. Places instruments in cassette.									
3. Locks lid on cassette and places it in the ultrasonic cleaner.									
4. Turns timer on ultrasonic to 12 minutes.									
5. Runs instruments in ultrasonic for 12 minutes.									
6. Removes cassette and ensures bioburden removal is complete.									
7. Rinses cassette with tap water and drains.									
8. Wraps cassette in airtight package style.									
9. Secures wrap with masking tape.									
10. Labels tape with pencil; applies small piece of autoclave tape on wrap.									
11. Places cassette in sterilizer.									
12. Disinfects utility gloves and washes hands.									

Courtesy of University of Cincinnati, Raymond Walters College Dental Hygiene Program

37

STERILIZER MONITORING PROCEDURES SKILL SHEET

Student _____

Date _____

Instructor _____

Re-evaluation

Instr: _____   Instr: _____

Date _____   Date _____

	S	U	Comments	S	U	Comments	S	U	Comments
Vials									
1. Labels one vial as control and the other as test.									
2. Places test vial in sterilizer with items to be sterilized.									
3. Crushes both test and control vials at completion of cycle.									
4. Incubates vials for 24 to 48 hours.									
5. Examines vials for color change.									
a. Test vial remains purple.									
b. Control vial turns yellow.									
6. Recognizes the need for corrective procedures if the color change is not appropriate.									
7. Sterilizes the control and properly disposes of both vials.									
8. Records testing results on a tracking sheet and keeps information of file.									
9. Indicates sterilizers need to be tested on a weekly basis.									
Strips									
1. Obtains three test strips.									
2. Keeps one strip in the envelope and places the other two into instrument packs.									
3. Sterilizes instrument packs with test strips inside.									
4. Sends all three strips to the testing agency for verification.									
5. Records information from the testing agency on a tracking sheet and keeps information on file.									
6. Verbalizes that a negative report indicates adequate sterilization occurred and a positive report indicates corrective procedures must be made immediately.									

Courtesy of University of Cincinnati, Raymond Walters College Dental Hygiene Program

AUTOCLAVE PERFORMANCE SKILL SHEET

Student _____

Date _____

Instructor _____

Re-evaluation
Instr: _____
Date _____

Instr: _____
Date _____

	S	U	Comments	S	U	Comments
Pre-Sterilization Procedures/Loading Trays:						
1. Covers bottom of metal trays with paper towels.						
2. Arranges cassettes and/or paper/plastic bags (paper side up) in single layer on separate tray.						
3. Arranges plastic (nyclave tubing) pouches on tray (may be stacked double).				∴		
***Tuttnauer* Autoclaving Procedures:**						
1. Turns on autoclave using start button.						
2. Checks water level at opening in reservoir on top of autoclave.						
3. Adds **distilled water,** if needed.						
4. Sets temperature at 273° F.						
5. Turns control knob to "Fill Water".						
6. Turns control knob to "STE" when water touches indicator groove in chamber.						
7. Closes door tightly.						
8. Sets timer for appropriate sterilization time: 30 minutes.						
9. After autoclaving, turns control knob to "EXH. DRY".						
10. When pressure gets to "0", opens door slightly to vent autoclave.						
11. Sets timer for 30 minute drying cycle.						
12. Turns control knob to "O" when drying cycle is completed.						
***Midmark* Autoclave Procedures:**						
1. Turns on autoclave using "On/Standby" padswitch.						
2. Checks water level at colored (red/green) indicator inside the door.						
3. Adds **distilled water,** if needed.						
4. Closes door tightly making sure door handle is latched and secured down.						
5. Presses appropriate category on padswitch.						
6. Presses "start" padswitch.						

Courtesy of Indiana University Purdue University Fort Wayne Dental Hygiene Program

Chapter 2

Medical and Dental Histories

William A. Johnson, DMD, MPH

MediaLink

A companion CD-ROM, included free with each new copy of this book, supplements the procedures presented in each chapter. Insert the CD-ROM to watch video clips and view a large collection of color images that is also included. This multimedia library is designed to help you add a new dimension to your learning.

KEY TERMS

adverse reaction. Undesired effect as a result of drug therapy.

allergy. Overreaction by the immune system to a foreign substance, characterized by itching, redness, and difficulty in breathing.

antibiotic premedication. Pretreatment antibiotic therapy to prevent possible infection caused by bacteremia.

bacteremia. Introduction of bacteria into the bloodstream, which can lead to treatment complications in certain circumstances.

chief complaint. Principle reason for seeking dental treatment.

closed-ended question. A question whose answer requires no explanation; a yes-or-no question.

course of action. A planned response after analyzing pertinent information.

disease-oriented question. A question requesting specific information about past or present diseases experienced by the patient.

hyperventilation. An increased rate of breathing, often as a response to stress, that can cause an unwanted patient response.

immunosuppressed. A term describing a patient with an immune system unable to respond at its maximum potential.

infective endocarditis. Infection of the heart's lining, often as a result of a bacteremia.

informed consent. An agreement, signed by the patient, to proceed with treatment after all possible treatment outcomes are revealed.

medical alert. A process to warn healthcare providers that a patient may respond to treatment in a life-threatening manner.

medical consultation. A request for further information from a dental patient's physician to clarify responses to the questionnaire.

mitral valve prolapse. Abnormal closure of the valve between the heart's left atrium and ventricle.

objective symptom. A patient's response to a medical or dental condition that can be readily observed or measured by the healthcare provider.

over-the-counter (OTC). A drug that can be purchased without a prescription.

open-ended question. A question whose answer requires an explanation.

Physicians' Desk Reference (PDR). A publication that describes the purpose, dosage, contraindications, and side effects of drugs.

side effect. A predictable, unwanted reaction (e.g., nausea and diarrhea) to a drug by a body system.

subjective symptom. A patient's response (to a medical or dental condition) that cannot be easily measured or readily observed.

symptom-oriented questions. A question concerning any response a patient may be experiencing to a medical or dental condition.

syncope. Temporary unconsciousness (fainting) resulting from decreased oxygen to the brain.

LEARNING OBJECTIVES

After reading this chapter, the student will be able to:

- list the components and purposes of a comprehensive medical/dental history;
- identify conditions that require immediate treatment modification or medical consultation;
- recognize conditions that may complicate dental hygiene care;

- determine systemic signs and symptoms that require medical follow up;
- utilize interview techniques for gathering additional information from patients;
- plan a course of action based on the results of the questionnaire and interview.

I. **Introduction**

A. Medical/dental history

The medical/dental history provides critical information, from the patient's point of view, that may affect diagnosis and treatment. The healthcare provider has the responsibility to interview the patient to verify the accuracy of the information obtained as well as gather additional information that may have been omitted by the patient. The medical/dental history is a legal document that must be completed and signed by the patient, legal guardian or designee, in indelible ink, and should be updated and signed at each consecutive appointment.

1. Objectives of the medical/dental history are to

a. Define the physical and mental health status of the patient

b. Identify conditions that may cause an office emergency

c. Determine conditions requiring antibiotic premedication

d. Suggest etiologies for existing dental conditions

e. Recognize conditions that may compromise treatment procedures and outcomes

f. Delineate symptoms of systemic disorders that require medical follow-up

g. Provide information upon which the healthcare provider bases further questions regarding the patient's health

h. Determine a course of action based on information obtained from the questionnaire and interview

2. Important considerations regarding the medical/dental history

a. Avoid treatment, including emergency care or examination procedures, until an adequate history has been taken

b. Certain medical conditions preclude any dental care until additional information is received or precautions are taken; those medical conditions may not be recognized until the history is taken

c. Update medical/dental history at each visit by asking the patient if any changes have occurred since the last visit

d. When making corrections on the medical/dental history, or any other patient document, draw one line through the incorrect information, then date and initial

II. **Components of a Comprehensive Medical/Dental History—consists of three parts: questionnaire, interview, and course of action**

A. Questionnaire consists of a written document used to gather specific medical and dental information from the patient

1. Purpose: To gather information quickly and easily regarding the patient's past and present medical and dental conditions

2. Completed as a written form prior to receiving care

a. Forms vary, since there is no accepted standard

b. May range from simple to complex, depending on the needs of the dental care facility

c. American Dental Association (ADA) form is an example of a comprehensive questionnaire[1] (Figure 2–1)

3. Questions: Often require *yes* or *no* answers that are either checked or circled; *yes* answers usually require additional follow-up dialogue during the interview process

---

PRECLINICAL TIP

Investigating Your Knowledge:
Example: *Have you had rheumatic fever?*
☐ Yes ☐ No
A checked yes box requires follow-up. *Good questionnaires are organized so* yes *responses are obvious.*

| Medical Alert: | Condition: | Premedication: | Allergies: | Anesthesia: | Date: |

ADA. American Dental Association
www.ada.org

HEALTH HISTORY FORM

Name: _____ Home Phone: ( ) _____ Business Phone: ( ) _____
　　　LAST　　　　FIRST　　　　MIDDLE
Address: _____ City: _____ State: _____ Zip Code: _____
　　P.O. BOX or Mailing Address
Occupation: _____ Height: _____ Weight: _____ Date of Birth: _____ Sex: M ❑ F ❑
SS#: _____ Emergency Contact: _____ Relationship: _____ Phone: ( ) _____

If you are completing this form for another person, what is your relationship to that person? _____
　　　　　　　　　　　　　　　　　　　　　　　　　NAME　　　　　　　　　RELATIONSHIP

For the following questions, please (X) whichever applies, your answers are for our records only and will be kept confidential in accordance with applicable laws. Please note that during your initial visit you will be asked some questions about your responses to this questionnaire and there may be additional questions concerning your health. This information is vital to allow us to provide appropriate care for you. This office does not use this information to discriminate.

DENTAL INFORMATION

	Yes	No	Don't Know
Do your gums bleed when you brush?	❑	❑	❑
Have you ever had orthodontic (braces) treatment?	❑	❑	❑
Are your teeth sensitive to cold, hot, sweets or pressure?	❑	❑	❑
Do you have earaches or neck pains?	❑	❑	❑
Have you had any periodontal (gum) treatments?	❑	❑	❑
Do you wear removable dental appliances?	❑	❑	❑
Have you had a serious/difficult problem associated with any previous dental treatment?	❑	❑	❑
If yes, explain:			

How would you describe your current dental problem? _____

Date of your last dental exam: _____

Date of last dental x-rays: _____

What was done at that time? _____

How do you feel about the appearance of your teeth? _____

MEDICAL INFORMATION

	Yes	No	Don't Know
If you answer yes to any of the 3 items below, please stop and return this form to the receptionist.			
Have you had any of the following diseases or problems?			
Active Tuberculosis	❑	❑	❑
Persistent cough greater than a 3 week duration	❑	❑	❑
Cough that produces blood	❑	❑	❑
Are you in good health?	❑	❑	❑
Has there been any change in your general health within the past year?	❑	❑	❑
Are you now under the care of a physician?	❑	❑	❑
If yes, what is/are the condition(s) being treated?			

Date of last physical examination: _____

Physician:
NAME _____ PHONE _____
ADDRESS _____ CITY/STATE _____ ZIP _____

NAME _____ PHONE _____
ADDRESS _____ CITY/STATE _____ ZIP _____

	Yes	No	Don't Know
Have you had any serious illness, operation, or been hospitalized in the past 5 years?	❑	❑	❑
If yes, what was the illness or problem?			

	Yes	No	Don't Know
Are you taking or have you recently taken any medicine(s) including non-prescription medicine?	❑	❑	❑
If yes, what medicine(s) are you taking?			

Prescribed: _____

Over the counter: _____

Vitamins, natural or herbal preparations and/or diet supplements: _____

	Yes	No	Don't Know
Are you taking, or have you taken, any diet drugs such Pondimin (fenfluramine), Redux (dexphenfluramine) or phen-fen (fenfluramine-phentermine combination)?	❑	❑	❑
Do you drink alcoholic beverages?	❑	❑	❑
If yes, how much alcohol did you drink in the last 24 hours?			
In the past week?			
Are you alcohol and/or drug dependent?	❑	❑	❑
If yes, have you received treatment? (circle one) Yes / No			
Do you use drugs or other substances for recreational purposes?	❑	❑	❑
If yes, please list:			
Frequency of use (daily, weekly, etc.):			
Number of years of recreational drug use:			
Do you use tobacco (smoking, snuff, chew)?	❑	❑	❑
If yes, how interested are you in stopping? (circle one) Very / Somewhat / Not interested			
Do you wear contact lenses?	❑	❑	❑

PLEASE COMPLETE BOTH SIDES

Figure 2–1　ADA Medical History Questionnaire

Are you allergic to or have you had a reaction to?   Yes No Don't Know

Local anesthetics ☐ ☐ ☐
Aspirin ☐ ☐ ☐
Penicillin or other antibiotics ☐ ☐ ☐
Barbiturates, sedatives, or sleeping pills ☐ ☐ ☐
Sulfa drugs ☐ ☐ ☐
Codeine or other narcotics ☐ ☐ ☐
Latex ☐ ☐ ☐
Iodine ☐ ☐ ☐
Hay fever/seasonal ☐ ☐ ☐
Animals ☐ ☐ ☐
Food (specify) _____ ☐ ☐ ☐
Other (specify)_____ ☐ ☐ ☐
Metals (specify)_____ ☐ ☐ ☐

To yes responses, specify type of reaction.
_____
_____
_____
_____

Have you had an orthopedic total joint   Yes No Don't Know
(hip, knee, elbow, finger) replacement?   ☐ ☐ ☐
If yes, when was this operation done? _____

If you answered yes to the above question, have you had
any complications or difficulties with your prosthetic joint?
_____
_____

Has a physician or previous dentist recommended
that you take antibiotics prior to your dental treatment?   ☐ ☐ ☐
If yes, what antibiotic and dose? _____
Name of physician or dentist: _____
Phone: _____

WOMEN ONLY

Are you or could you be pregnant? ☐ ☐ ☐
Nursing? ☐ ☐ ☐
Taking birth control pills or hormonal replacement? ☐ ☐ ☐

Please (X) a response to indicate if you have or have not had any of the following diseases or problems.

Yes No Don't Know

Abnormal bleeding ☐ ☐ ☐
AIDS or HIV infection ☐ ☐ ☐
Anemia ☐ ☐ ☐
Arthritis ☐ ☐ ☐
Rheumatoid arthritis ☐ ☐ ☐
Asthma ☐ ☐ ☐
Blood transfusion. If yes, date: _____ ☐ ☐ ☐
Cancer/ Chemotherapy/Radiation Treatment ☐ ☐ ☐
Cardiovascular disease. If yes, specify below: ☐ ☐ ☐
____ Angina   ____Heart murmur
____ Arteriosclerosis   ____High blood pressure
____ Artificial heart valves ____Low blood pressure
____ Congenital heart defects ____Mitral valve prolapse
____ Congestive heart failure ____Pacemaker
____ Coronary artery disease ____Rheumatic heart
____ Damaged heart valves   disease/Rheumatic fever
____ Heart attack
Chest pain upon exertion ☐ ☐ ☐
Chronic pain ☐ ☐ ☐
Disease, drug, or radiation-induced immunosuppression ☐ ☐ ☐
Diabetes. If yes, specify below: ☐ ☐ ☐
____ Type I (Insulin dependent)   ____Type II
Dry Mouth ☐ ☐ ☐
Eating disorder. If yes, specify: _____ ☐ ☐ ☐
Epilepsy ☐ ☐ ☐
Fainting spells or seizures ☐ ☐ ☐
Gastrointestinal disease ☐ ☐ ☐
G.E. Reflux/persistent heartburn ☐ ☐ ☐
Glaucoma ☐ ☐ ☐

Yes No Don't Know

Hemophilia ☐ ☐ ☐
Hepatitis, jaundice or liver disease ☐ ☐ ☐
Recurrent Infections ☐ ☐ ☐
If yes, indicate type of infection: _____
Kidney problems ☐ ☐ ☐
Mental health disorders. If yes, specify: _____ ☐ ☐ ☐
Malnutrition ☐ ☐ ☐
Night sweats ☐ ☐ ☐
Neurological disorders. If yes, specify: _____ ☐ ☐ ☐
Osteoporosis ☐ ☐ ☐
Persistent swollen glands in neck
Respiratory problems. If yes, specify below: ☐ ☐ ☐
____ Emphysema   ____ Bronchitis, etc.
Severe headaches/migraines ☐ ☐ ☐
Severe or rapid weight loss ☐ ☐ ☐
Sexually transmitted disease ☐ ☐ ☐
Sinus trouble ☐ ☐ ☐
Sleep disorder ☐ ☐ ☐
Sores or ulcers in the mouth ☐ ☐ ☐
Stroke ☐ ☐ ☐
Systemic lupus erythematosus ☐ ☐ ☐
Tuberculosis ☐ ☐ ☐
Thyroid problems ☐ ☐ ☐
Ulcers ☐ ☐ ☐
Excessive urination ☐ ☐ ☐

Do you have any disease, condition, or problem
not listed above that you think I should know about?   ☐ ☐ ☐
Please explain: _____

NOTE: Both Doctor and patient are encouraged to discuss any and all relevant patient health issues prior to treatment.

I certify that I have read and understand the above. I acknowledge that my questions, if any, about inquiries set forth above have been answered to my satisfaction. I will not hold my dentist, or any other member of his/her staff, responsible for any action they take or do not take because of errors or omissions that I may have made in the completion of this form.

_____   _____
SIGNATURE OF PATIENT/LEGAL GUARDIAN   DATE

FOR COMPLETION BY DENTIST

Comments on patient interview concerning health history:
_____

Significant findings from questionnaire or oral interview:
_____

Dental management considerations:
_____

Health History Update: On a regular basis the patient should be questioned about any medical history changes, date and comments notated, along with signature.

Date	Comments	Signature of patient and dentist

S500

Figure 2–1   (Continued)

a. Types of questions[2]
   (1) Disease-oriented questions
      (a) Consist of objective questions about specific diseases a patient has had or currently has
      (b) Interviewer can usually use closed-ended questions during follow-up evaluation
   (2) Symptom-oriented questions
      (a) Deal with subjective symptoms the patient may be experiencing
      (b) Interviewer can usually use open-ended questions during follow-up evaluation
   (3) Personal information: Obtained not only to identify the patient but also to gain insight into the overall health status; questions include
      (a) Patient's name, age, gender, height, weight, occupation, and whether the patient is currently under the care of a physician (note that height to weight ratios outside of normal ranges could indicate the need for nutritional counseling or reveal a predisposition for high blood pressure and/or diabetes)
      (b) Personal habits, such as smoking, drinking, eating patterns, and drug use
        • Excessive tobacco, alcohol, and drug use could have a bearing on treatment success due to the condition of oral tissues and a compromised healing process; a correlation exists between tobacco use and periodontal disease and heart disease
   (4) Dental history questions include
      (a) Reason for patient's visit
      (b) Description of chief complaint
      (c) Description of any present dental symptom(s) (e.g., pain, sensitive teeth, bleeding on brushing)
      (d) Information about previous dental care, including periodontal, orthodontic, prosthodontic, and endodontic treatment
      (e) Name, address, and telephone number of the patient's previous dentist, needed in order to request radiographs or other information
      (f) Patient's attitude toward receiving dental care in order to judge level of apprehension
   (5) Medical history questions are concerned with the patient's
      (a) Past and present medical treatment
      (b) Symptom(s)
      (c) Medication(s) and dosage(s)
      (d) Allergies

B. Interview: Purpose is to clarify information provided on the questionnaire and confirm its accuracy; it should
  1. Encompass an important component of the medical/dental history and *not* be underestimated
  2. Help determine, together with the questionnaire, a course of action
  3. Use techniques that will invoke trust and confidence from the patient[3]

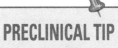

PRECLINICAL TIP

Investigating Your Knowledge: A *chief complaint* is the oral condition that brought the patient to the office. Treat it first! Then focus on the other aspects of dental hygiene care.

PRECLINICAL TIP

Investigating Your Knowledge: A patient who has had periodontal surgery may have areas of recession. Active orthodontic patients may need additional plaque control instruction. Prosthetic appliances may need special cleaning.

a. Conduct in a comfortable location that affords privacy, especially if potentially sensitive questions are to be asked or addressed

    b. If privacy is not entirely possible, the interviewer should speak softly, yet clearly, so nearby persons cannot hear

    c. Interviewer should

       (1) Sit at eye level, not above the patient, and make eye contact when asking questions

       (2) Speak in a confident, matter-of-fact manner and phrase all questions tactfully

       (3) Use terms appropriate to patient's level of understanding

C. Course of Action: Purpose is to achieve the objectives of the medical/dental history by altering treatment in response to the results of the questionnaire and interview

   1. Can be determined after a history is completed; determines options to

    a. Proceed with treatment with no modifications

    b. Proceed with treatment with modifications

    c. Affix a medical alert to the health history form and proceed with treatment

    d. Proceed with treatment after prophylactic premedication is received by the patient

    e. Request a medical consultation—treatment will depend on the physician's response

    f. Postpone treatment until physician examines patient or until symptoms subside

III. Accomplishing Medical/Dental History Objectives

Medical/dental history objectives include outcomes that are expected to occur if the process is comprehensive; objectives include

A. Define the patient's physical and mental health status

   1. Questionnaire: Sample questions include the following

    a. *Are you in good health?*

    b. *Have there been any changes in your general health in the last year?*

    c. *Are you currently under the care of a physician?*

   2. Information gathered includes

    a. Physician's name, address, and phone number

    b. Date of last physician visit

    c. Reason for the visit

   3. Interview

    a. Health status is relative and requires additional information from the patient; for example, an 80-year-old patient recovering from a recent heart transplant may indicate he/she is in good health

    b. If a patient has seen a physician recently, still inquire about the visit even though the reason may have been indicated on the questionnaire

   4. Course of action

    a. Estimate medical risk of patient to receive dental care according to the American Society of Anesthesiologists, or ASA (Table 2–1)

       (1) ASA I: Normal, healthy patient with no apparent systemic disease

Table 2–1   Patients for ASA Classifications

ASA Classification	Examples of Patients
ASA II	1. Well-controlled NIDDM, epilepsy, asthma, hyper- and hypothyroid disorders (with normal thyroid function) 2. Healthy pregnant women 3. Healthy patients with allergies, especially to drugs 4. Healthy patients with extreme dental fears 5. Healthy patients over 60 years old 6. B.P. between 140 and 160 mmHg systolic and/or 90 and 94 mmHg diastolic
ASA III	1. Stable angina pectoris 2. Well-controlled IDDM 3. Exercise-induced asthma 4. Symptomatic hyper- and hypothyroid disorders 5. Status post-CVA and postmyocardial infarction more than 6 months before treatment with no residual signs and symptoms 6. Emphysema or chronic bronchitis 7. B.P. between 160 and 200 mmHg systolic and/or 94 and 114 mmHg diastolic
ASA IV	1. Unstable angina pectoris 2. CVA within the past 6 months 3. Uncontrolled IDDM and epilepsy 4. Severe CHF or COPD 5. B.P. greater than 220 mmHg systolic or 115 mmHg diastolic
ASA V	End-stage • Cancer • Cardiovascular disease • Hepatic disease • Infectious disease • Renal disease • Respiratory disease

NIDDM = Noninsulin-dependent diabetes mellitus
B.P. = Blood pressure
IDDM = Insulin-dependent diabetes mellitus
CVA = Cardiovascular accident
CHF = Congestive heart failure
COPD = Chronic obstructive pulmonary disease

       (2) ASA II: Patient with a mild systemic disease
       (3) ASA III: Patient with a severe but not incapacitating systemic disease
       (4) ASA IV: Patient with a life-threatening, incapacitating systemic disease
       (5) ASA V: Patient *not* expected to survive 24 hours (not applicable in dentistry)
       (6) If an emergency situation exists, add an *E* before the ASA classification
    b. Proceed with treatment if a patient indicates good health and nothing on the health history indicates otherwise (ASA I and II)
    c. Encourage patients who have not been to a physician recently to practice preventive medicine
    d. If patient is an ASA III or IV, determine reason(s) patient is in poor health, then decide whether treatment should proceed; a medical consultation may be necessary in many cases
B. Identify conditions that may cause an office emergency[5]
    1. Questionnaire: Sample questions include the following:
       a. *Have you had any problems with any previous dental care?*

(1) Patients may indicate that dental procedures make them extremely nervous; this should alert the healthcare provider to a potential problem, and precautions should be taken

(2) Anxiety can lead to an emergency situation for patients with certain medical conditions, including angina, asthma, hypertension, and seizure disorders

(3) Most common emergencies that occur in the dental office are related to anxiety and include

    (a) Syncope/psychogenic shock (fainting): Result of insufficient oxygen to the brain causing temporary loss of consciousness

    (b) Hyperventilation: Result of rapid breathing due to excessive oxygen in the blood; causes tingling in extremities and potential loss of consciousness

    (c) Panic: Denotes uncontrolled fear precipitating a need to escape

    (d) Hypoglycemia: Indicates low blood sugar resulting from increased demand for insulin caused by stressful situations

b. *Are you allergic to any of the following?*

(1) List of allergens, which include medications, foods, latex, animals, and so on

(2) Ask patient if he/she has been diagnosed with an allergy—some self-diagnose; note what types of symptoms and signs are experienced with allergic reaction

(3) Allergic responses to medications can be life-threatening; for example

    (a) Allergy to PABA (sunscreen) may indicate an allergy to benzocaine; therefore, topical lidocaine must be used

    (b) Allergy to tropical fruits, such as papaya and kiwi, could indicate an allergy to latex[6]

c. *Do you have any of the following conditions: angina, asthma, epilepsy?*

(1) Each of these conditions can lead to a medical emergency

(2) May require specific medications to control symptoms

2. Interview

a. Ask patient about past dental experiences; be reassuring and sensitive if patient is anxious about dental care

b. Ask patient if prescribed medications have been taken for medical conditions exacerbated by anxiety

c. Determine if dental care has triggered previous attacks

d. Discuss all allergies, since a person sensitive to one allergen may be sensitive to others

e. Be thorough! Patients often confuse allergic reactions with side effects; whereas side effects are inconvenient, they are not as serious as an allergic response

3. Course of action

a. Use a calm approach and constant reassurance to help the anxious patient

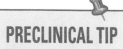

PRECLINICAL TIP

Investigating Your Knowledge: *Allergic reactions* may include itching, rash, and shortness of breath. *Side effects* may include nausea, diarrhea, and constipation. Both are *adverse reactions,* but an allergic reaction is more dangerous.

b. Make sure asthma, cardiac, and seizure patients have medications handy in case of an attack; often they are placed on the bracket tray or nearby to assure easy access; if patient forgets to bring inhaler, use one from the emergency drug cart

c. If a true allergy exists, affix a medical alert to the patient's record according to established office/clinic protocol

C. Identify conditions requiring antibiotic premedication (Table 2–2)

1. Questionnaire: Sample questions include the following

a. *Have you been diagnosed with any of the following: mitral valve prolapse, rheumatic fever, inborn heart defects, heart murmur, lupus erythematosus?*

    (1) Patients with any of these conditions may have damaged heart valves or damaged lining of the heart

    (2) If heart damage is present, a bacteremia is more likely to lead to infective endocarditis (inflammation of the lining of the heart)

    (3) Use antibiotic premedication prior to dental care to prevent bacteremia-induced endocarditis

b. *Have you had a joint replacement in the past year?*

    (1) Bacteremia-induced vegetations may grow on recently placed joint replacements

    (2) Some physicians request antibiotic premedication for patients with a joint replacement

c. *Are you receiving chemotherapy for cancer?*

    (1) Patients receiving chemotherapy may have a low white blood cell count and are therefore susceptible to infections

    (2) Usually treatment would be postponed, but premedication may still be indicated

2. Interview

a. If patient indicates a mitral valve prolapse condition, be sure it is "with regurgitation", which may require antibiotic premedication

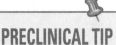

PRECLINICAL TIP

Investigating Your Knowledge: If a true allergy exists, avoid patient contact with the allergen.

PRECLINICAL TIP

Investigating Your Knowledge: Bacteremia is an introduction of bacteria into the bloodstream that can lead to bacterial growths (vegetations) on damaged heart valves or joint replacements.

PRECLINICAL TIP

Investigating Your Knowledge: *Mitral valve prolapse* is the improper closing of the mitral valve of the heart. This results in backwards flow of blood into the left atrium (regurgitation). Prolapse without regurgitation does *not* require premedication.

Table 2–2   Medical Conditions Requiring Antibiotic Premedication or Physician Consultation

1. Cardiac-related conditions
   - Congenital heart disease/congenital heart defect
   - Rheumatic heart disease/rheumatic fever (valve damage)
   - Some heart murmurs, such as organic
   - Prosthetic heart valves
   - History of infective endocarditis
   - Temporary pacemaker
   - Heart bypass surgery (premedicate for first 6 months)
   - Mitral valve prolapse with regurgitation
   - Heart transplant
   - Shunts
2. Other medical conditions
   - Chemotherapy
   - Kidney transplant
   - Renal disorders, including dialysis
   - Shunts common with kidney dialysis or with patients with spina bifada (hydrocephalic conditions)
   - Uncontrolled/poorly controlled diabetes
   - Immunosuppressive therapy
   - Blood disorders (e.g., leukemia, sickle cell anemia)
   - Total prosthetic joint replacement (within last 2 years)

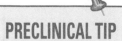

PRECLINICAL TIP

Investigating Your Knowledge:
The *American Heart Association* recommends 2 gms of Amoxicillin one hour before the appointment. If the patient is allergic to penicillin, 600 mg of Clindamycin or 2 gms of Cephalexin is substituted.[7]

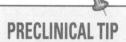

PRECLINICAL TIP

Investigating Your Knowledge:
Three categories of drugs, phenytoin (Dilantin) for seizures, calcium channel blockers (nifedipine) for high blood pressure, and cyclosporine for the prevention of transplant rejection, can cause gingival enlargement.[8]

    b. Ask patient if the physician has indicated need for premedication

    c. Ask patient if premedication, before dental visits, has been indicated in the past

    d. If premedication is indicated, ask if medication has been taken

3. Course of action

    a. Patients requiring premedication should take the antibiotic as prescribed *before* any invasive procedure is performed that could create a bacteremia; such procedures include

      (1) Probing

      (2) Debridement

      (3) Polishing that extends subgingivally

      (4) Extractions

    b. Seek medical consultation if patient is unsure whether premedication is necessary before proceeding

    c. Postpone treatment if medication is necessary and has not been taken

D. Suggest possible etiologies for dental conditions

1. Questionnaire: Sample questions include the following

    a. *Are you presently taking any prescribed or over-the-counter (OTC) medications?*

      (1) Gingival enlargement can be an inherited trait, but it can also be caused by drug therapy—specifically, phenytoin for seizures, calcium channel blockers for cardiovascular conditions, and cyclosporine for transplant rejection

      (2) Many OTC medications (*not* requiring a prescription), like antihistamines and weight loss medications, can lead to xerostomia (dry mouth)

    b. *What is your age, gender, weight, height? Are you pregnant?*

      (1) Disproportionate height/weight ratios may indicate anorexia nervosa, an eating disorder; some anorexics practice bulimia (purging after eating), which can lead to eroded dentition caused by stomach acid

      (2) Changes in female hormone levels during puberty, menopause, and pregnancy can exacerbate clinical signs of gingivitis[9]

    c. *Are you receiving chemotherapy cancer treatments?*

      (1) Anticancer drugs can cause oral lesions

      (2) White blood cell (WBC) count may be necessary before treatment

2. Interview

    a. Ask patients who are taking any drugs with possible oral side effects if they have noticed any unusual oral conditions

    b. Ask female patients if they have noticed any changes in their oral tissues during their menstrual cycle

    c. Question pregnant patients about any oral changes

3. Course of action

    a. Research all drugs in reference guides such as the *Physicians' Desk Reference (PDR)* and/or *Medline,* because information can change

    b. Educate patients exhibiting exaggerated gingival response to bacterial plaque

    c. Verify WBC count is at acceptable levels

E. Identify conditions that may compromise treatment procedures and outcomes

1. Questionnaire: Sample questions include the following

   a. *Are you presently taking any prescribed or over-the-counter medications?*

      (1) Prescription drugs for hypertension, anxiety, and psychological disorders can also cause xerostomia, as can OTC drugs for weight management and the treatment of cold and allergy symptoms; xerostomia can lead to plaque accumulation, resulting in increased periodontal disease and caries

      (2) Common OTC drugs, such as aspirin and ibuprofen, can lead to prolonged bleeding if taken often for such conditions as arthritis or chronic pain; prolonged bleeding can be caused by anticoagulant drugs such as Coumadin and medical conditions such as hemophilia

   b. *Do you use tobacco products?*

      (1) Poor wound healing due to increased plaque accumulation and smoke irritants can be caused by excessive tobacco use

      (2) Additional stain removal procedures may be necessary for heavy smokers

   c. *Do you have diabetes? Describe your nutritional status. Are you immunosuppressed due to medications, disease, or age?*

      (1) Uncontrolled diabetes and improper nutrition can lead to poor wound healing

      (2) Immunosuppressed patients may have an exaggerated response to plaque and extreme gingivitis or periodontal disease

   d. *Do you have any of the following contagious diseases: tuberculosis, herpes labialis, impetigo?*

      (1) Tuberculosis is an airborne disease that can spread through aerosols in the dental office

      (2) Herpes labialis (commonly known as a cold sore) is a viral infection on the lips that can easily spread

      (3) Impetigo is a highly contagious skin infection that is easily spread through contact

2. Interview

   a. Patients often believe OTC drugs, such as aspirin or diet supplements, are *not* necessary to list because they are harmless; question patients about their use of OTC drugs

   b. Ask immunosuppressed patients if they have noticed any changes in their oral health

   c. Ask diabetic patients if medication is taken regularly and when and what they last ate; have appropriate medical treatment, such as juice and canned frosting, readily available in emergency drug cart in case of hypoglycemia

   d. Ask patients with an infectious disease how long they have had the symptoms and whether they are receiving medical care; for example, patients with tuberculosis must be on medication for several months to *not* be infectious

   e. Question patients about their diet, especially if they appear malnourished; diets low in protein and zinc lead to slow wound healing[10]

3. Course of action
   a. Warn patients taking excessive amounts of aspirin or ibuprofen that they may experience prolonged bleeding; in most circumstances care can proceed, but caution is advised
   b. Recommend a saliva substitute for patients experiencing xerostomia; be prepared to rinse their mouths more frequently during polishing procedures; xerostomia and immunosuppressed patients usually require more plaque removal instruction
   c. Medical consultation is necessary, before proceeding, for a patient who
      (1) Has recently contracted tuberculosis; postpone treatment until the physician indicates a noncontagious status
      (2) Is taking an anticoagulant, such as Coumadin
   d. Nutritional counseling may be necessary for patients with signs of an unbalanced diet

F. Delineate symptoms of systemic disorders that require medical follow-up
   1. Questionnaire: Sample questions include the following:
      a. *Are you experiencing any abnormal breathing? Do you have chest pain upon exertion? Have you had a change in your sleeping patterns?*
         (1) Certain questions ask patients about symptoms they may be experiencing
         (2) Some questions ask about changes in normal patterns of behavior
      b. *Have you had recent rapid weight loss? Are you experiencing excessive urination?*
         (1) Some questions are intended to identify signs of potentially serious medical conditions that necessitate physician follow-up
         (2) It is the responsibility of all healthcare providers to be familiar with these signs and refer accordingly
   2. Interview
      a. Any symptom marked yes on a medical history requires interview follow-up; some offices mark yes answers in red
      b. Use open-ended questions when asking patient to describe his or her symptoms
   3. Course of action
      a. Review the questionnaire and determine if the patient has recently seen a physician
      b. If the patient is presently experiencing life-threatening symptoms, postpone care until medical attention is sought
      c. If symptoms are not clinically evident, encourage the patient to seek a medical evaluation as soon as possible

IV. **Conclusion**

The health history consists of the questionnaire, interview, and course of action, and is an integral part of total patient care. No care should be provided until an adequate health history is completed. To accomplish the objectives of the medical/dental history, interview the patient about all questions marked yes on the questionnaire and determine a course of action before proceeding. Do not assume, because the questionnaire doesn't have yes responses, that there are no medical/dental complications. It is

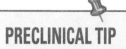

PRECLINICAL TIP

Investigating Your Knowledge: Signs of cardiovascular disease include chest pain on exertion, shortness of breath, and swelling of the extremities.

PRECLINICAL TIP

Investigating Your Knowledge: Early signs of diabetes include frequent thirst, urination, and excessive hunger.

the responsibility of the healthcare provider to always interview the patient and affirm the questionnaire is correct.

QUESTIONS

1. In which of the following situations does a medical/dental history NOT have to be taken?
   a. An examination is going to be performed.
   b. The patient is in pain and needs immediate attention.
   c. The patient refuses to give a medical history.
   d. The patient is a minor.
   e. All situations require a medical/dental history.

2. All of the following are purposes of a medical/dental history EXCEPT one. Which one is the EXCEPTION?
   a. Identify conditions that will require the use of universal precautions.
   b. Identify conditions that may precipitate an emergency during treatment.
   c. Determine conditions that require premedication before treatment.
   d. Recognize situations that may require medical follow-up.
   e. Suggest etiologies for existing dental conditions.

3. Which of the following is an example of an open-ended question?
   a. What is your date of birth?
   b. When was your last visit to a dentist?
   c. Do your gums bleed when you brush?
   d. What do you feel are good qualities of a dental hygienist?
   e. Do you have any hobbies?

4. Which of the following courses of action would be LEAST appropriate for a patient who is not sure if premedication is needed for an existing heart murmur?
   a. Request a medical consultation.
   b. Proceed with scaling and root planing on the condition the patient bring a statement from the physician to next appointment.
   c. Postpone care until a medical consultation is obtained.
   d. Avoid invasive procedures until a medical consultation is obtained.

5. Which of the following conditions is MOST indicative of an allergic response?

   a. Diarrhea
   b. Xerostomia
   c. Itching
   d. Nausea
   e. Constipation

6. Which of the following conditions does NOT require antibiotic premedication before proceeding with invasive dental treatment?
   a. Heart valve replacement
   b. Mitral valve prolapse without regurgitation
   c. Hip replacement 2 months previously
   d. Rheumatic fever resulting in a heart murmur

7. According to the American Heart Association, which of the following is the appropriate antibiotic premedication for an adult with no known allergies?
   a. 2 gm Amoxicillin 1 hour preoperatively
   b. 600 mg of Erythromycin 6 hours preoperatively
   c. 2 gm Amoxicillin 1 hour preoperatively and 1 gm 6 hours postoperatively
   d. 2 gm Clindamycin 1 hour preoperatively

8. A scheduled patient is taking Dilantin, an anticonvulsive drug for seizures; Procardia, a calcium channel blocker, and Lasix, a diuretic, both for high blood pressure; and Neoral, a cyclosporine for rheumatoid arthritis. Which of these drugs is LEAST likely to cause gingival enlargement?
   a. Dilantin
   b. Procardia
   c. Lasix
   d. Neoral

9. A scheduled patient suffers from xerostomia because of recent head and neck radiation treatment for cancer. Which of the following would you LEAST likely include in your course of action for your patient because of xerostomia?
   a. Recommend a saliva substitute.
   b. Spend additional time on plaque-control measures.
   c. Rinse frequently during polishing procedures.
   d. Suggest mouth rinses that contain fluoride and alcohol.
   e. Avoid tobacco use.

10. Which of the following is the MOST common medical emergency situation that occurs in the dental office?
    a. Heart attack
    b. Anaphylactic shock
    c. Stroke
    d. Seizure
    e. Syncope

REFERENCES

1. American Dental Association. Medical History Form (S-500), ADA Department of Salable Materials, 211 East Chicago Ave., Chicago, IL 60611.

2. Wiles, C. B., & W. J. Ryan. *Communication for Dental Auxiliaries.* Reston, Virginia, 1982.

3. Wittmann, K. J. & S. H. Kass. Communications. In S. J. Daniels & S. A. Harfst (Eds.), *Dental Hygiene, Concepts, Cases, and Competencies.* St. Louis: Mosby, 2002, pp. 57–71.

4. American Society of Anesthesiologists, New Classification of Physical Status, *Anesthesiology,* 24, 111, January–February 1963.

5. Malamed, Stanley F. *Medical Emergencies in the Dental Office,* 5th ed. St. Louis: Mosby, 2000, pp. 13–49.

6. Roy, A. Epstein, J, Onno, E. Latex Allergies in Dentistry, Recognition and Recommendations, *Journal of the Canadian Dental Association,* 63, 297, April 1997.

7. Dajani, A. S., Taubert, K. A, Wilson, W. Prevention of Bacterial Endocarditis. Recommendations by the American Heart Association. *Journal of the American Medical Association,* 277, 1794, June 11, 1997.

8. Seymour, R. A., Thomason, J. M., Ellis, J. S. The Pathogenesis of Drug-Induced Gingival Overgrowth, *Journal of Clinical Periodontology,* 23, 165, March 1996.

9. Wilkins, E. M. *Clinical Practice of the Dental Hygienists,* 8th ed. Philadelphia: Lippincott, Williams & Wilkins, 1999.

10. Davis, J. R., & C. A. Stegeman. *The Dental Hygienist's Guide to Nutritional Care.* Philadelphia: Saunders, 1998.

Chapter 3

Vital Signs

Mary D. Cooper, RDH, MSEd

MediaLink

A companion CD-ROM, included free with each new copy of this book, supplements the procedures presented in each chapter. Insert the CD-ROM to watch video clips and view a large collection of color images that is also included. This multimedia library is designed to help you add a new dimension to your learning.

KEY TERMS

aneroid. A device that consists of a circular gauge with a needle that moves as pressure rises during cuff inflation when taking a blood pressure.

antipyretic. A substance or procedure used to reduce fever.

ausculatory gap. Silent interval between the true systolic and diastolic pressures.

binaurals. Connects ear pieces to tubing.

bradycardia. Slow pulse rate.

bradypnea. Slow respiration (breathing).

diaphragm. Connected to tubes to carry sound to the earpieces of the stethoscope.

diastolic pressure. The lower number recorded when taking a blood pressure; occurs when the heart relaxes between beats.

hypertension. Elevated blood pressure persistently measuring over 140/90mm Hg.

hypotension. A blood pressure measuring lower than the norm.

Korotkoff sounds. Sharp tapping or knocking sounds heard during each contraction of the heart while taking a blood pressure.

opioid. Possessing some properties characteristic of opiate narcotics.

pulse. Represents the beating of the heart.

respiration. Inhaling and exhaling.

respiratory alkalosis. Result of an excess loss of carbon dioxide, which can be caused by hyperventilation.

sphygmomanometer. Device used to measure arterial blood pressure.

systolic pressure. The upper number recorded when taking a blood pressure; occurs when the heart beats (contracts).

tachycardia. Rapid pulse rate.

tachypnea. Rapid respiration (breathing).

LEARNING OBJECTIVES

Upon reading this chapter, the student should be able to:

- take the following vital signs: blood pressure, heart rate, respiratory rate, and temperature;
- identify the armamentarium of the stethoscope, sphygmomanometer, and inflatable cuff;
- discuss the importance of using a properly fitting blood pressure cuff;
- determine, from the blood pressure reading, when a patient should be referred to a physician;
- compare and contrast the aneroid and mercury manometers;
- list factors that cause hypertension and hypotension;
- determine the factors that affect the performance of taking a blood pressure reading;
- recall the normal resting pulse for adults, children, and well-trained athletes;
- recall the normal temperature and respiratory rates for children and adults.

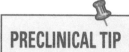

I. Introduction

Obtaining vital signs implies the measurement of vital or critical physiologic functions. It is essential to secure and record vital signs before performing any dental treatment. This information helps determine the patient's ability to tolerate stress during treatment and gives the healthcare provider comparison readings for managing emergency situations.

Four main vital signs should be obtained and recorded at the initial appointment before dental treatment begins.[1]

1. Blood pressure
2. Heart rate (pulse)
3. Respiratory rate
4. Temperature

However, other measures, such as smoking status, should also be evaluated, since this information can alter the practice of healthcare providers. Some healthcare providers view tobacco assessment as a vital sign.[1] Evaluating this information establishes an opportunity to increase counseling and promote smoking cessation programs.

In addition, obtain the height and weight of the patient. An increase or decrease in weight may indicate other health problems.

II. Blood Pressure (B.P.)

Blood pressure is the force exerted by the circulating blood against the walls of the arteries, veins, and chambers of the heart.[3] Monitoring blood pressure helps minimize acute complications associated with high blood pressure, such as strokes, coronary heart disease, congestive heart failure, renal failure, and peripheral vascular disease.

A. Values obtained to measure blood pressure: Systole, diastole, and pulse; most commonly measured by auscultation (hearing) using a sphygmomanometer

1. Systolic pressure: Highest pressure; ventricles contract to send blood into circulation; normal reading is less than 140mm Hg
2. Diastolic pressure: Lowest pressure; ventricles relax to fill with blood returned by the circulation; normal reading is less than 85mm Hg
3. Pulse pressure: Difference between systolic and diastolic pressures; normally around 50mm Hg

B. Armamentarium: Stethoscope, sphygmomanometer, and inflatable bladder

1. Stethoscope (sensing microphone for detection of Korotkoff sounds): Amplifies body sounds; placed lightly over the brachial artery in the antecubital space; (Figure 3–1)

    a. Earpieces: Insert snuggly into ears in an anterior direction
    b. Binaurals: Connects two earpieces to tubing
    c. Diaphragm: Bell-shaped or flat-end piece connected by tubes to carry sound to the earpieces; placed on antecubital space—bend in elbow (Figure 3–2)

        (1) Bell-shaped piece (low-frequency filter): Permits more accurate auscultation of the Korotkoff sounds than does the flat-end piece, especially with diastolic pressure
        (2) Flat-end piece: Most commonly used side due to convenience and easy placement

    d. Rubber tubing: Connects binaurals to diaphragm; should be 12 to 15 inches in length, with airtight connections and not in the way of operator during procedure

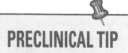

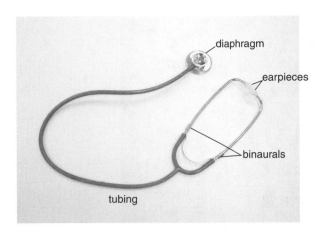

Figure 3–1   Parts of the stethoscope.

2. Sphygmomanometer: Device used to measure arterial blood pressure; consists of manometer (gauge) and inflatable cuff
   a. Marked with lines; short lines are positioned at 2-mm intervals between each long line, which are at 10mm Hg (millimeters of mercury); calibration scale is usually from 0 to 300mm Hg
   b. Types
      (1) Mercury gravity: Contains mercury in a column that rises when pressure is created from inflating the cuff and lowers when pressure is released from cuff (Figure 3–3)
         (a) Most accurate and reliable
         (b) Includes several models, such as freestanding on wheels and top- or wall-mounted units
         (c) Caution: Handle with care to avoid breakage; mercury spills have toxic effect on environment
      (2) Aneroid: Consists of a circular gauge with needle that moves as pressure rises during cuff inflation; most frequently used (refer to Figure 3–4)

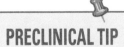

PRECLINICAL TIP

Measuring Your Knowledge: There are several automatic and semiautomatic machines that facilitate self-measurement. Some give a digital printout. They should be periodically calibrated.

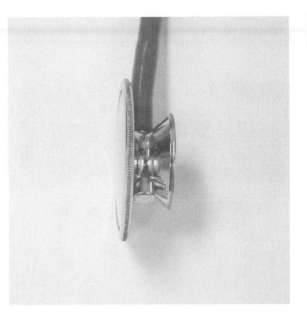

Figure 3–2   Diaphragm (flat-end piece and bell-shaped piece).

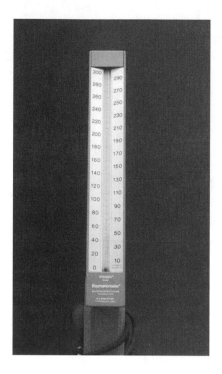

Figure 3–3   Mercury manometer.

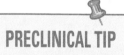
3. Inflatable cuff (bladder): Consists of a nonelastic cloth that houses the inflatable bladder; encircles the arm and is fastened by Velcro
   a. Parts (Figure 3–4)
      (1) Rubber bulb: Connects to tubes; inflates cuff by squeezing
      (2) Control valve: Attaches to rubber bulb; tighten when inflating cuff and loosen when deflating cuff
      (3) Two tubes: One connects to the hand control bulb and the other connects to manometer (pressure gauge)
   b. Size selection: Determined by size of patient's arm
      (1) Compare length of bladder inside the cuff with the circumference of patient's arm—bladder should be at least 80% of the circumference of arm[3] (Figure 3–5)
      (2) Width should be 20% greater than diameter of the limb[3]
      (3) Available in many sizes—most common are child, regular, adult, and thigh

Figure 3–4   Parts of the inflatable cuff.

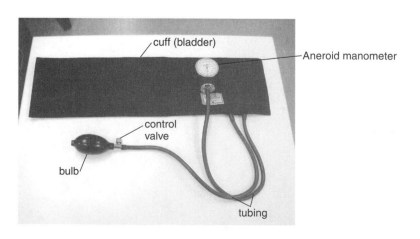

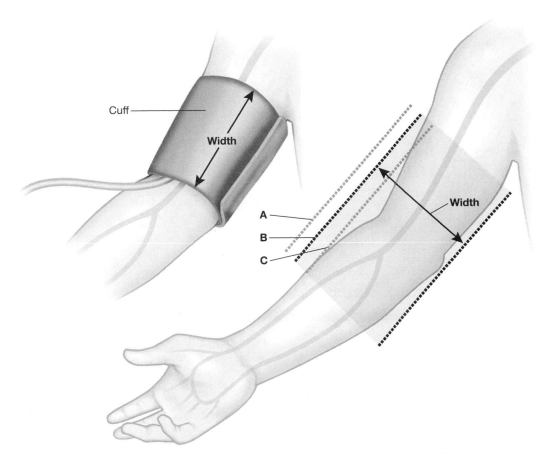

Figure 3–5   Selection of cuff size. A) Too wide; B) Proper width—20% greater than diameter of arm; C) Too narrow.

C. Procedure
1. Patient preparation
   a. Explain procedure to patient
   b. Seat patient in an upright position with legs and feet uncrossed
   c. Rest patient's arm at level of heart, slightly flexed, and re-laxed—if arm is below heart level, reading will be high; if above heart level, reading will be low; support comfortably on a firm surface[7]
   d. Permit patient to rest 5 minutes prior to taking blood pressure and keep the environment peaceful[5]
2. Taking B.P.
   a. Have paper and pen available for recording B.P. in legal docu-ment (medical/dental history or patient chart)
   b. Palpate brachial artery in upper arm near inner bend in elbow (Figure 3–6)
   c. Wrap cuff evenly and snugly around bare upper arm with center of bladder over brachial artery—some cuffs have an arrow to show point of placement (readings will not be accurate other-wise); lower edge of cuff should be 1 inch above antecubital space where bell of stethoscope will be placed

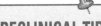

PRECLINICAL TIP

Measuring Your Knowledge: Sometimes different seating posi-tions must be used, which can af-fect B.P. readings. Be sure to document patient's position—sit-ting, lying, or standing—when recording measurement in chart. An average difference in systolic pressure of 11mm Hg and diastolic pressure of 12mm Hg can occur with different positions.[6]

PRECLINICAL TIP

Measuring Your Knowledge: A relaxed patient and quiet environ-ment will give more accurate base-line results. Disturbances, emotions, and surroundings can affect the B.P. reading.

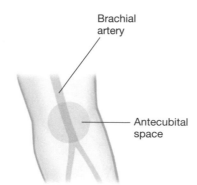

Figure 3–6   Palpate brachial artery.

PRECLINICAL TIP

Measuring Your Knowledge: No clothing should be under the cuff. This may also yield inaccurate B.P. readings.[3]

PRECLINICAL TIP

Measuring Your Knowledge: When a wrong sized cuff is used, results can be erroneous. A normal sized cuff placed on an obese patient produces elevated readings. A normal sized cuff placed on a child produces falsely decreased readings.

PRECLINICAL TIP

Measuring Your Knowledge: Steps for taking B.P. on the thigh:
1. Have patient lying face down.
2. Apply cuff with center of inflatable bladder over posterior aspect of midthigh.
3. Place head of stethoscope over artery in the popliteal fossa (behind the knee).

(1) Proper fit is essential to obtain accurate reading[3]
    (a) Too tight (small): If two fingers cannot fit under edge of cuff, produces an overestimation of B.P.
    (b) Too loose (large): Slips off arm: produces an underestimation of B.P.
    (c) Too narrow: Will result in overestimation of B.P. reading
(2) Special situations
    (a) Obese or muscular patients: Use a longer and wider cuff for adequate compression of the brachial artery; too small a cuff will produce a falsely elevated reading
    (b) Pregnant patients: Position can alter B.P. reading, especially in third trimester; sit patient with arm at heart level for more accurate measurement
    (c) Women who have had mastectomy: Measure B.P. in opposite arm from mastectomy due to removal of lymph; if a double mastectomy has been performed, B.P. should be taken on thigh with a thigh cuff; this is usually performed in a medical office
    (d) Dialysis patients: If shunt is in one arm for dialysis, take B.P. in other arm
d. Place manometer at eye level
e. Obtain palpatory systolic pressure: Cuff is inflated to point where the circulation has stopped and no pulsations can be felt; provides a preliminary estimation of the systolic B.P. to ensure an adequate level of inflation
    (1) Locate radial pulse (in the pocket in the wrist below thumb) by placing index and middle fingers on pulse (Figure 3–7)
    (2) Palpate pulse while inflating cuff until no pulse is felt (systolic pressure at which radial pulse disappears—artery is occluded); note the reading on the manometer when the pulse could not be felt and add 30mm Hg
f. Place earpieces of stethoscope into ear canals, angled forward for a snug fit
g. Tap stethoscope head to confirm setting

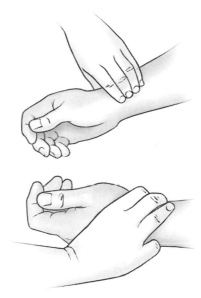

Figure 3–7   Locating radial pulse.

h. Place the head of the diaphragm over the brachial artery pulsation in the antecubital space, below the lower edge of the cuff—hold firmly in contact with skin (Figure 3–8)

i. Secure the valve ("righty tighty") and inflate the bladder rapidly to a pressure 30mm (or 15%) above the previously determined palpatory systolic pressure

j. Partially loosen valve ("lefty loosy") and deflate bladder at a rate of 2mm/second

k. As pressure in bladder falls, listen for Korotkoff sounds; note the manometer readings at the first appearance of sound (phase 1) and the disappearance of sound (phase 5)

l. Slowly deflate the cuff for the next 10mm to ensure that no further sounds are audible, then rapidly deflate the cuff

m. Remember the systolic pressure (phase 1) and diastolic pressure (phase 5) to the nearest 2mm Hg, the position patient was in, and which arm reading was taken

n. Have the patient rest for 30 seconds and repeat the procedure in the opposite arm; record the measurement from the arm with the higher reading[5]

o. Clean earpieces, according to manufacturer's directions, before putting equipment away

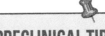

PRECLINICAL TIP

Measuring Your Knowledge: Determining the palpatory systolic pressure helps avoid underinflation in those with auscultatory gap and overinflation in those with low B.P.[8]

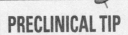

PRECLINICAL TIP

Measuring Your Knowledge: Avoid placing or wedging the head of the stethoscope under the cuff—results in extraneous noise.

Korotkoff sounds are caused by turbulent bloodflow through a constricted artery. As pressure is reduced during deflation of the cuff, sounds change in quality and intensity.[3, 5, 9] Five phases of changes are characterized as follows:

Phase 1 corresponds to systolic pressure	First sound heard; caused by blood blocked proximal to the cuff pushing its way through the artery; sound is clear tapping
Phase 2	Sounds are softer and longer
Phase 3	Sounds become crisper
Phase 4	Sounds are less distinct and muffled; results when cuff pressure is almost the same as arterial pressure
Phase 5 corresponds to diastolic pressure	Sound disappears, artery is no longer compressed, and blood flow is restored

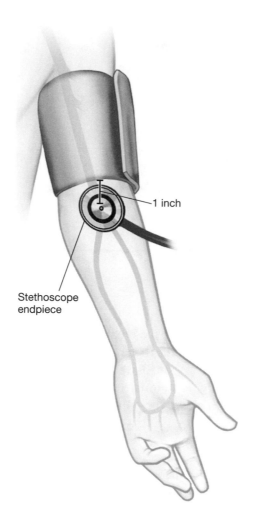

1 inch

Stethoscope
endpiece

Figure 3–8   Application of
diaphragm.

D. Normal/average blood pressure readings (mm Hg)[10]

	Age					
	0–1 yr.	1–6 yrs.	6–11 yrs.	11–16 yrs.	Adult	Elderly
Systolic	74–100	80–112	84–120	94–120	90–140	100–150
Diastolic	50–70	50–80	54–80	62–88	60–90	60–90

E. Classification of blood pressure for adults aged 18 years or older[11]

B.P. Classification	Systolic B.P., mm Hg[*]		Diastolic B.P., mm Hg[*]
Normal	<120	and	<80
Prehypertension	120–139	or	80–89
Stage 1 hypertension	140–159	or	90–99
Stage 2 hypertension	≥160	or	≥100

[*]Treatment determined by highest B.P. category

F. Factors that affect blood pressure
1. Elevated B.P. (hypertension): Exercise, emotional stress, diabetes, kidney disease, obesity, pregnancy, increasing age, high salt intake, and some medications

    2. Decreased B.P. (hypotension): After meals, change in posture (orthostatic), and some medications

Blood Pressure Disorder	Signs and Symptoms
Hypertension	Headache, edema, vision changes, and nose bleeds
Orthostatic hypotension	Dizziness, blurred vision, and fainting

G. Factors that affect the performance of the technique: Readings may be inaccurate due to instruments, operator, and/or patient factors[5, 12, 13, 14]

    1. Instruments

        a. Stethoscope

            (1) Check tubing for holes

            (2) Plugged earpieces results in poor sound transmission; clean earpieces after each use with gauze sprayed with disinfectant

        b. Sphygmomanometer: Manometers include

            (1) Mercury

                (a) Check for loss of mercury, presence of dirt, and signs of oxidation—cloudiness in the chamber; loss of mercury impairs reading

                (b) Clogging in an air vent at the top of the tube will cause mercury column to respond sluggishly to pressure from the bulb, causing an erroneous reading

                (c) Meniscus (curved upper surface of mercury) not at 0 at rest results in an inaccurate reading

            (2) Aneroid: May not be accurate if not calibrated with mercury manometer

                (a) If needle doesn't rise as the bulb is pumped, check for a leak

                (b) Always check that needle is at the 0 mark at the start and end of measurement; otherwise, an inaccurate reading results

        c. Rubber tubing: Check for leaks caused by cracked or perished rubber; results in inaccurate reading

        d. Cuff: Check control value for leakage; leads to difficulty in inflating and deflating bladder; causes underestimation of systolic and overestimation of diastolic pressures

    2. Operator: Poor technique due to inadequate training and/or development of bad habits; common operator errors include the following:

        a. Cuff

            (1) Selection of incorrect cuff size

                (a) If too small, the cuff will squeeze off a portion of the artery, requiring overinflation to hear the pulse, resulting in a false-high systolic reading[12]

                (b) If too wide results in a low reading

            (2) Cuff not completely emptied before use: Blood is trapped in lower arm, raising pressure there, thus requiring higher blood pressure in the upper arm to open vessels; results in a false-high systolic reading[12]

            (3) Deflation rate: Deflate cuff at 2mm Hg per second

                (a) Too fast results in too low systolic pressure reading and too high diastolic pressure reading[14]

(b) Too slow results in too high diastolic pressure reading (same as previous)

   b. Stethoscope
      (1) Improper placement of stethoscope
         (a) Diaphragm
            • If not in contact with skin or touching cuff, causes extraneous noise
            • If applied too firmly, results in too low diastolic reading[14]
            • Avoid placing thumb on diaphragm, since it has a pulse; use index and middle fingers on sides of diaphragm
         (b) Ear tips need to place snuggly forward into ear canals; if not, results in auditory impairment
   c. Avoid being biased; if a patient has had a normal B.P. reading in the past, don't assume subsequent readings will be the same
   d. Position patient properly
      (1) Make sure midpoint of arm is at heart level and supported; placement below and above heart level produce high and low readings respectively
      (2) Arm restricted by tight clothing can result in false reading
      (3) Legs crossed can cause possible error
3. Patient and environmental factors
   a. If room is too cold or patient too anxious, arm muscles tense resulting in a false-high diastolic reading[12]
   b. Talking, pain, or discomfort can produce a false-high reading
   c. Drinking beverages that contain caffeine and using tobacco and alcohol prior to the exam can alter readings, causing an increase in the reading

III. **Pulse (heart) rate**
   A. Pulse represents the beating of the heart; pulse rate is the number of times per minute the heart beats
   B. Recorded as beats per minute (bpm)
   C. Evaluate heart rhythm (regular or irregular) and pulse quality (thready, strong, bounding, or weak)
   D. Points of reference for palpation (Figure 3–9)
      1. Radial artery: Most common point to take a pulse; located on the thumb side of the inside wrist
      2. Brachial artery: Located on inside of upper arm; best to use on small children and infants
      3. Carotid artery: Supplies blood to head and neck; located along outer edge of trachea; often used in emergency situations
   E. Taking pulse on radial artery
      1. Hold patient's arm straight out, with elbow slightly bent, palm relaxed and facing up
      2. Elevate patient's thumb slightly upward by putting thumb in air or turning arm
      3. Locate and apply gentle pressure on radial pulse with index and middle fingers (on pocket under thumb); *do not* use thumb—it also has a pulse
      4. Count number of beats felt for 60 seconds
      5. Note any irregularities, including beats that come closer to preceding beats and any unwavering beats

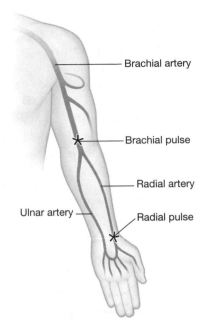

Figure 3–9   Points of reference for palpation.

    a. Determine heart rhythm—rhythmic beats that follow each other
      (1) Regular: Evenly spaced beats
      (2) Regularly irregular: Overall regular pattern with skipped beats
      (3) Irregularly irregular: No real pattern; difficult to measure rate
    b. Determine pulse quality, rate, and rhythm
      (1) Normal: Pulse is felt when applying light pressure to artery
      (2) Strong and bounding: Pulse is felt with definite pulsations; often associated with hypertension
      (3) Weak and thready: Pulse is difficult to feel; suggests that cardiac output and blood pressure are low
      (4) Tachycardia: Denotes a rapid pulse rate; over 100 beats per minute; associated with exercise, hyperthyroidism, and elevated temperature
      (5) Brachycardia: Denotes a slow pulse rate, below 50 beats per minute; can be normal or associated with conditions such as hypothyroidism or hypoadrenalism
  6. Record rate, rhythm, and quality of pulse

F. Factors that influence pulse (heart) rate
  1. Size; for example, children have a faster pulse rate than adults
  2. Age; for example, infants have a much faster pulse rate
  3. Medications; certain medications alter the pulse
  4. Gender; for example, women usually have a faster pulse rate than men
  5. Temperature; elevated temperatures alter pulse rate
  6. Overactive thyroid alters pulse rate
  7. Emotional excitement; for example, anger and fear increase the pulse rate

G. Normal resting pulse: Recorded in beats per minute (bpm)
  1. Infants less than 1 year old: 100 to 160 bpm
  2. Children between 1 and 10 years of age: 70 to 120 bpm

3. Teenagers and adults: 60 to 100 bpm
4. Well-trained athletes: 40 to 60 bpm

IV. **Body Temperature**

Denotes the balance between the heat lost and heat produced by the body; usually recorded when patient has febrile signs or symptoms.

A. Measured by
1. Oral: Most commonly used in dentistry; placed in right/left sublingual pocket under the tongue; contraindicated for those who are unconscious, restless, unable to follow instructions, infants, and young children
2. External: Axillary and groin positions; least accurate
3. Rectal: Used when oral thermometer cannot be used
4. Aural (ear)

B. Types of thermometers
1. Disposable: Use once to eliminate cross-contamination; generally made of thin plastic strips with a specially treated dot or strip indicator that changes color; readings are not as accurate
2. Electronic: Provides digital readout when the heat-sensitive tip is placed in mouth or ear
3. Glass-bulb: Thin glass tube with alcohol- or mercury-filled bulb at end; body temperature heats mercury to register with a silver streak, and alcohol is tinted red for easy readability
4. Tympanic (infrared): Consists of a probe that is placed in ear; measures infrared energy from eardrum (tympanic membrane)

C. Factors that change oral temperature measurements
1. Decrease of temperature: Cold drinks (wait 15 to 20 minutes after consumption to ensure accuracy)
2. Increase of temperature: Eating (diet high in protein increases the metabolism and produces heat), hot drinks, smoking, environmental temperature, physical activity, infection, and hyperthyroidism
3. Time of day: Increased temperatures in afternoon and early evening; decreased temperatures during sleep and early morning

D. Normal temperature
1. Adult: 98.6° F (37° C), but can vary as much as 1° F plus or minus over the course of the day
2. Child: 98.5° F

E. High temperature: Above 99.6° F (37.5° C); above 101°F (38.3°C) usually indicates presence of an active pathologic process
1. Treat immediately, since it can lead to dehydration and delirium; if related to dental infection, treat patient immediately with antibiotic and antipyretic therapy
2. If temperature is 104° F or higher, contact physician
3. Elective dental care is contraindicated

F. Procedure for taking oral temperature
1. Cover thermometer with disposable sheath
2. Place bulb under right or left posterior sublingual pocket of tongue
3. Ask patient to gently hold remaining portion of thermometer with lips—avoid biting with teeth
4. Remove thermometer after 3 minutes; hold thermometer by the stem and find column of mercury; reevaluate if temperature is high
5. Record temperature in patient's chart (medical/dental history)

6. Disinfect thermometer, if no sheath was used, according to manufacturer's directions

V. Respirations

Involves inspiration and expiration (inhaling and exhaling); monitored by observing the movement of the chest and abdomen in the quietly breathing patient.[15]

A. Normal respirations

1. Adult: 16 to 18 breaths per minute
2. Child: 16 to 40 breaths per minute

B. Factors that affect respiration

1. Increased respiration: Usually seen with fever and alkalosis; anxiety and obesity
2. Decreased respiration: May be produced by opioid administration

C. Technique

1. *Do not* announce you are measuring respirations, because the patient's breathing changes; perform immediately after taking a patient's pulse
2. Begin to observe patient's breathing with fingers still on pulse site—observe if it is labored or normal
3. Count breaths for 15 seconds and multiply by 4

D. Variable respirations

1. Tachypnea (rapid respiration): Most common form is hyperventilation; can result in lowered carbon dioxide levels (respiratory alkalosis) and includes such symptoms as tingling in toes and fingers and nausea; observed during times of exercise, stress, and fever
2. Bradypnea (slow respiration): May be caused by opioid administration

As healthcare providers, it is essential to measure vital signs—blood pressure, respiration, temperature, and pulse rate—during an initial examination appointment. This information provides a baseline normal value for each patient and should be recorded on the medical/dental history. Baseline vital signs provide a standard comparison in the event of an emergency within the clinical or office setting. If an emergency occurs, the vital signs will be taken and compared to the normal values initially recorded. Obtaining vital signs can also help identify possible abnormalities. If the healthcare provider notes a high blood pressure reading, referral should be made to the patient's physician so a further evaluation can be performed and a proper diagnosis established.

Table 3–1   Vital Signs[10]

Vital Signs	Age					
	0–1 year	1–6 years	6–11 years	11–16 years	Adult	Elderly
Temperature (°F)	96–99.5	98.5–99.5	98.5–99.6	98.6–100.6	98.6–100.6	97.2–99.6
Pulse (beats per minute)	80–160	70–120	70–120	60–100	60–100	60–100
Respirations (per minute)	40–60	25–40	18–25	16–25	16–18	12–25
Blood pressure (mm Hg)						
Systolic	74–100	80–112	84–120	94–120	90–140	100–150
Diastolic	50–70	50–80	54–80	62–88	60–90	60–90

QUESTIONS

1. Which of the following Korotkoff sounds (phases) denotes the systolic pressure?
   a. 1
   b. 2
   c. 3
   d. 4
   e. 5

2. All of the following are possible operator errors performed during the taking of a blood pressure EXCEPT one. Which one is the EXCEPTION?
   a. Improper placement of stethoscope
   b. Incorrect selection of cuff size
   c. Deflating the cuff too slowly
   d. A cold room

3. Which of the following, in beats per minute (bpm), is the normal resting pulse for an adult?
   a. 45 to 60
   b. 60 to 110
   c. 70 to 130
   d. 80 to 160

4. A standard adult cuff can be used to take blood pressure on a child. However, the blood pressure results would be falsely high.
   a. Both first and second statements are TRUE.
   b. Both first and second statements are FALSE.
   c. The first statement is TRUE. The second statement is FALSE.
   d. The first statement is FALSE. The second statement is TRUE.

5. An increase in pulse rate is
   a. tachycardia.
   b. tachypnea.
   c. brachycardia.
   d. bradypnea.

6. Which of the following is TRUE regarding arm positioning when taking a blood pressure?
   a. If the arm is positioned above the heart level, the blood pressure reading will be high.
   b. If the arm is positioned above the heart level, the blood pressure reading will be low.
   c. If the arm is positioned below the heart level, the blood pressure reading will be low.
   d. The position of the arm while taking the blood pressure does not affect the reading.

7. Normal respiration rate for an adult, in breaths per minute, is
   a. 26 to 40.
   b. 20 to 30.
   c. 12 to 24.
   d. 14 to 20.

8. Causes of hypertension include all of the following EXCEPT one. Which one is the EXCEPTION?
   a. Exercise
   b. Postural change
   c. Obesity
   d. Pregnancy

9. The MOST common artery to palpate when taking and evaluating the pulse (heart) rate is
   a. radial.
   b. brachial.
   c. carotid.
   d. inferior alveolar.

10. When taking a blood pressure reading, all of the following techniques should be performed EXCEPT one. Which one is the EXCEPTION?
    a. Rest patient's arm at heart level.
    b. Wrap cuff evenly and snugly around bare upper arm.
    c. Insert earpieces in a posterior direction.
    d. Deflate the bladder at a rate of 2 mmHg/second.

REFERENCES

1. Daniels, S. J., & S. A. Harfst (Eds.). *Dental Hygiene Concepts, Cases, and Competencies,* St. Louis: 2002, Mosby.

2. Centers for Disease Control and Prevention. Annual Smoking-attributable mortality, years of potential life lost, and economic costs (United States, 1995–1999). MMWR 51(14) 300-3, April 18, 2002.

3. Jolly, A. Taking blood pressure. *Nursing Times* 87(15), 40–43, 1991.

4. Burt, V. L., P. Whelton, C., Brown, J. A., Cutler, M. J., Horan, M. Higgins, & D. Labarrhe, Prevalence of hypertension in the U.S. adult population: Results from the Third National Health and Nutrition Examination survey, 1988–1991. *Hypertension*, 25, 305–313, 1995.

5. Anderson, F. D., & J. P. Maloney. Taking blood pressure correctly—it's no off the cuff matter. *Nursing*, 24, 34–39, 1994.

6. Vital signs: Evidence-based practice information sheet for health professions. *Australian Nursing Journal*, 7(3), 1999. www.ipfw.edu/denthy/6-27-01

7. Manning, D. M. Miscuffing: Inappropriate blood pressure application. *Hypertension*, 765, 1993.

8. Beevers, G., G. Y. Lip, & E. O'Brien. ABC of hypertension: blood pressure measurement: Part II—Conventional sphygmomanometry: Technique of auscultatory blood pressure measurement. *British Medical Journal*, 322(7293), 1043, 2001.

9. McAlister, F. A., & S. E. Strauss. Evidence-based treatment of hypertension: Measurement of blood pressure; an evidence-based review. *British Medical Journal*, 322(7291), 908, 2001.

10. Brian, J. N., & M. D. Cooper. *Prentice Hall's Complete Review of Dental Hygiene.* Upper Saddle River, NJ: Prentice Hall, 2002.

11. http://jama.ama-assn.org/cgi/content/full/289.19.2560vl/ TABLEJSC 3009671 www.ipfw.edu/denthy/ 8-15-03

12. Karch, A. M., & F. E. Karch. When a blood pressure isn't routine. *American Journal of Nursing* 100(3), 23–24, 2000.

13. Perloff, D., C. Grim, J. Flack, E. D. Frohlich, M. Hill, M. McDonald, & B. Z. Morgenstern. Human blood pressure determination by sphygmomanometry. *Circulation*, 88, 2460–67, 1993.

14. American Heart Association. *Human blood pressure determination.* 1994.

15. Little, J. W. Falace, D. A., Miller, C. S., and Rhodus, N. L. *Dental Management of the Medically Compromised Patient.* St. Louis: Mosby, 1997.

BLOOD PRESSURE PERFORMANCE SKILL SHEET

Student _____

Date _____

Instructor _____

Patient _____

Re-evaluation

Instr: _____   Instr: _____

Date _____   Date _____

	S	U	Comments	S	U	Comments	S	U	Comments
1. Seats patient in upright position with legs uncrossed.									
2. Uses proper cuff size.									
3. Palpates brachial artery.									
4. Places center of bag over the brachial artery.									
5. Covers inner aspect of arm with inflatable bladder.									
6. Places bottom edge of cuff 1" above antecubital space.									
7. Makes sure no clothing is between the arm and the cuff.									
8. Applies cuff evenly and snugly.									
9. Palpates radial pulse.									
10. Places meniscus at eye level.									
11. Inflates cuff, palpates radial pulse until it disappears.									
12. Determines palpatory systolic reading. ____ mm Hg.									
13. Waits at least 30 seconds.									
14. Extends arm.									
15. Places diaphragm of stethoscope over artery just below cuff.									
16. Makes sure diaphragm is not in contact with clothing or cuff.									
17. Inflates cuff rapidly 30 mm Hg. per above the systolic pressure.									
18. Deflates cuff at a rate of 2mm Hg per second.									
19. Deflates cuff until all sounds cease.									
20. Records the systolic/diastolic blood pressure ____/____ mm Hg.									
21. Cleans earpieces with disinfectant/gauze sponge and wraps cuff properly.									

Courtesy of Indiana University Purdue University Fort Wayne Dental Hygiene Program

Chapter 4

Extraoral and Intraoral Examinations

Nancy Cuttic, RDH, BSDH, MEd

MediaLink

A companion CD-ROM, included free with each new copy of this book, supplements the procedures presented in each chapter. Insert the CD-ROM to watch video clips and view a large collection of color images that is also included. This multimedia library is designed to help you add a new dimension to your learning.

KEY TERMS

auscultation. Listening for sounds.

autoimmune disease. Any disorder that arises from and causes destruction of an individual's own body.

basal cell carcinoma. Slow-growing, usually non-metastatic cancer of the skin that often occurs in sun-damaged skin of the elderly or fair-skinned.

bilateral. Both sides.

congenital. Defect or disorder present at birth.

endocarditis. Inflammation of the inner tissue of the heart.

edema. Swelling.

gingiva. Gum tissue.

glossitis. Inflammation of the tongue.

hyperkeratosis. Thickening of the outer layer of the epidermis or mucous membrane.

indurations. Underlying hardened area detected during palpation.

lesion. A wound, injury, or pathological change in the tissue.

lymphadenopathy. Swelling of lymph node(s).

mastication. Act of chewing.

melanoma. Highly metastatic skin cancer of the melanin-producing cells of the skin.

palpate. Examine by pressing and feeling.

sclera. White portion of the eye.

stippling. "Orange-peel" texture found on areas of normal masticatory mucosa.

stomatitis. Inflammation of the mucous membranes of the mouth (stoma).

systemic disease. Generalized and relating to the entire body system, not one part.

unilateral. One side.

LEARNING OBJECTIVES

After reading this chapter, the student will be able to:

- perform the different palpation methods used to complete extraoral and intraoral examinations;
- recall proper patient and operator positions to be used while performing extraoral and intraoral examinations;
- identify the overall general appearance of the patient, including stature, skin coloring, physical characteristics, and demeanor or emotional state;
- identify deformities in the patient's extremities that can indicate systemic diseases;
- identify certain ophthalmic changes, which can indicate other problems;
- locate the sinuses, muscles, salivary glands, and lymph nodes, which are checked during the extraoral and intraoral examinations;
- demonstrate proper evaluation of the temporomandibular joint (TMJ);

- demonstrate a sequential pattern for extraoral and intraoral examinations;
- identify fordyce granules, parotid papilla, linea alba, and caliculus angularis;
- list and identify four types of papillae found on the tongue;

- list and identify parts of the floor of the mouth and palate;
- compare and contrast normal and diseased gingiva.

I. Introduction

The extraoral and intraoral examinations, often referred to as an oral cancer screening, are critical assessment components performed as part of a routine prophylaxis. They help establish a basis for the most suitable home care and treatment plans for the patient. They are also used to detect abnormalities, disease, and oral cancer, and to educate the patient about oral abnormalities and benign deviations from the norm. There is growing evidence of the link between oral health/disease and systemic health/disease.[1] Prevention of disease, through early recognition, is most desirable.

A. Oral cancer considerations
1. Approximately 30,000 new cases of oral cancer are diagnosed each year in the United States[2]
2. Oral cancer claims around 9,000 lives in the U.S. each year[2]
3. Most common sites are the lateral borders of the tongue and the floor of the mouth; other areas include the palate, tonsils, salivary glands, oropharynx, gingiva, and lips[3]
4. Early detection is critical and translates to improved survival rates[2, 4]

B. Diseases and disorders

Extraoral and intraoral examinations also assist the clinician in identifying systemic diseases, nutritional deficiencies, and various abnormalities such as

1. HIV/AIDS: Various lesions associated with conversion from HIV to AIDS are often seen orally before systemic symptoms present and thus can serve to alert the patient of health problems
2. Systemic diseases: Autoimmune and similar diseases, endocrine disorders, diabetes, leukemia, and infections are often manifested in the oral cavity in the form of lesions, swellings, and abnormalities in tissue color, shape, size, and texture
3. Nutritional deficiencies: Sometimes visible orally, especially on the tongue and gingiva such as glossitis, stomatitis, and bleeding
4. Various abnormalities: Developmental disorders, benign tumors, growths, salivary gland stones, traumatic injuries, and injuries related to abuse

II. Relevant Information Regarding Extraoral and Intraoral Examinations

A. Sequencing: Sequence of steps performed during the examinations varies from one clinician to the next
1. Extraoral examination
    a. Involves examining the outer structures of the head and neck
    b. Usually performed first, since the patient is already seated in an upright position after vital signs are taken
    c. Follow a logical sequence that progresses from one area in close proximity to another area; for example, before or after ex-

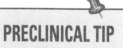

PRECLINICAL TIP

Inspecting Your Knowledge: The dental hygienist's role in reducing the number of oral cancer deaths has been recognized by leading health advocates.[4]

PRECLINICAL TIP

Inspecting Your Knowledge: Whichever sequential order the dental hygienist chooses to use, it is important that the approach be systematic and consistent from one patient to the next to ensure a thorough examination.

amining the lymph nodes around the neck area, it is logical to examine the thyroid gland of the neck

2. Intraoral examination
   a. Involves examining the inner structures of the mouth
   b. Follows the extraoral examination

B. Methods

1. Visual inspection
   a. Observe head and neck area
   b. Perform with adequate illumination
   c. Record observations in the patient's chart

2. Palpation methods (Figure 4–1)
   a. Digital palpation: Use one finger (digit) to feel and press against the tissue

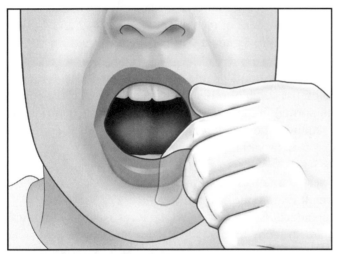

A. Digital palpation—Use index finger. Example—detect the presence of exostosis on the border of the mandible.

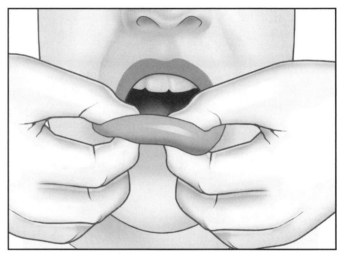

B. Bidigital palpation—Use finger and thumb of same hand. Example—Palpate the lips.

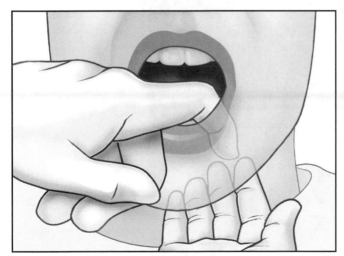

C. Bimanual palpation—Use finger(s) and/or thumb from each hand. Example—palpate floor of mouth.

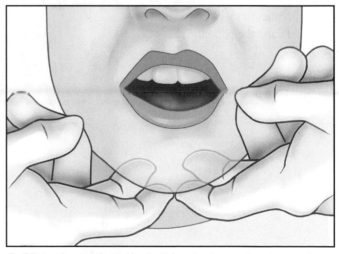

D. Bilateral palpation—Use both hands at same time to examine corresponding structures on opposite sides of body. Example— examine submental nodes.

Figure 4–1 Palpation methods. A. Digital palpation—using the index finger to detect the presence of exostosis on the border of the mandible. B. Bidigital palpation—palpating the lips. C. Bimanual palpation—palpating the floor of the mouth with the index finger of one hand while pressing the same area extraorally with the finger of the opposite hand under the chin. D. Bilateral palpation—using both hands to examine the submental nodes.

  b. Bidigital palpation: Use finger and thumb (two digits) to manipulate tissue

  c. Bimanual palpation: Use finger(s) and thumb of both hands to compress and feel the tissue—one hand supports the tissue extraorally while the other hand palpates structures intraorally

  d. Bilateral palpation: Use all fingers of both hands simultaneously to press and manipulate tissue on both sides of the face

  e. Circular compression: Use fingertips in a circular motion while applying pressure to feel the underlying tissue

 3. Auscultation: Listen for sounds, such as popping of the temporomandibular joint

 4. Smell: Observe and note foul or abnormal malodor of oral cavity

C. Patient position

 1. Extraoral examination: Conduct with patient seated in a comfortable upright position and examiner seated facing the patient or standing behind or in front of the patient (Figures 4–2 and 4–3)

 2. Intraoral examination: Conduct with patient placed in a fully supine position

D. Normal versus abnormal limits (Table 4–1 and Table 4–2)

 1. The clinician must be able to distinguish findings that are considered "within normal limits" from those that are abnormal or suspicious; this requires knowledge of normal anatomic structures and landmarks, as well as variants of normal

 2. Examples

  a. Normal versus traumatized torus

   (1) Normal: Extra bone covered by mucosa

   (2) Traumatized: Can occur when the torus is large and injured by hard, crunchy foods

Figure 4–2 Performing an extraoral examination with the examiner seated facing the patient.

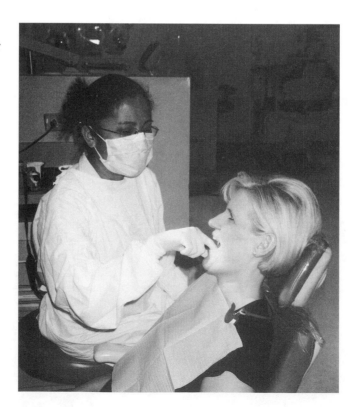

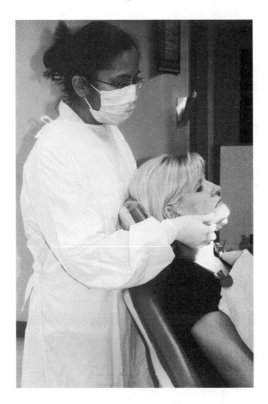

Figure 4–3   Performing an extra-oral examination with the examiner standing behind the patient.

    b. Fordyce granules versus lipoma: Both can manifest as soft, yellow elevations of the mucosa
      (1) Fordyce granules: Tiny clusters are a variant of normal
      (2) Lipoma: Indicates a tumor of adipose tissue
    c. Melanin pigmentation versus nevus versus melanoma: All usually manifest as brown pigmentation
      (1) Melanin pigmentation: Normal for dark-skinned individuals
      (2) Nevus: Mole, which can be seen intraorally and is a variant of normal
      (3) Melanoma: Can also appear as a concentrated area of melanin; however, it is a malignancy
  3. Documentation
    a. Note all findings from inspection in patient's chart
    b. Record suspicious lesions, indicating five key components: location, color, size (in millimeters), shape, and texture/consistency
    c. Note any associated symptoms as well
E. Instructions, prior to the examination:
  1. Loosen clothing around patient's neck for comfort
  2. Remove eyeglasses
  3. Remove dentures and prosthetic appliances—removal of appliances allows for all tissues to be visible for accurate evaluation, revealing possible lesions that may be concealed

III. Extraoral Clinical Examination

The following sequence of the extraoral examination is adapted from *Oral Diagnosis, Oral Medicine and Treatment Planning,* by Bricker, Langlais, and Miller,[6] and *Detecting Oral Cancer,* available from the National Institutes of Health.[7]

Table 4–1   Lesion Categories

	Lesion	Description	Size	Example
Lesion Categories				
Macule	Macule	Circumscribed, change in color without elevation or depression	< 1 cm	Freckle
Papule	Papule	Superficial, solid elevation	< 1 cm	Mole or elevated freckle
Nodule	Nodule	Solid, elevated mass with depth	< 1 cm	Wart
Tumor	Tumor	Solid, elevated mass extending deep into the tissue	> 1 cm	Neurofibroma
Wheal	Wheal	Superficial, elevated area of edema varying in size and shape	varies	Hives
Plaque	Plaque	Flat, raised area	> 1 cm	Candidiasis

Table 4–1 (Continued)

		Lesion Categories			
	Lesion	Description	Size	Example	
Vesicle	Vesicle	Circumscribed, fluid-filled elevation	< 1 cm	Herpes labialis	
Bulla	Bulla	Large, fluid-filled elevation containing serum or mucin	> 1 cm	Burn lesion	
Pustule	Pustule	Circumscribed, pus-filled lesion	< 1 cm	Acne	
Cyst	Cyst	Encapsulated, fluid-filled mass located in the dermis or subcutaneous tissue	varies	Sebaceous cyst	

					Size in Millimeters					
1 mm	2 mm	3 mm	4 mm	5 mm	6 mm	7 mm	8 mm	9 mm	1 cm	

A. General appearance of the patient
  1. Gait: Refers to the way one walks (observation)
    a. Observe the patient walk from the reception area to the operatory—a cautious gait may require different patient management, necessitating the use of stress reduction techniques
    b. Observe functional movement of body parts; patients with limited mobility and those in wheelchairs may require altered management to make the appointment as comfortable as possible or may need adaptive aids for oral hygiene use; note in the patient's chart the reason for difficulty in mobility
  2. Overall appearance (visual inspection)
    a. General appearance: Begin assessing general appearance of patient upon the escort to the operatory; includes the patient's stature, skin coloring, physical characteristics, and demeanor or emotional state

Table 4–2   Lesion Descriptors

Descriptive Colors	
pink	red
purple	brown
blue	grey
yellow	black
white	

Descriptive Texture/Consistency Terminology	
indurated	soft, spongy
firm	fluctuant
smooth	verrucose
crusted	exophytic
pseudomembranous	fissured
cratered	corrugated

Descriptive Shape Terminology	
flat	irregular
elevated (papillary)	depressed (ulcer-like)
pedunculated	sessile
descrete	confluent
lobulated	

(1) Skin coloring
  (a) Patients with pallor (skin paleness) may be ill or weak
  (b) Yellow skin coloring may indicate liver dysfunction and/or jaundice
  (c) Flushed appearance or clammy skin can indicate diabetic distress
(2) Physical characteristics: Bruising may indicate leukemia or abuse
(3) Observe patient's demeanor—often determines how patient is feeling and will affect the treatment plan; for example, a highly anxious patient may have difficulty getting through standard treatment without adaptations
  b. Extremities, hands, and nails
  (1) Note loss of digits—may impact choice for oral hygiene aids
  (2) Note deformities in the extremities for indicators of systemic health, such as
    (a) Joint enlargement—may indicate arthritis or one of many systemic inflammatory diseases of the connective tissue
    (b) Skin changes, such as bruising—can indicate physical abuse or systemic illness such as leukemia or Kaposi's sarcoma associated with AIDS
    (c) Braised/callused knuckles—may indicate self-induced vomiting of a bulimic
    (d) Pigmentation
      • Loss of pigmentation: Autoimmune condition called vitiligo
      • Excessive pigmentation: Red pigment could indicate port wine stain, whereas brown areas of pigmentation could indicate moles, melanoma, or café au lait spots associated with systemic disease

(e) Yellowing (jaundice) or pallor of cyanosis

(f) Loss of function—Possibly due to stroke, advanced Lyme disease, or one of many systemic connective tissue or joint inflammatory diseases

(3) Nailbeds: Inspect for abnormality in texture and color

(a) Blue nail beds may indicate circulatory problems

(b) Bleeding can indicate endocarditis

(c) Pitting can be seen with psoriasis

(d) Grooving is the result of trauma

B. Examination of the head and neck

1. Evaluate all structures of the head and neck for abnormalities that may indicate systemic, genetic, or oral problems

2. Problematic symptoms with the temporomandibular joint, sinuses, and salivary glands are somewhat similar, thus necessitating thorough examination of these areas

3. Facial form and symmetry (visual inspection)

a. Evaluate overall shape of face for symmetry

(1) Swelling in any area indicates inflammation or possibly a tumor

(2) Unilateral swelling occurs on one side

(3) Bilateral swelling indicates swelling on both sides

b. Examine facial profile for proper growth and positioning of maxilla and mandible; refer to Chapter 5, "Examination and Charting of Hard and Soft Tissues"

4. Skin, ears, hair, and eyes (visual inspection)

a. Observe skin and ears for color changes or crusts, fissures, scars or growths; patients often may be unaware of the presence of these changes; may observe cancer of the head and neck

(1) Basal cell carcinoma, a form of skin cancer, may be suspected (Figure 4–4)

(2) Melanoma is the deadliest form of skin cancer

b. Insufficient hair in large patches, as well as skin discolorations, can indicate ectodermal (skin) disorders, a psychological condition in which the patient pulls out own hair, or may be a sign of abuse

c. Examination of the eyes is important because many conditions can include opthalmic changes, such as

(1) Yellowing of the sclera (whites of the eyes) can indicate jaundice

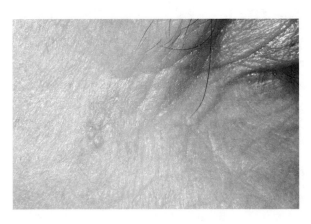

Figure 4–4   Basal cell carcinoma.

(2) Redness in the sclera can indicate eye infection or conjunctivitis

(3) Bluish sclera of the eyes indicates thinning of the sclera, often seen with genetic bone or dentin developmental disorders

(4) Uneven or dilated pupils can indicate neurologic dysfunction

(5) Pinpoint pupils may indicate drug abuse

5. Nose (visual inspection)
   a. Observe for congenital and acquired variations; cartilage can be fractured, causing a deviation (bending) of the nasal septum, which may lead to mouth breathing and its associated oral conditions
   b. Note loss of nasal septum—may be indicative of cocaine abuse

6. Lips and labial mucosa (visual inspection); the lips form the external border of the oral cavity; the labial mucosa lines the internal portion of the lip
   a. Lip position: At rest, the lips normally touch; if apart, it can indicate conditions such as:
      (1) Mouth breathing—involves breathing through the mouth instead of the nose; often causes irritation of the facial gingiva and chapped lips
      (2) Tongue thrusting—involves abnormal movement of the tongue during swallowing; tongue is forced forward during swallowing instead of towards the palate
      (3) Nasal obstruction—sinus problems, cold, allergies, or deviated septum are often causes for nasal obstruction, which leads to mouth breathing
   b. Vermillion border: The exposed red portion where the lip, covered by mucosa but with no mucous glands, meets the skin; evaluated for color, texture, and fissuring; enlargements can be unilateral or bilateral (Figure 4–5); abnormalities include
      (1) Junction of the lip becomes less distinct, caused by advanced age and/or prolonged sun exposure
      (2) Fissures and cracks can be seen when exposed to the elements, constant licking, or nutritional deficiencies
      (3) Blisters or vesicles, caused by sun exposure and/or systemic illness such as herpes labialis (Figure 4–6)

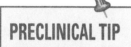

PRECLINICAL TIP

Inspecting Your Knowledge: An anterior openbite can result from tongue thrusting.

Figure 4–5   Normal lips.

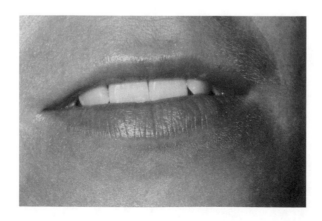

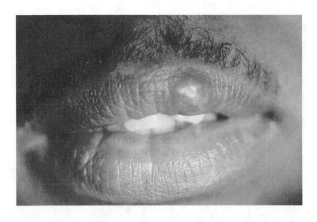

Figure 4–6 Herpes labialis.

7. Muscles (bilateral palpation and circular compression from behind the patient); note deviations between the two sides as well as swellings, indurations, and abnormalities in function
   a. Mentalis muscle
      (1) Located on the chin
      (2) Technique: Begin palpating at the center (symphasis), working along the border of the mandible toward the angle (Figure 4–7)
   b. Masseter muscle
      (1) Major muscle of each cheek
      (2) Technique (Figure 4–8)
         (a) Place fingers of each hand from the angle of the mandible onto the cheek
         (b) Ask patient to clench teeth, causing muscle to contract
         (c) Observe the function and note any deviations
   c. Temporalis muscle
      (1) Fan-shaped muscle radiating from the zygomatic arch superiorly across the area of the temples to the parietal area

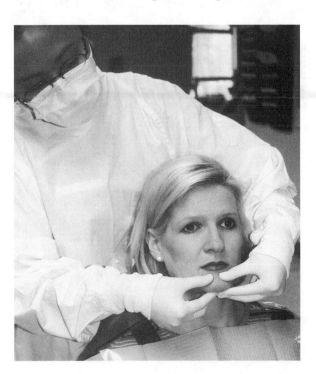

Figure 4–7 Palpating submental nodes and mentalis.

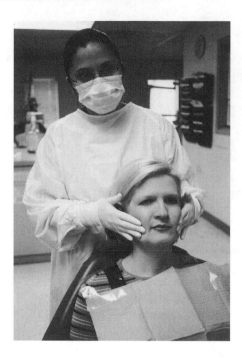

Figure 4–8   Palpating masseter muscles.

(2) Technique: Place fingers of each hand just above the zygomatic process of the mandible, moving superiorly over the temporal area

8. Paranasal sinuses (bimanual palpation and circular compression); two major bilateral sinuses in the frontal and maxillary areas; pain or discomfort can indicate sinusitis, an inflammation and/or infection of the sinuses

  a. Frontal sinuses

    (1) Located in the midline above the eyes

    (2) Technique: Palpate both sinuses simultaneously with the index and middle fingers (Figure 4–9)

Figure 4–9   Palpating frontal sinuses.

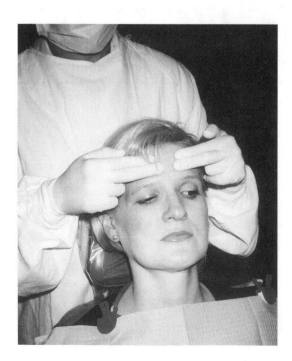

b. Maxillary sinuses
   (1) Located below the orbital bones of the eyes
   (2) Technique: Palpate simultaneously with the index and middle fingers (Figure 4–10)
9. Lymph nodes (Figure 4–11) and salivary glands (Figure 4–12) (bilateral palpation and circular compression); depending on the glands and lymph nodes being palpated, the examiner may palpate from behind or in front of the patient; note any deviations in density or size and note any discomfort
   a. Lymph nodes are bean-shaped organs found in clusters along lymph channels
   b. Function is to remove toxic products from lymph and prevent their entry into systemic circulation
   c. Normal lymph nodes are not visible or palpable
   d. Regional lymph nodes—each group drains lymph fluid from specific areas; palpate to detect enlarged nodes, which often indicate increased immune system activity
   e. Palpable lymph nodes
      (1) Must be larger than 1 cm in diameter to be palpable
      (2) Feel like peas or grapes under the skin
      (3) Note location, size, tenderness, mobility, and attachment to surrounding tissue
         (a) Inflammatory condition—usually soft and tender, enlarged, and freely moveable
         (b) Malignant disease—usually hard, nontender, and fixed to surrounding tissues
   f. Specific salivary glands/lymph nodes
      (1) Submental lymph nodes/sublingual gland (see Figure 4–12)
         (a) Located inferior to the chin

PRECLINICAL TIP

Inspecting Your Knowledge: When palpating the maxillary sinuses, if gentle pressure does not produce discomfort, the percussion technique can be used. Leaving fingers in the same position and thumping with the middle finger of the opposite hand can accomplish this.[6]

PRECLINICAL TIP

Inspecting Your Knowledge: Lymph nodes associated with malignancies are often hard, nontender, and nonmoveable.

PRECLINICAL TIP

Inspecting Your Knowledge: A localized infection such as a dental abscess would manifest unilaterally. A systemic infection such as tuberculosis would likely manifest bilaterally.

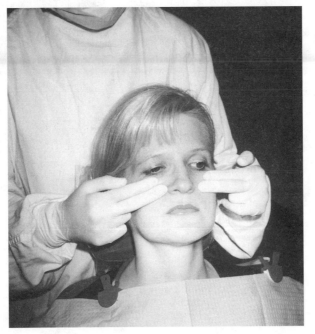

Figure 4–10   Palpating maxillary sinuses.

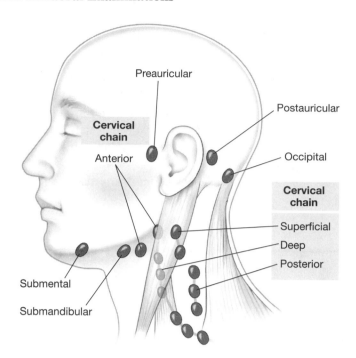

Figure 4–11   Lymph nodes palpated during head and neck examination.

Figure 4–12   Salivary glands.

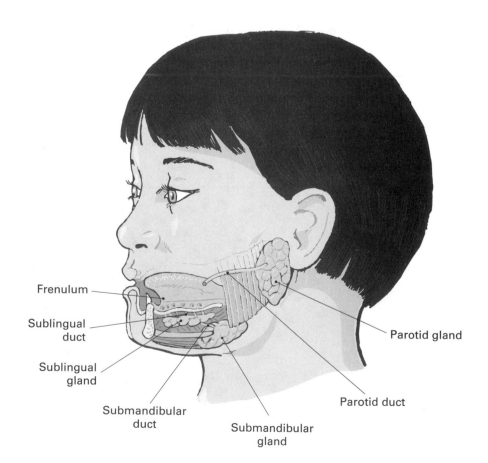

(b) Technique
- May be palpated from behind the patient
- Tip patient's head slightly toward the chest
- Cup fingers and gently press tips against the floor of the mouth, with a focus on the submental area

(c) Lymphadenopathy (lymph node swelling) in this area can indicate infection in mandibular incisors, tip of tongue, floor of mouth, midline of lower lip, and/or chin;[8, 9] swelling may indicate a blocked salivary gland duct—Bartholin's duct

(2) Submandibular gland/submandibular nodes

(a) Located under the border of the mandible just below the skin surface

(b) Technique (Figure 4–13)
- May be palpated from behind patient
- Tip patient's head slightly toward the chest
- Cup fingers and lightly press up into the floor of the mouth
- Roll tissue across the inferior border of the mandible

(c) Lymphadenopathy in this area can indicate inflammation of cheeks, nasal cavity, maxillary teeth with the exception of third molars, mandibular teeth except incisors, floor of mouth, tongue, sublingual and submandibular glands, upper lip, or hard palate;[8, 9] swelling may indicate a blocked salivary gland duct—Wharton's duct

(3) Parotid gland—a triangular-shaped salivary gland, includes parotid nodes

(a) Located under the skin of the cheek and in front of the ear

(b) Technique (bilateral palpation)

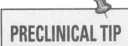

PRECLINICAL TIP

Inspecting Your Knowledge: The sublingual gland branches into smaller ducts called ducts of Rivinius.

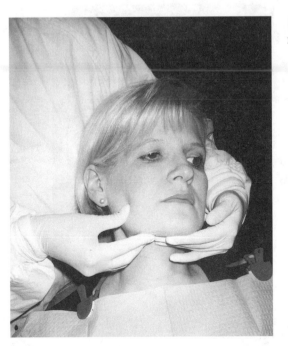

Figure 4–13   Palpating submandibular nodes.

- With both hands, bilaterally compress in a circular motion the area anterior to the tragus of the ear
- Move inferiorly to the angle of the mandible feeling for enlargements or nodules

(c) Swelling in this area indicates inflammation/infection of the parotid gland (e.g., mumps) or a blocked salivary gland duct—Stensen's duct

(4) Preauricular nodes

    (a) Located in front of the ears (auricles)

    (b) Technique: Palpate area directly in front of the ears simultaneously using bimanual palpation and circular compression (Figure 4–14)

    (c) Lymphadenopathy in this area may be due to infection of the scalp, temporal or frontal areas, or eyes[6]

(5) Postauricular nodes

    (a) Located behind the ears

    (b) Technique: Palpate area directly behind the ears bimanually and simultaneously by moving the fingertips in a circular motion (Figure 4–15)

    (c) Lymphadenopathy in this area may be due to infection of the scalp, temporal or frontal areas, or eyes[6]

(6) Occipital nodes

    (a) Located under the occipital bone at the base of the skull

    (b) Technique

- Tip patient's head forward
- Palpate the base of the head bimanually in small circular motions (Figure 4–16)

    (c) Lymphadenopathy in this area can indicate infection in the occipital part of the scalp[9]

Figure 4–14   Palpating preauricular nodes.

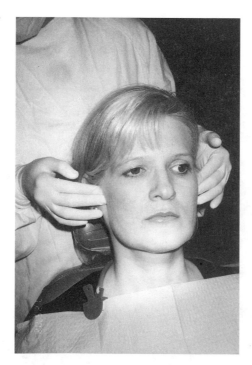

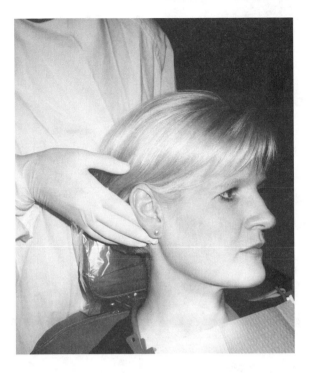

Figure 4–15   Palpating postauricular nodes.

(7) Posterior cervical nodes—part of the cervical chain of nodes that falls into three categories: anterior or posterior, superior or inferior, superficial or deep[8]
  (a) Located behind the sternocleidomastoid muscle of the neck; superior nodes are found in the upper neck area while inferior nodes are found closer to the clavicles; superficial component is along external jugular vein; deep component is along carotid artery deep to the sternocleidomastoid muscle
  (b) Technique (Figure 4–17)

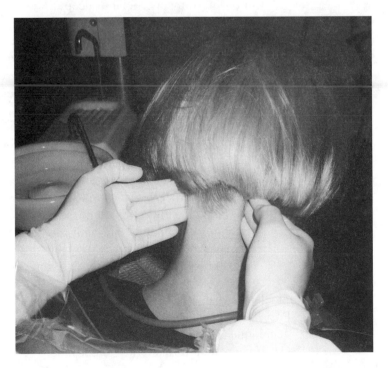

Figure 4–16   Palpating occipital nodes.

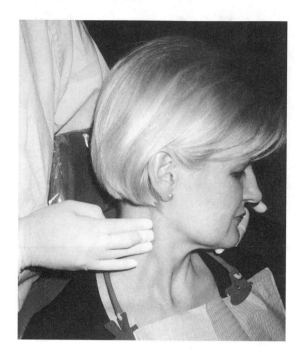

Figure 4–17   Palpating posterior cervical nodes.

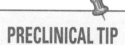
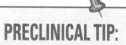
- Tip and turn patient's head slightly away from the side being palpated
- Palpate nodes unilaterally by placing the fingertips behind the muscle beginning at the base of the neck and moving upward

(c) Lymphadenopathy can indicate an infection of the posterior two-thirds of the scalp or thyroid gland, as well as the ear, parotid gland, or associated structures[8, 9]

(8) Anterior cervical nodes—part of the cervical chain of nodes that falls into three categories: anterior or posterior, superior or inferior, superficial or deep[8]

(a) Located in front of the sternocleidomastoid muscle of the neck; superior nodes are found in the upper neck area, while inferior nodes are found closer to the clavicles; superficial component is along external jugular; deep component is along carotid artery deep to the sternocleidomastoid muscle

(b) Technique (Figure 4–18)
- Tip patient's head slightly forward and away from the side being palpated
- Use tips of fingers to unilaterally palpate in front of the sternocleidomastoid muscle, pressing fingers along the entire length of the muscle

(c) Lymphadenopathy can indicate inflammation of the anterior third of the scalp, facial structures, or thyroid gland; often associated with a sore throat and/or oral infection[6, 8]

10. Sternocleidomastoid muscle
   a. Prominent muscle along the side of the neck
   b. Technique (figures 4–19a and 4–19b)
      (1) Have patient turn slightly to one side

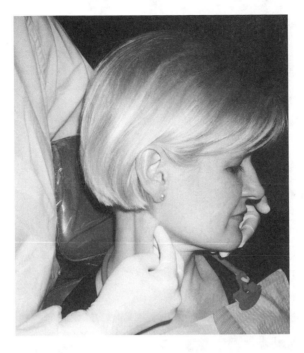

Figure 4–18 Palpating anterior cervical nodes.

(2) Bidigitally palpate the muscle on that side of the neck, grasping the muscle between the thumb and fingers

(3) Begin at the angle of the mandible and progress to the clavicle

11. Thyroid gland (bimanual palpation)

    a. Located in the midline of the neck below the thyroid cartilage and bilaterally above the larynx

    b. Technique (Figure 4–20)

       (1) Palpate the area, with the patient's chin slightly lowered

PRECLINICAL TIP

Inspecting Your Knowledge: A healthy thyroid gland is not visible and should move vertically as the patient swallows. An enlarged thyroid gland, often called a goiter, may feel hard and lose its ability to ascend and descend during swallowing.

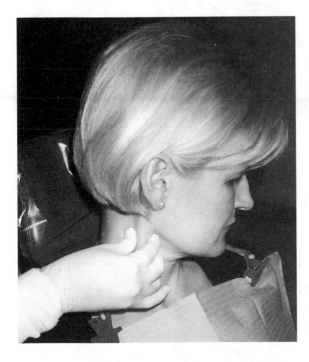

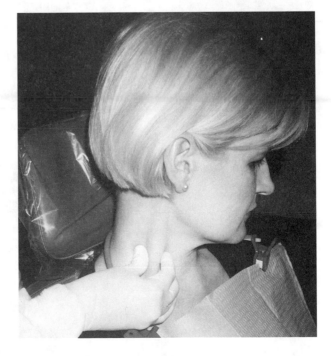

Figure 4–19 Palpating sternocleidomastoid muscle

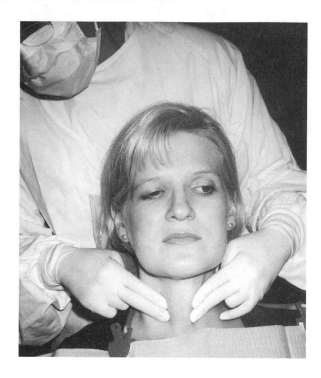

Figure 4–20   Palpating thyroid gland.

(2) Place fingers on either side of the trachea and ask the patient to swallow several times—gland should move vertically as the patient swallows
(3) With one hand, gently displace the thyroid tissue to one side of the neck while the other hand palpates the misplaced thyroid tissue
(4) Repeat to the opposite side and compare the two lobes
(5) Evaluate the size of the thyroid as well as enlargement, growths or nodules, or lack of movement during swallowing

12. Larynx
   a. Located below the thyroid cartilage and gland
   b. Technique (Figure 4–21)
     (1) Palpate bidigitally, positioned in front of patient
     (2) Place fingertips of one hand bilaterally over the larynx, applying gentle pressure
     (3) Ask patient to swallow

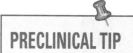

PRECLINICAL TIP

Inspecting Your Knowledge: A normal larynx will move vertically during swallowing.

Figure 4–21   Palpating the larynx.

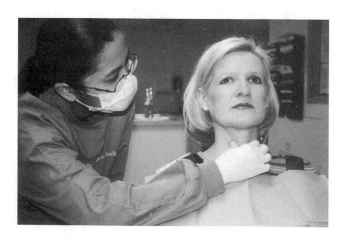

13. Temporomandibular joint (bilateral palpation and auscultation); TMJ connects the mandible to the maxilla
    a. Located in front of the patient's ears
    b. Technique: Examiner can be positioned in front or behind the patient (Figure 4–22)
       (1) Locate joint by placing the fingertips in front of the patient's ear
       (2) Ask patient to open and close mouth
    c. Assessment
       (1) Place index and middle fingers of each hand just anterior to the tragus of the ear simultaneously on both sides
       (2) Ask the patient to open and close slowly several times, as well as protrude and retrude the mandible, and perform lateral excursions (moving the jaw from side to side)
       (3) Observe deviations in the gliding during movement; one side may move forward before the other, which can indicate dysfunction of the muscles of mastication
       (4) Auscultation: Listen for sounds like popping, clicking, or grating; these abnormal noises can indicate masticatory muscle dysfunction or internal problems within the joint capsule; grating noise (called *crepitus*) indicates irreversible, more advanced derangement of the joint capsule and deterioration of the membrane, causing bone-to-bone contact
       (5) Evaluate maximum opening distance
          (a) Normal distance from maxillary incisors to mandibular incisors should be the distance of three fingers end-on-end[6]
          (b) Two fingers end-on-end indicates a reduction in opening, but not necessarily a reduction in function
          (c) One finger opening reveals reduced function[6]

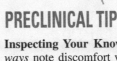

PRECLINICAL TIP

Inspecting Your Knowledge: *Always* note discomfort when examining the TMJ. Since this is a joint, inflammation and arthritis are possible.

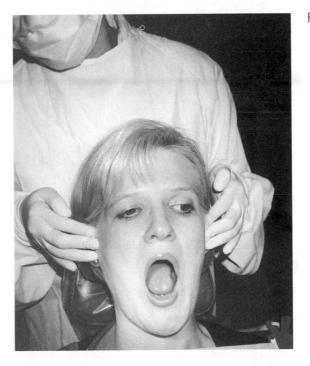

Figure 4–22   Palpating the TMJ.

IV. Intraoral Clinical Examination

The examination of the oral cavity includes the methodic inspection of the lips, buccal mucosa, mucobuccal fold, hard and soft palates, uvula, oropharynx, tongue, floor of the mouth, and periodontium. Before beginning the intraoral examination, a cursory inspection of the oral cavity should be performed to determine if any lesions or problems exist that might prevent the examination from proceeding. Do this with a mirror prior to placing fingers in the patient's mouth.

A. Internal surface of the lip
1. Technique
   a. Retract lips, first the upper, then the lower, to observe labial gingiva and mucosa (Figures 4–23 and 4–24)
   b. Use bidigital palpation (Figure 4–25) to examine lips for submucosal nodules, bullae, and other abnormalities such as a hemangioma, which is a blood blister (Figure 4–26)
2. Landmarks to evaluate
   a. Accessory salivary glands: Numerous small mucous glands appear and feel as small nodules but are normal anatomy
   b. Frena (*frenum* = singular): String-like attachments of the lip to maxilla and mandible; evaluate by gently pulling on the upper and lower lips
      (1) Locations
         (a) Maxillary labial frenum is located between the maxillary central incisors, approximately 4 to 7 mm apical to interdental region
         (b) Mandibular labial frenum is located slightly below and between mandibular central incisors within alveolar mucosa
         (c) Maxillary and mandibular buccal frenae are located adjacent to maxillary and mandibular premolars respectively
      (2) Size of attachments vary among individuals; tight and low attachments may lead to the development of diastemas or mucogingival junction problems

B. Buccal mucosa (visual inspection with mirror and bidigital or bimanual palpation)
1. The buccal mucosa is the inner lining of the cheeks; it is made up of smooth epithelium and resembles the labial mucosa in appearance

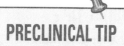

PRECLINICAL TIP

Inspecting Your Knowledge: It is critical to thoroughly dry the labial mucosa to view the accessory salivary ducts and observe if they secrete saliva.

Figure 4–23   Retracting upper lip.

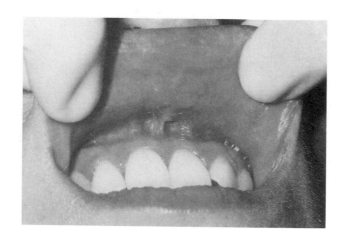

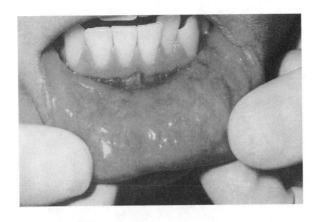

Figure 4–24   Retracting lower lip.

2. Technique
   a. Dry the mucosa with air or gauze for maximum visibility and inspect tissue (Figures 4–27 and 4–28)
   b. Retract with mouth mirror or tongue blade to observe the area
   c. Bimanually palpate the buccal tissue (Figure 4–29)
3. Normal structures or variants of normal (common deviations) include the following:
   a. Fordyce granules: Ectopic sebaceous glands appear as yellow clusters of nodules frequently found on the buccal mucosa and lips; occurs in 80% of adults[2] (Figure 4–30)
   b. Parotid papilla: Pad of tissue near the maxillary second molar containing the opening of the parotid gland—Stensen's duct
   c. Linea alba: White line of hyperkeratotic tissue corresponding to the occlusion of the teeth; caused by pressure of the buccinator muscle on the maxillary teeth
   d. Caliculus angularis: Hyperkeratotic palpable nodule of tissue at the anterior termination of linea alba at the inner commissures

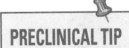

PRECLINICAL TIP

Inspecting Your Knowledge: Dry mucosa with air syringe to ensure all structures are clearly visible and salivary ducts are not blocked.

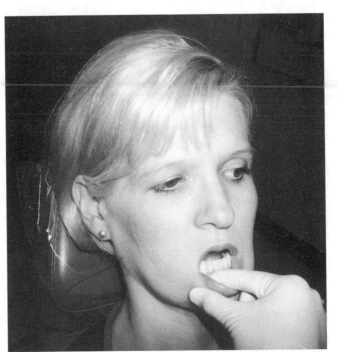

Figure 4–25   Palpating labial mucosa.

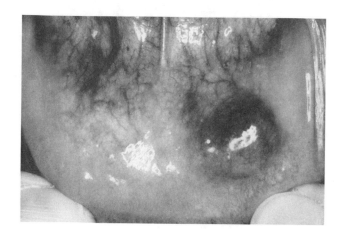

Figure 4–26   Hemangioma.

C. Tongue
   1. The tongue is a muscular organ covered by stratified squamous epithelium; the dorsal side is covered with four papillae: filiform, fungiform, circumvallate, and foliate
   2. Technique (visual inspection)
      a. Have patient open wide for maximum visibility of the tongue
      b. Use a gauze square to gently pull tongue forward, to the left, right, and upward, to inspect the posterior lateral borders; this is done because many lesions are not visible until the tongue is moved (Figure 4–31)
      c. Palpate entire body of tongue, using the bidigital method, to feel for indurations and abnormalities; avoid areas near the base where the gag reflex can be stimulated (Figure 4–32)
   3. Parts of the tongue
      a. Dorsal surface (top) (Figure 4–33)
         (1) Papillae: Dorsum is covered by four types of papillae
            (a) Filiform papillae
               • Small, hairlike projections
               • Most numerous, covering most of the dorsum and giving it a velvety appearance
               • Subject to being discolored, elongated, and denuded (stripped of tissue)
               • Do not contain taste buds

PRECLINICAL TIP

Inspecting Your Knowledge: Significance of evaluating the papillae of the tongue is to determine normal conditions versus abnormal conditions, which affect the appearance of the papillae. Such abnormalities include geographic tongue, nutritional disorders, black hairy tongue, and hairy leukoplakia, among others.

Figure 4–27   Right buccal mucosa.

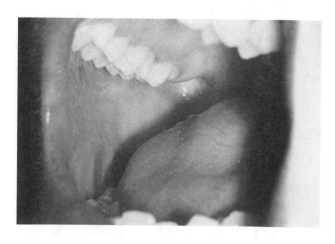

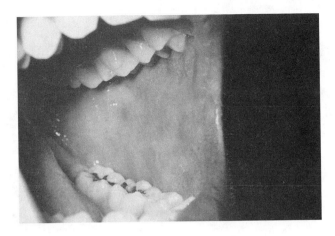

Figure 4–28   Left buccal mucosa.

(b) Fungiform papillae
  • Small, mushroom-shaped elevations
  • Second most numerous papillae on the tongue—lateral border and anterior tip
  • Redder in color than filiform papillae
  • Contain taste buds
(c) Circumvallate or vallate papillae
  • Contain 8 to 12 large, round elevations with a groove around them—divides the tongue into the anterior two-thirds and posterior third
  • Located posteriorly, along the sulcus terminalis, in a V-shape
  • Contain some taste buds
(d) Foliate papillae
  • Located on lateral borders
  • Appear as vertical, leaflike folds
  • Contain taste buds

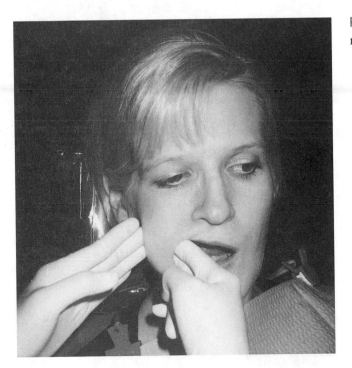

Figure 4–29   Palpating buccal mucosa.

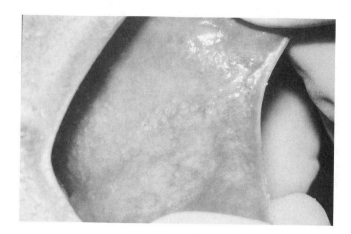

Figure 4–30   Fordyce granules.

- Often lymphoid tissue in the area is mistaken for foliate papillae
(2) Median sulcus
  (a) Depression in midline of the tongue
  (b) Ends in the terminal sulcus, which separates the dorsum of the tongue from the base or root
  (c) Foramen ceacum is located at the apex of the terminal sulcus
(3) Lingual tonsils (*lingual* refers to tongue): Elevations of lymphoid tissue; located on base of tongue posterior to terminal sulcus; should have similar color and texture as the pharynx
(4) Common deviations
  (a) Fissured tongue (Figure 4–34)
    - Deep grooves seen on the tongue
    - Often seen with nutritional deficiencies and Down syndrome patients

Figure 4–31   Inspecting right lateral border of tongue.

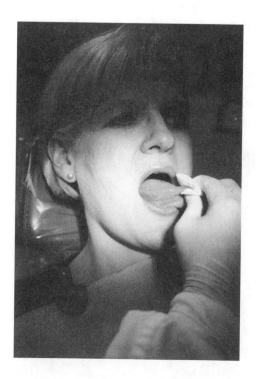

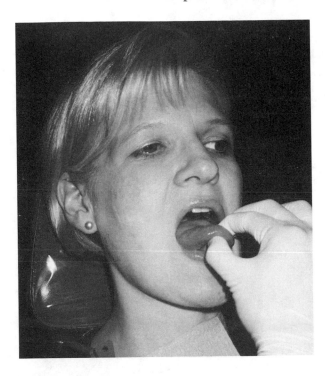

Figure 4–32   Palpating body of tongue.

(b) Black hairy tongue (Figure 4–35)
   • Filiform papillae become elongated and dark in color
   • Caused by chromogenic (color-producing) bacteria
(c) Geographic tongue (benign migratory glossitis) (Figure 4–36)
   • Multiple areas of denuded filiform papillae appearing red and surrounded by yellow-white borders

Figure 4–33   Parts of the tongue.

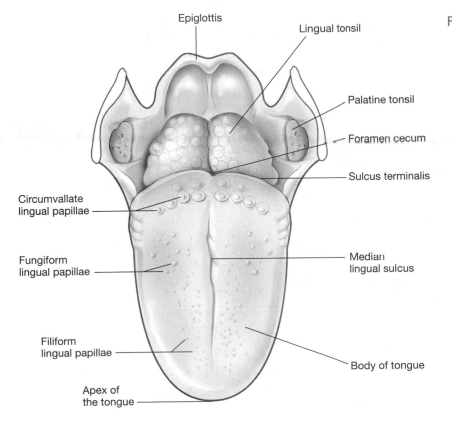

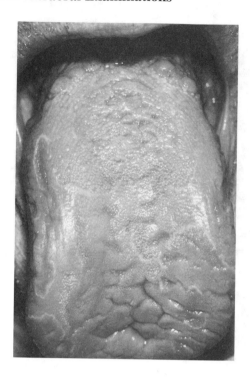

Figure 4–34   Fissured tongue.

- Areas heal and move to other locations of the tongue
- Unknown etiology, believed to be associated with stress

b. Ventral surface (underside) (Figure 4–37)
    (1) Technique: To view, ask patient to lift the tip of tongue to roof of mouth
    (2) Landmarks and normal structures of the ventral surface of the tongue include
        (a) Lingual frenum—attaches the tongue to the floor of the mouth
            - Length of the frenum varies; when it is short or not present, it is termed *ankyloglossia* (tongue-tied), causing inability of the tip of the tongue to move freely, which can affect proper pronunciation of sounds requiring the tongue to touch the anterior palate and resulting in a nasal tone

Figure 4–35   Black hairy tongue.

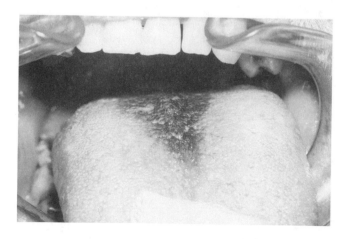

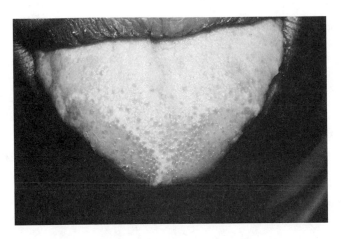

Figure 4–36   Geographic tongue.

      (b) Plica fimbriata—tiny tissue projections located on ei-
ther side of the frenum; contain minor gland duct openings

      (c) Lingual veins or varicosities
- Raised bluish-purple veins
- Typically become more evident with age

D. Floor of mouth (visual inspection and bimanual palpation) (Figure
4–38)

  1. Technique

    a. Lift patient's tongue to the roof of the mouth

    b. Reflect light from the mouth mirror

    c. Place index finger of one hand on the floor of the mouth while
the fingertips of the opposing hand are placed externally in the
submandibular area; NOTE: Using only one hand to palpate can
displace any indurations or growths, which is why two hands
are necessary for detection (Figure 4–39)

    d. Palpate entire floor of the mouth, beginning in the posterior of
one side, then move anteriorly and to the other side

  2. Landmarks of the floor of the mouth

    a. Sublingual fold

      (1) Elevations located from the posterior of one side to the lin-
gual frenum and back to the posterior of the other side

      (2) Contains Bartholin's ducts, which are sublingual salivary
gland ducts

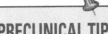

PRECLINICAL TIP

Inspecting Your Knowledge: The
patient may need to be seated upright for this inspection, since lesions can "disappear" if patient is
in a supine position during examination.

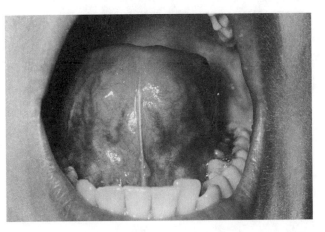

Figure 4–37   Ventral surface of
tongue.

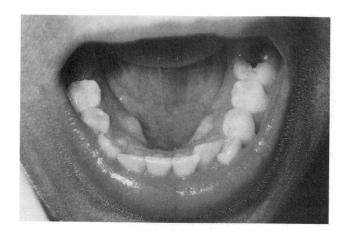

Figure 4–38   Floor of mouth.

  b. Sublingual caruncle
   (1) Two small spherical projections located on either side of the lingual frenum
   (2) Site of Wharton's ducts, which are submandibular salivary gland openings
  c. Mandibular torus (tori)—extra bone commonly found on the lingual to the mandibular premolars; may be unilateral or bilateral
 E. Hard palate
  1. The hard palate appears pink because it is covered with a thin layer of keratinized, stippled tissue covering bone; it is critical to thoroughly dry the hard palate to observe if accessory salivary ducts secrete saliva
  2. Technique: Visual inspection and use of one finger to palpate (Figures 4–40 and 4–41)
  3. Landmarks of the hard palate (Figure 4–42)
   a. Incisive papilla
    (1) Elevation of tissue directly behind the central incisors
    (2) Site for injection of the nasopalatine nerve
    (3) Often this area sustains trauma such as thermal burns from hot foods and beverages or abrasions from hard, crunchy, or coarse foods
   b. Midpalatine suture (median palatine raphe; midline palatal suture)
    (1) Located in the midline of the palate

Figure 4–39   Palpating floor of mouth.

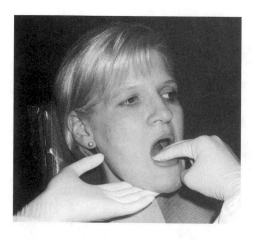

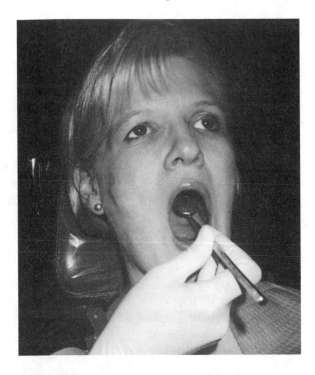

Figure 4–40   Visual inspection of the hard palate.

    (2) Line running anteriorly from the incisive papilla and becoming indistinct in the soft palate area posteriorly
    (3) Represents the joining of the palatal shelves during palate formation
    (4) Palatal (maxillary) torus—exostosis commonly seen in the midline of the palate
  c. Palatine rugae
    (1) Ridges of tissue radiating outward from midpalatine suture
    (2) Aid in mastication
    (3) Should feel dense and firm

Figure 4–41   Palpating the hard palate.

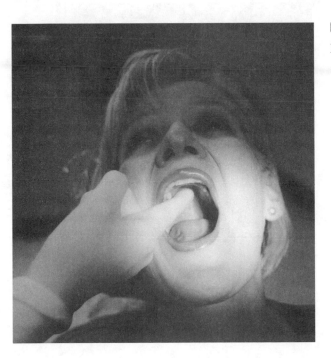

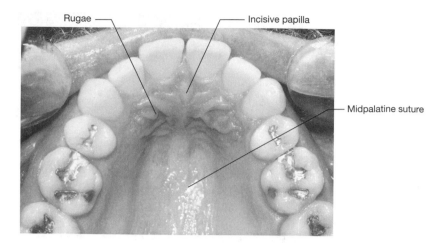

Rugae — Incisive papilla

Midpalatine suture

Figure 4–42 Landmarks of the hard palate.

d. Palatine fovea
(1) Located on either side of the median palatine raphae
(2) Two small, centrally located openings for the palatine glands
F. Soft palate
1. Located posterior to the hard palate and lacks bony support
2. Technique: Visual inspection (ask patient to say *ahh*) and digital palpation; use caution not to touch base of tongue, which activates the gag reflex
3. Appearance
a. Thin, muscular tissue separating mouth from nose
b. Appears redder than the hard palate due to thick vascular connective tissue; yellowish appearance often seen is considered normal and due to underlying adipose tissue
4. Uvula: Projection of vertical tissue extending from the soft palate

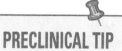

PRECLINICAL TIP

Inspecting Your Knowledge: Bifurcated uvula is a congenital deformity causing the uvula to be divided or bifurcated.

Figure 4–43 Inspecting the oropharynx.

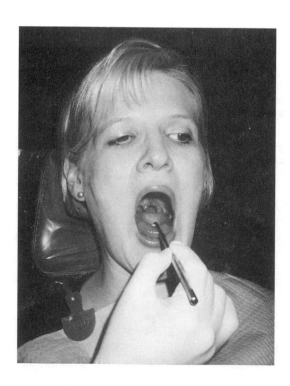

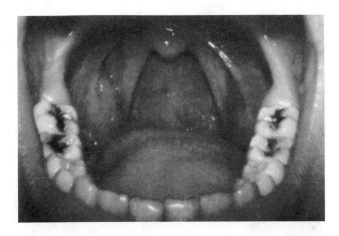

Figure 4–44   Palatine tonsils.

G. Oropharynx
1. The oropharynx, as its name implies, is the transitional area from the oral cavity to the pharynx, composed of the anterior and posterior tonsillar pillars and palatine tonsils
2. Technique: Visual inspection (ask patient to say *ahh*) and depress the mirror or tongue blade on the dorsum of the tongue to examine the oropharynx area (Figure 4–43)
3. Landmarks
   a. Anterior and posterior pillars (fauces)—two arches found bilaterally in the soft palate complex
      (1) Anterior pillar is formed by the palatoglossus muscle
      (2) Posterior pillar is formed by the palatopharyngeal muscle
   b. Palatine tonsils (Figure 4–44)
      (1) Pad of lymph tissue located between anterior and posterior pillars
      (2) Size varies from small papules to large masses that fill the oropharynx
      (3) Observations
         (a) Tonsilitis is an inflammation of the palatine tonsils
         (b) Inflamed tonsils appear red and swollen and may be covered with pus
         (c) Tonsils may *not* be present; some patients have had them surgically removed (tonsillectomy)

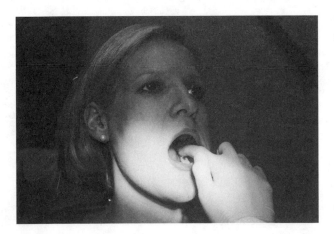

Figure 4–45   Palpating the retromolar pad.

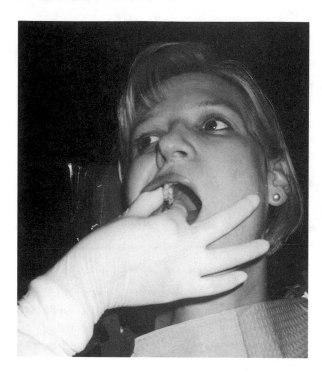

Figure 4–46   Palpating the gingiva.

H. Maxillary tuberosity and retromolar pad
1. The maxillary tuberosity and retromolar pad (triangle) are located directly distal to the most posterior tooth in the maxilla and mandible respectively
2. Technique: Visual inspection and digital palpation; examine bony areas covered by gingival tissue (Figure 4–45)

I. Periodontium
1. The periodontium is the tissue that surrounds and supports the teeth; it consists of the alveolar bone, periodontal ligament, cementum, and gingiva; gingiva is attached to the teeth and alveolar bone
2. Technique: Visual inspection (direct and indirect) and digital palpation (Figure 4–46)
3. Gingiva is first viewed from facial and lingual aspects
   a. Gingiva should be palpated to assess consistency; palpation may reveal edema, bleeding, or pus, or may cause discomfort, indicating gingival inflammation and possible periodontal disease

Figure 4–47   Gingivitis.

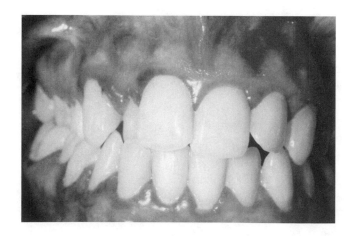

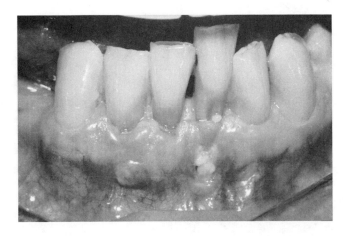

Figure 4–48   Recession, plaque, and purulis.

(1) Normal gingiva includes the following characteristics:
   (a) Color—coral pink, pink, or pigmented melanin
   (b) Texture—stippled and tightly bound to the underlying alveolar bone
   (c) Contour—firm against the tooth; interdental papilla fills the interdental space, giving it a knifelike adaptation
(2) Diseased gingiva may appear swollen, shiny, and red; bleeding and foul odor often accompany the inflammation (Figures 4–47, 4–48, and 4–49); characterisitics of diseased gingiva include
   (a) Color—red
   (b) Texture—affected, causing it to lose its knifelike adaptation and stippling, giving it a shiny appearance
   (c) Contour—puffy or swollen
     • Fistula, also called a *gum boil,* appears as a raised enlargement on the mucosa, often the gingiva; results from an infected (abscessed) tooth and a path of drainage bored by the body through solid tissue from the apex of the tooth to the surface of the mucosa; pus often extrudes from the hole in the center (Figure 4–50)
     • Exostosis—areas of extra bone not confined to the maxillary and mandibular tori; can be found on gingival ridges within the oral cavity, most notably the buccal surfaces of maxillary and posterior gingiva

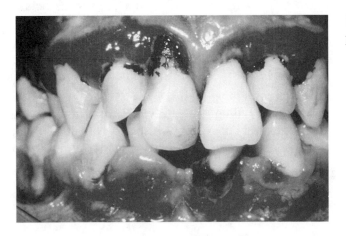

Figure 4–49   Progressed periodontitis.

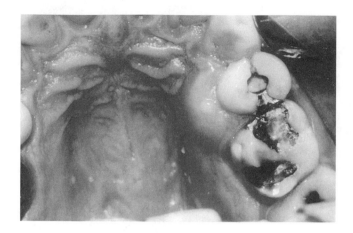

Figure 4–50   Fistula.

Performing thorough extraoral and intraoral examinations on patients is essential to help provide a basis for treatment and recognition of abnormalities, disease, and oral cancer. Early detection is the key to prevention. As healthcare professionals, it is our responsibility to provide a thorough assessment on every patient.

QUESTIONS

1. Which of the following is essential when performing the extraoral and intraoral examinations?
   a. Begin with the intraoral examination.
   b. Perform muscle palpation first.
   c. Use the same sequence each time.
   d. Position the patient in a supine position for both.

2. Which of the following palpation methods involves the use of finger and thumb to manipulate tissue?
   a. Digital
   b. Bidigital
   c. Bimanual
   d. Bilateral

3. Which of the following lymph nodes are located in front of the ears?
   a. Preauricular
   b. Postauricular
   c. Submandibular
   d. Anterior cervical

4. Which lymph nodes are palpated by pressing the fingers against the floor of the mouth and rolling the tissue across the inferior border of the mandible?
   a. Submandibular
   b. Anterior cervical
   c. Submental
   d. Posterior cervical

5. Which of the following statements about lymph nodes is TRUE?
   a. Palpable nodes often indicate decreased immune system activity.
   b. Normal nodes are visible and palpable.
   c. Nodes associated with malignancies are often soft, tender, and moveable.
   d. Palpable nodes may be enlarged.

6. In which of the following lymph node groups can a sore throat and/or oral infection result in lymphadenopathy?
   a. Preauricular
   b. Postauricular
   c. Anterior cervical
   d. Posterior cervical

7. Name the duct associated with the parotid gland.
   a. Stensen's
   b. Bartholin's
   c. Wharton's
   d. There is no duct associated with the parotid gland.

8. Which of the following palpation techniques is used to palpate the sinuses during the extraoral examination?
   a. Digital
   b. Bidigital
   c. Bimanual
   d. Bilateral

9. Which of the following lists the five *key* elements that should be used when describing a lesion?
   a. Color, odor, shape, size, location
   b. Appearance, texture, size, color, shape
   c. Color, size, shape, consistency, location
   d. Palpability, consistency, texture, shape, size

10. When examining a patient's eyes, the dental hygienist notes yellowing of the sclera. This can indicate
    a. drug abuse.
    b. neurological dysfunction.
    c. conjunctivitis.
    d. jaundice.

11. All of the following structures should be bilaterally palpated EXCEPT one. Which one is the EXCEPTION?
    a. Temporomandibular joint
    b. Parotid glands
    c. Masseter muscle
    d. Posterior cervical nodes

12. Which palpation technique is used to palpate the floor of the mouth?
    a. Digital
    b. Bidigital
    c. Manual
    d. Bimanual

13. Which of the four types of papillae on the dorsal surface are located on the lateral borders of the tongue?
    a. Filiform
    b. Fungiform
    c. Foliate
    d. Circumvallate

14. Which of the following tissues is found between the anterior and posterior pillars of the soft palate complex?
    a. Palatine tonsils
    b. Lingual tonsils
    c. Plica fimbriata
    d. Palatine rugae

REFERENCES

1. Perno, M. The dental hygienist: Our role in women's health—Management of the female client. *Compendium of Continuing Education in Dentistry,* 22(1), 2001.

2. Centers for Disease Control. Preventing and controlling oral pharyngeal cancer recommendations from a national strategic planning conference. *MMWR* 47, August 28, 1998.

3. Silverman, S. *Oral Cancer,* 4th ed. St. Louis: Mosby Yearbook, 1998.

4. Goldie, M. P. Oral and pharyngeal cancer: The role of the oral health-care professional. *RDH,* 22(7), July 2002.

5. Johns, S. The extraoral examination from the perspective of the patient. *Journal of Dental Hygiene,* 25(4), Fall 2001.

6. Bricker, S. L., R. P. Langlais, & C. S. Miller. *Oral Diagnosis, Oral Medicine and Treatment Planning.* Philadelphia: Lea & Febiger, 1994.

7. Detecting Oral Cancer; A Guide for Health Care Professionals. U.S. Department of Health and Human Services, Public Health Service, National Institutes of Health, National Institute of Dental Research, 1996.

8. Fehrenbach, M. J., & S. W. Herring. *Illustrated Anatomy of the Head and Neck.* Philadelphia: W.B. Saunders, 2002.

9. Hiatt, J. L., & L. P. Gartner. *Textbook of Head and Neck Anatomy,* 3rd ed. Philadelphia: Lippincott Williams & Wilkins, 2001.

INTRAORAL EXAMINATION TASK SHEET

Student _____

Date _____

Instructor _____

Re-evaluation
Instr: _____
Date _____

Instr: _____
Date _____

	S	U	Comments	S	U	Comments	S	U	Comments
Internal Surface of the Lip and Labial Mucosa									
1. Accessory salivary glands									
Frena									
1. Midline upper lip									
2. Midline lower lip									
3. Adjacent to maxillary and mandibular premolars									
4. Buccal mucosa									
Tongue									
1. Dorsal surface									
2. Ventral surface									
Floor of mouth									
1. Sublingual fold									
2. Sublingual caruncles									
3. Underlying tissues and musculature									
Hard Palate									
1. Incisive Papilla									
2. Median palatine raphae (midline palatine suture)									
3. Palatine rugae									
4. Palatine fovea									
Soft Palate/Uvula									
Oropharynx									
1. Anterior and posterior pillars (fauces)									
2. Palatine tonsils									
Maxillary tuberosity									
Retromolar pad									
Gingiva and periodontium									
Occlusion									

EXTRAORAL EXAMINATION TASK SHEET

Student _____
Date _____
Instructor _____

Re-evaluation
Instr: _____
Date _____

Instr: _____
Date _____

General Appearance	S	U	Comments	S	U	Comments	S	U	Comments
1. Gait									
Overall appearance									
Examination of the Head and Neck									
1. Facial form and symmetry									
2. Skin, Ears, Hair and Eyes									
3. Nose									
4. Lips and Labial Mucosa									
Muscles									
1. Mentalis									
2. Masseter									
3. Temporalis									
Paranasal Sinuses									
1. Frontal									
2. Maxillary									
Lymph nodes and Salivary Glands									
1. Submental gland									
2. Sublingual lymph glands									
3. Submandibular gland									
4. Submandibular lymph nodes									
5. Parotid gland									
6. Preauricular lymph nodes									
7. Postauricular lymph nodes									
8. Occipital lymph nodes									
9. Posterior cervical lymph nodes									
10. Anterior cervical lymph nodes									
Sternocleidomastoid muscle									
Thyroid gland									
Larynx									
TMJ									

Chapter 5

Examination and Charting of the Hard and Soft Tissues

Lauri Wiechmann, RDH, MPA

MediaLink

A companion CD-ROM, included free with each new copy of this book, supplements the procedures presented in each chapter. Insert the CD-ROM to watch video clips and view a large collection of color images that is also included. This multimedia library is designed to help you add a new dimension to your learning.

KEY TERMS

abfraction. A noncarious lesion resembling cracks, notches, or lines around the cervical third of the tooth.

abrasion. Mechanical wearing away of the tooth.

Angle's classification. Most commonly used classification system for determining occlusion of permanent teeth.

arrested caries. Remineralized area of the tooth structure that was once demineralized.

attrition. Wearing of incisal biting surfaces.

dental caries. Decalcified enamel due to acid exposure; also known as cavity or decay.

dental prosthesis. Functional, artificial replacement for one or more teeth; may be fixed or removable.

erosion. Loss of tooth structure as a result of chemical action.

extrinsic stain. Pigmented deposits that can be removed during instrumentation and/or polishing.

facial profile. Classification of a visual observation of the profile of the patient; provides information on the relationship between the maxillary and mandibular arches.

furcation. Loss of attachment between the furca of multirooted teeth.

incipient lesion. Beginning of a carious lesion without cavitation.

intrinsic stain. Stain within the tooth that cannot be removed; also known as endogenous stain.

malocclusion. Abnormal tooth alignment when teeth are together.

mesognathic (pronounced *mesonathic*). A classification of facial profile; maxilla and mandible appear to be in the same relation to each other.

mobility. Involves the extent of movement of a tooth in either a horizontal and/or apical direction.

occlusion. Tooth-to-tooth relationship of the maxilla and mandible when the mouth is closed.

prognathic (pronounced *pro-nathic*). A classification of facial profile; mandible appears to be protruded in relation to the maxilla.

recession. Apical migration of the marginal gingiva resulting in exposure of the root surface.

recurrent caries. Occurs around an already existing restoration (filling); also known as secondary caries

retrognathic (pronounced *retro-nathic*). A classification of facial profile; mandible appears to be retruded in relation the maxilla.

LEARNING OBJECTIVES

After reading this chapter, the student will be able to:

- differentiate between a geometric and anatomic chart used in charting the hard tissues of the oral cavity;
- discuss the purposes of charting the hard and soft tissues of the oral cavity;
- explain the difference between the types of restorative materials listed;
- compare and contrast an onlay, inlay, and crown;
- discuss the findings of the hard tissue examination, which may have an impact on the periodontal health;
- distinguish between the types of prostheses listed;
- discuss centric relation;

- determine the occlusal classification of both permanent and primary dentitions using Angle's classification from a given case study and from study models;
- discuss the causes for malocclusions;
- give details of the following malocclusions: crossbite, openbite, overjet, overbite, midline deviation, end-to-end, edge-to-edge;
- using pictures, diagrams, or definitions, determine the facial profile and relate it to the respective occlusal classification;
- discuss G. V. Black's classification for dental caries and restorations and determine, from a description, picture, or drawing, the appropriate classification for the carious lesion or restoration present;

- compare and contrast intrinsic and extrinsic stains, evaluating source of stain, area of presence on the tooth, and color;
- describe the difference between abrasion and attrition;
- explain the significance of utilizing radiographs during the charting of the hard tissues of the oral cavity;
- discuss the factors affecting the color, contour, and consistency of the gingival tissue;
- compare and contrast the color, contour, and consistency of the gingival tissue in both health and disease;
- discriminate between a gingival pocket and a periodontal pocket;
- explain the classifications for mobility and furcation and the techniques for determining the status of them;
- discuss the PSR system.

I. Introduction

Examination of the hard and soft tissues is a vital component of the assessment data collected and recorded for each patient. Initial findings serve as baseline information, and findings at subsequent appointments may determine a significant change in health. It is important to note even the smallest finding regardless of how insignificant it may seem. Sometimes even the smallest change can be serious to the health of the patient.

II. Dental Charting Hard Tissues

A. Purposes of charting
   1. Legal documentation: Dental records serve as a legal document and may be utilized in case of litigation
   2. Accurate baseline of dental status: Aids in preparing treatment plan, reviewing radiographs, and providing services at a recare appointment
   3. Dialogue with insurance company: Dentition chart demonstrates to the insurance company the condition of the patient's hard tissues—information that may be required to determine eligibility of services
   4. Forensic identification: Charting the hard tissues aids in postmortem dental examination, especially when radiographs are not available

B. Types of charting (Figure 5–1)
   1. Geometric: Each tooth represented by a circular grid with each section representing an area of the tooth
   2. Anatomic: Each tooth represented by a schematic drawing of the actual tooth

C. Components of charting: Required information includes
   1. Tooth numbering systems: A numerical or alphabetical means of identifying each specific tooth (Figure 5–2)
      a. Universal notation labels each permanent tooth from 1 through 32 and each primary tooth from A through T
      b. Federation Dentaire Internationale (FDI) notation labels each tooth by the quadrant it is in and its location from the midline
      c. Palmer notation labels each tooth using a symbol to designate which quadrant the tooth is in and its location from the midline; labels each permanent tooth 1 through 8 and each primary tooth A through E
   2. Charting locations: Numerous terms used to describe the various areas of the mouth and specific locations on the teeth (Figure 5–3)

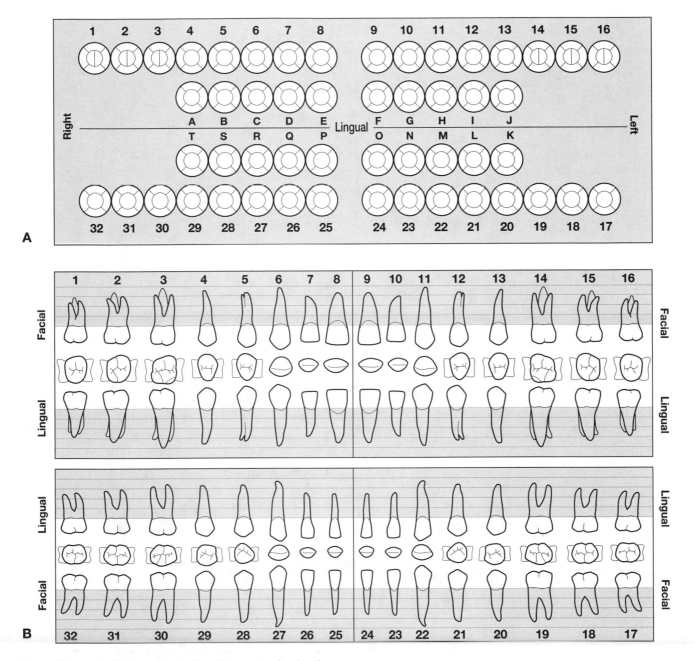

Figure 5–1   A. Geometric charting. B. Anatomic charting.

a. *Arch* denotes the division of the mouth into two parts—the maxillary (upper) and the mandibular (lower)

b. Quadrant is a method of dividing the mouth into fourths from the midline posteriorly
   (1) Labeling begins from the maxillary right and follows clockwise, finishing at the mandibular right
   (2) Two quadrants make up an arch; four quadrants per mouth

c. Sextant is a method of dividing the mouth into sixths
   (1) Four permanent posterior sextants include two premolars and three molars
   (2) Two anterior sextants include two canines and four incisors

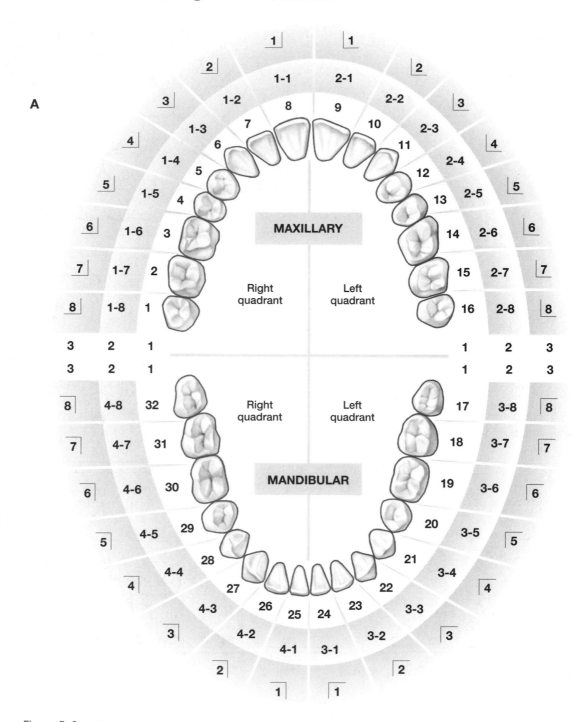

Figure 5–2   Tooth numbering systems. A. Permanent dentition.

(3) Labeling begins with maxillary right posterior sextant (1) and follows clockwise, finishing with the mandibular right posterior sextant (6)

(4) Three sextants per arch; six sextants per mouth

d. Directional terms identify specific areas of the tooth; commonly used to describe the location of restorations (fillings) or carious lesions (cavities)

(1) Mesial: Toward the midline

(2) Distal: Away from the midline

B

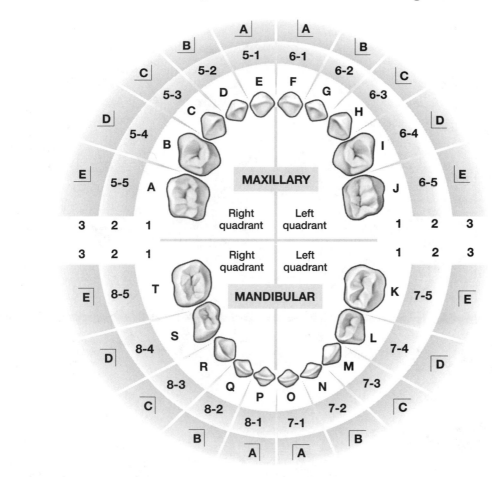

Figure 5–2   B. Primary dentition. Tooth numbering systems.

(3) Lingual: Toward the roof of the mouth or tongue
(4) Facial: Toward the cheek; *buccal* refers to posterior teeth, *labial* refers to anterior teeth
(5) Occlusal: Chewing surface of posterior teeth
(6) Incisal: Biting edge of anterior teeth
(7) Tooth divisions (Figure 5–4)
   (a) Horizontal
      • Cervical/gingival third: Portion of the tooth closest to the gingival/cervical area
      • Middle third: Portion in the middle of the tooth
      • Incisal/occlusal third: Portion of the tooth closest to the biting/chewing surface
   (b) Vertical
      • Distal third: Portion of the tooth farthest away from the midline
      • Middle third: Portion in the middle of the tooth
      • Mesial third: Portion of the tooth closest to the mid-line
3. Missing teeth are teeth not present in the oral cavity; may be unerupted, congenitally missing, or previously extracted; radiographs are necessary to determine the presence and status of missing teeth

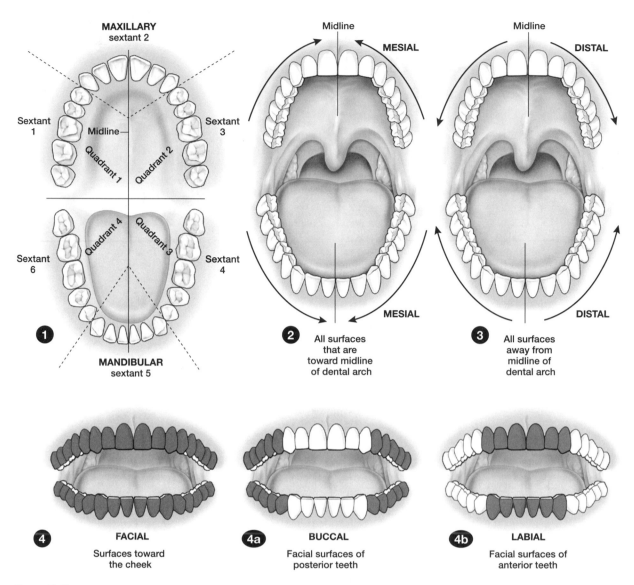

Figure 5–3   Charting locations.

   a. Typically recorded schematically on chart; teeth that have been extracted are charted differently from those that are unerupted

   b. Knowing whether a tooth has been extracted or is unerupted may assist in the differential diagnosis of oral pathology findings

4. Extruded teeth (supraversion, supraerupted, extruded) are teeth that are moved out of the alveolar bone beyond the line of occlusion

   a. Noted on chart in writing or schematically

   b. Tend to occlude prematurely, interfering with the way the teeth contact during chewing and grinding

   c. Commonly results in trauma to the supporting periodontium, possibly causing a deeper periodontal pocket

5. Intruded teeth (infraversion, intrusion) are teeth that are *not* erupted to the line of occlusion

   a. Typically noted on chart in writing or schematically

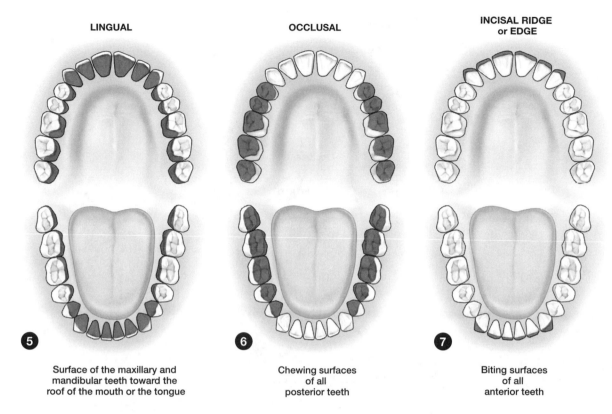

LINGUAL   OCCLUSAL   INCISAL RIDGE or EDGE

⑤ Surface of the maxillary and mandibular teeth toward the roof of the mouth or the tongue

⑥ Chewing surfaces of all posterior teeth

⑦ Biting surfaces of all anterior teeth

Figure 5–3   Charting locations.

    b. Do *not* contribute in chewing or grinding; can result in damage to the periodontal structure

6. Drifted teeth are teeth that have drifted or moved into the adjacent space once occupied by a tooth; may result from the premature loss of a primary tooth or extraction of an adjacent tooth
    a. Typically noted on chart in writing or schematically
    b. Excess plaque accumulation may result in these areas
    c. If drifting is caused by premature loss of a primary tooth, the erupting permanent tooth may not have enough space for full eruption; a space maintainer is commonly placed

7. Impacted teeth are imbedded in the bone

8. Restorations are areas on the tooth that have been replaced with some type of restorative material (e.g., amalgam or composite); typically noted schematically on chart; visually indicates extent of past caries activity; restorative materials include
    a. Amalgam—composed of a blend of various metals and mercury; usually silver or dark gray in color[1]
    b. Composite—tooth-colored resin material; commonly used in anterior restorations for esthetic value; growing in use in posterior teeth
    c. Sealant—plastic resin most commonly placed in the pits and fissures of posterior teeth; may be opaque, pink, white, yellow, or translucent in color
    d. Gold-yellow or white in color; commonly used in cast crowns, inlays, or onlays

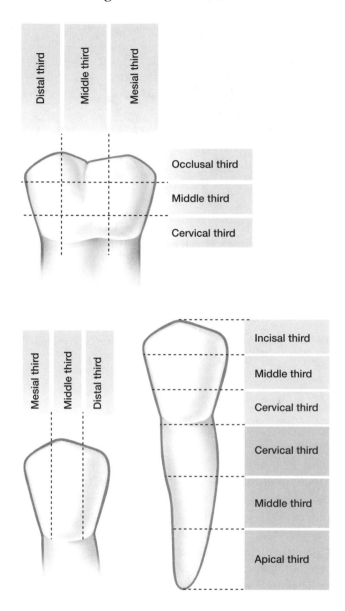

Figure 5–4   Tooth divisions.

(1) Cast crown: Custom-made tooth-shaped cap that covers the crown of a tooth; replicated in a laboratory and cemented onto the prepared crown of the tooth

(2) Inlay: Cast replication of a portion of the tooth; when cemented in place it is confined within the marginal ridges of the occlusal surface[2]

(3) Onlay: Cast restoration, when cemented in place, covers the marginal ridges of the occlusal surface and one or more cusps of a posterior tooth[2]

e. Temporary restoration—material intended for short-term placement, usually while laboratory work is being completed; usually a soft, pliable material (composed of aluminum or acrylic for a crown), which is compacted into the prepared area and hardens upon setting

f. Veneer—made up of thin resin composite or porcelain surface bonded onto the facial surface of a tooth; similar to a false fingernail

g. Porcelain—white ceramic material commonly used to make crowns, inlays, and veneers; most common crown fabricated is porcelain fused-to-metal

9. Overhanging restoration is a projection of restorative material extending beyond the curvature of the tooth; may be detected with an instrument or radiographically
   a. Typically noted on chart in writing or schematically
   b. Creates an area for excess plaque/food accumulation, which affects the health of periodontium
   c. Interferes with interproximal cleaning aids (e.g., shreds floss)

10. Existing prosthesis is a functional, artificial replacement for one or more teeth; may be fixed (e.g., bridge, implant) or removable (denture)
   a. Typically noted on chart in writing or schematically
   b. May be an area for excess plaque accumulation (e.g., as may occur with a bridge)
   c. May cause gingival irritation (e.g., as may occur with poorly fitting denture)
   d. May alter instrument selection (e.g., plastic instruments for use with implant)
   e. Types of common prostheses
      (1) Dentures (partial or full): "False teeth"; may replace one tooth to a full arch of teeth; removable
      (2) Bridge: Replaces one or more missing teeth; consists of abutment(s)—natural teeth that act as the anchor to hold or support the bridge and pontic(s)—artificial tooth that replaces the missing tooth; fixed
      (3) Implants: Surgical implantation of post(s) or a prepared frame to support a prosthetic appliance[1]

11. Supernumerary teeth are extra teeth; may need radiographs to verify
   a. Typically recorded on chart pictorially or in writing
   b. May cause crowding, pathology (e.g., dentigerous cysts), displacement of permanent teeth, failure of eruption of adjacent teeth[3]

12. Rotated teeth are teeth that are rotated either mesially or distally in relation to the long axis of the tooth; torsoversion
   a. Typically recorded on chart pictorially or in writing
   b. Can create an area for plaque accumulation; patient may have difficulty removing plaque, which can cause gingival inflammation

13. Occlusion is the tooth-to-tooth relationship of the maxilla and mandible when the mouth is closed; typically noted on the chart in writing; occlusal classifications (Figure 5–5) include
   Note: Two methods of determining the occlusion for permanent teeth are given; Method 1 uses the permanent maxillary first molar or canine as the determinant; Method 2 uses the permanent mandibular first molar or canine as the determinant; both methods result in the same classification
   a. Centric occlusion: Ideal occlusion; relation of the mandible to the maxilla when the teeth are in maximum intercuspation; tooth-to-tooth relationship[4]

PRECLINICAL TIP

Assessing Your Knowledge: Males are twice as likely as females to have supernumerary teeth in their permanent dentition.[3]

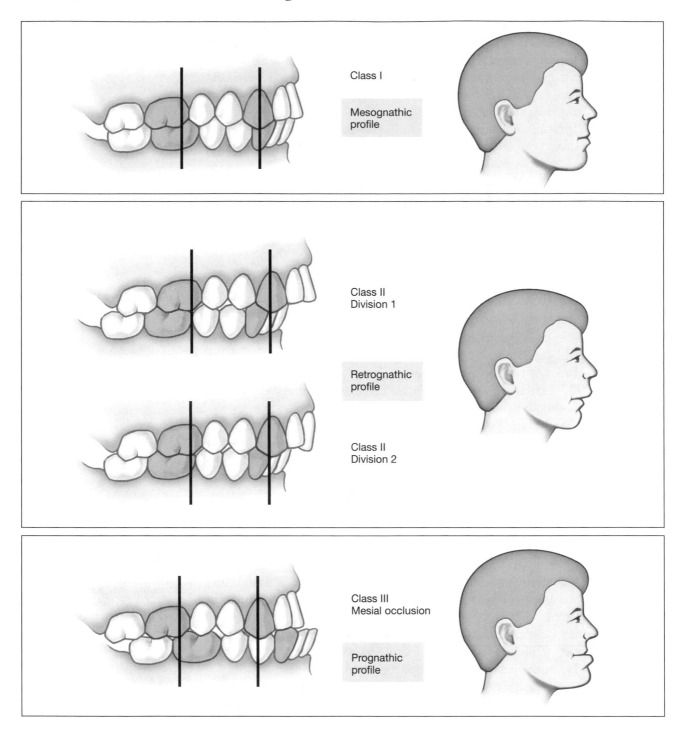

Figure 5–5   Occlusal relationships: Class I (*top*); class II, division 1 (*middle top*), class II, division 2 (*middle bottom*); class III (*bottom*).

(1) Molar relationship
    (a) Method 1: Mesiobuccal cusp of the permanent maxillary first molar is in alignment with the buccal groove of the permanent mandibular first molar
    (b) Method 2: Buccal groove of the permanent mandibular first molar is in alignment with the mesiobuccal cusp of the permanent maxillary first molar

(2) Canine relationship
   (a) Method 1: Permanent maxillary canine occludes with the distal half of the permanent mandibular canine and the mesial half of the permanent mandibular first premolar
   (b) Method 2: Distal half of the permanent mandibular canine and the mesial half of the permanent mandibular first premolar occlude with the permanent maxillary canine
   (c) Other: All teeth are in maximum intercuspation with the respective teeth in the opposite arch with no malposition
b. Permanent dentition: Most commonly classified using Angle's classification
   (1) Class I (neutrocclusion)
      (a) Molar relationship
         • Method 1: Mesiobuccal cusp of the permanent maxillary first molar is in alignment with the buccal groove of the permanent mandibular first molar
         • Method 2: Buccal groove of the permanent mandibular first molar is in alignment with the mesiobuccal cusp of the permanent maxillary first molar
      (b) Canine relationship
         • Method 1: Maxillary permanent canine occludes with the distal half of the mandibular permanent canine and the mesial half of the mandibular first premolar
         • Method 2: Distal half of the permanent mandibular canine and the mesial half of the permanent mandibular first premolar occlude with the permanent maxillary canine
      (c) Other: Other malocclusion or positioning of individual teeth occurs; this differentiates Class I from centric occlusion
   (2) Class II (distocclusion)
      (a) Molar relationship
         • Method 1: Mesiobuccal cusp of the permanent maxillary first molar is mesial to the buccal groove of the permanent mandibular first molar by the width of a premolar
         • Method 2: Buccal groove of the permanent mandibular first molar is distal to the mesiobuccal cusp of the permanent maxillary first molar by the width of a premolar
      (b) Canine relationship
         • Method 1: Distal surface of the permanent maxillary canine is mesial to the mesial surface of the permanent mandibular canine by at least the width of a premolar
         • Method 2: Mesial surface of the permanent canine is distal to the distal surface of the permanent maxillary canine by at least the width of a premolar

(c) Class II, division I: Molar and canine relationship is the same as listed previously; one or more anterior incisors are facially inclined

(d) Class II, division II: Molar and canine relationship is the same as listed previously; one or more of the anterior incisors are lingually inclined

(e) Tendency toward Class II
- Molar relationship: Distance between the mesiobuccal cusp of the permanent maxillary first molar and the buccal groove of the permanent mandibular molar is less than the width of a premolar
- Canine relationship: Distance between the distal surface of the permanent maxillary canine and the mesial surface of the permanent mandibular canine is less than the width of a premolar

(3) Class III (mesiocclusion)
(a) Molar relationship
- Method 1: Mesiobuccal cusp of the permanent maxillary first molar is distal to the buccal groove of the permanent mandibular first molar
- Method 2: Buccal groove of the permanent mandibular first molar is mesial to the mesiobuccal cusp of the permanent maxillary first molar by at least the width of a premolar

(b) Canine relationship
- Method 1: Mesial surface of the permanent maxillary canine is distal to the distal surface of the permanent mandibular canine by the width of a premolar
- Method 2: Distal surface of the permanent mandibular canine is mesial to the mesial surface of the permanent maxillary canine by the width of a premolar

(c) Tendency toward Class III
- Molar relationship: Distance between the mesiobuccal cusp of the permanent maxillary first molar and the buccal groove of the permanent mandibular first molar is less than the width of a premolar
- Canine relationship: Distance between the mesial surface of the permanent maxillary canine and the distal surface of the permanent mandibular canine is less than the width of a premolar

c. Primary dentition[4] (Figure 5–6)
(1) Flush terminal plane: Primary molars are in an end-to-end relationship
(2) Mesial step: Distal surface of the primary mandibular second molar is mesial to the distal surface of the primary maxillary second molar
(3) Distal step: Distal surface of the primary mandibular second molar is distal to the distal surface of the primary maxillary second molar

d. Malocclusion denotes abnormal tooth alignment (see Figure 5–7)
(1) Causes

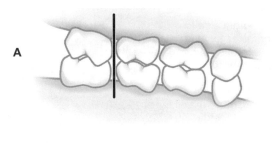

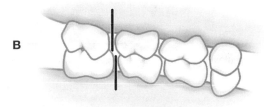

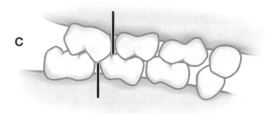

Figure 5–6   Occlusal relationships of the primary dentition: A. Flush terminal plane; B. Mesial step; C. Distal step.

    (a) Growth patterns: Determined by how the body grows during developmental years
    (b) Occlusal development: Determined by how the maxilla and mandible grow during developmental years[4]
    (c) Temporomandibular joint (TMJ) dysfunction: Caused by developmental changes occurring with the TMJ
    (d) Habits: Interaction with the teeth that causes them to move out of alignment; common habits include thumb sucking, tongue thrusting, lip biting, mouth breathing, and bruxism[5]
    (e) Local factors: Events occurring in the mouth affecting the alignment of the teeth; some factors include over-retained primary teeth, ectopic eruption of permanent first molars, congenitally missing teeth, and impacted teeth
(2) Midline deviation: Interproximals of the maxillary central incisors do not align with the interproximals of the mandibular central incisors
    (a) Assess the midline from behind the patient, using the philtrum, nasal septum, and frenum attachment as fixed points
    (b) Typically record, in millimeters, the direction to which the mandible deviates
    (c) Can cause possible TMJ trauma
(3) Crossbite: The facial surface(s) of one or more mandibular teeth are facial to the corresponding maxillary teeth
    (a) Note specific teeth (maxillary/mandibular) on chart

Crossbite	A. Unilateral crossbite—right side is normal, left side mandibular teeth facial to normal position; B. Bilateral crossbite 1— mandibular teeth facial to normal position; C. Bilateral crossbite 2— mandibular teeth lingual to normal position; D. Anterior crossbite—maxillary teeth lingual to mandibular teeth.	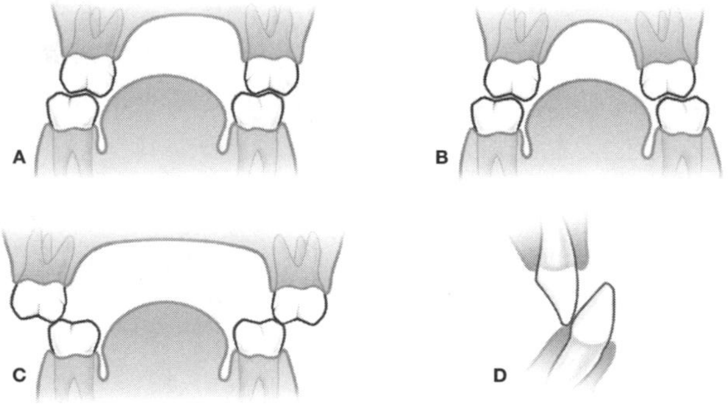
Overbite	Vertical overlap of the maxillary anterior teeth to the mandibular anterior teeth.	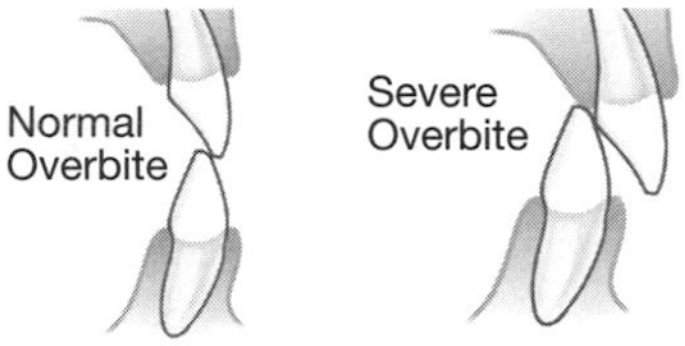
End-to-end	The relationship of the occlusal surface of a maxillary posterior tooth to its corresponding mandibular tooth; occlusal cusp to occlusal cusp.	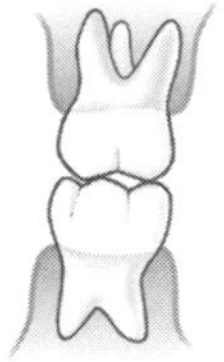
Edge-to-edge	The relationship of the incisal edge of a maxillary anterior tooth to its corresponding mandibular tooth, incisal edge to incisal edge.	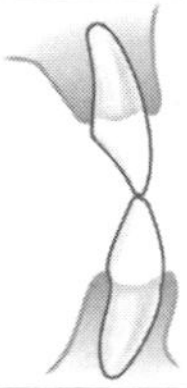
Overjet	The horizontal overlap of the maxillary teeth to the mandibular teeth.	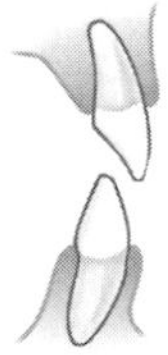
Openbite	Maxillary and mandibular teeth are not in exclusion, may include one or more teeth.	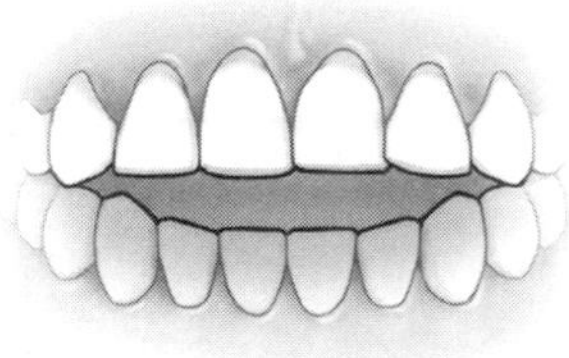

Figure 5–7   Malocclusion of individual or groups of teeth.

(b) Can affect TMJ as the mandible is forced to one side to provide a more functional bite

(c) Variations include[1, 4]

- Unilateral crossbite—only the right or left half of the mouth is in crossbite (refer to Figure 5–7)

- Bilateral crossbite 1—all of the surfaces of the maxillary teeth are positioned lingual to the lingual surfaces of the respective mandibular teeth; this occurs when the maxilla is extremely smaller than the mandible; known as acromegaly (refer to Figure 5–7)

- Bilateral crossbite 2—all of the facial surfaces of the mandibular teeth are positioned lingual to the lingual surfaces of the respective maxillary teeth; this occurs when the mandible is extremely smaller than the maxilla (refer to Figure 5–7)

(4) Overbite: Vertical overlap of the maxillary anterior teeth to the mandibular anterior teeth[4] (refer to Figure 5–7)
  (a) Commonly noted on the chart in writing
  (b) May cause mobility and/or trauma to palate and TMJ if severe
  (c) Classifications
    - Normal—maxillary incisal edge is within the incisal third of the mandibular anterior tooth
    - Moderate—maxillary incisal edge is within the middle third of the mandibular anterior tooth
    - Severe—maxillary incisal edge is within the cervical third of the mandibular anterior tooth

(5) End-to-end: Relationship of the occlusal surface of a maxillary posterior tooth to its corresponding mandibular tooth; occlusal cusp to occlusal cusp (refer to Figure 5–7)
  (a) Note specific teeth on chart in writing
  (b) May cause attrition to teeth or trauma to TMJ

(6) Edge-to-edge: Relationship of the incisal edge of a maxillary anterior tooth to its corresponding mandibular tooth; incisal edge to incisal edge (refer to Figure 5–7)
  (a) Note specific teeth on chart in writing
  (b) May cause attrition to teeth and/or trauma to TMJ
  (c) Patient commonly experiences posterior openbite

(7) Overjet: Horizontal overlap of the maxillary anterior teeth to the mandibular anterior teeth (refer to Figure 5–7)
  (a) Measured with probe and readings are noted in millimeters on chart (Figure 5–8)
  (b) May cause occlusal trauma

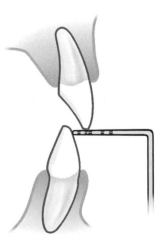

Figure 5–8   Measuring overjet with probe—measure horizontal distance between the facial of the mandibular anterior tooth to the lingual of the maxillary anterior tooth.

(8) Open bite: Maxillary and mandibular teeth are not in occlusion; may involve one or more teeth (refer to Figure 5–7)

    (a) Note specific teeth on chart in writing

    (b) May cause occlusal and TMJ trauma

(9) Wear facet: Worn and flattened area on a tooth surface of posterior teeth; usually occurs due to bruxism, attrition, or malocclusion[6]

    (a) Note area on chart in writing

    (b) May cause occlusal trauma and/or mobility of teeth

e. Checking occlusion

    (1) Have patient close together on posterior teeth while lifting tip of tongue to palate

    (2) Retract cheek with tongue depressor or mirror to examine occlusal relationship of posterior teeth (i.e., Angle's classification and malpositioned teeth)

    (3) Use direct vision and necessary instruments to determine occlusal relationships of anterior teeth (i.e., Angle's classification and malpositioned teeth)

    (4) Have patient open as you observe the occlusal and incisal edges for malpositioning or evidence of occlusal wear

f. Facial profile: Classification of a visual observation of the profile of the patient; provides information on the relationship between the maxillary and mandibular arches[2] (see Figure 5–5)

    (1) Mesognathic is affiliated with a Class I occlusion; maxilla and mandible appear to be in the same relation to each other

    (2) Retrognathic is affiliated with a Class II occlusion; the mandible appears to be retruded in relation to the maxilla

    (3) Prognathic is affiliated with a Class III occlusion; mandible appears to be protruded in relation to the maxilla

g. Caries: Decalcified enamel due to acid exposure; utilize radiographs to check for caries also;[5] demineralized areas can also be noted

    (1) Commonly recorded on the chart using colored pencil

    (2) Methods of detection include visual, tactile, and radiographic

        (a) Visual—use direct vision or transillumination; look for discoloration of enamel or cementum or a change in the density of tooth structure; fiber optic lights help with this process

        (b) Tactile—use explorer to apply pressure into pits and fissures and around margins of restorations

        (c) Radiographic—examine interproximal areas just apical to the contact point, dentinoenamel junction for evidence of possible occlusal caries, cementum and dentin just below the cervical area of the tooth for root caries, and adjacent to existing restorations for recurrent caries

    (3) Types of dental caries

        (a) Arrested: Remineralized area that was once demineralized; light brown to brown in color and feels smooth with an explorer

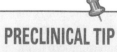

PRECLINICAL TIP

Assessing Your Knowledge: A sharp explorer used to check for caries can cause cavitation in areas that are remineralizing or could be remineralized. Note cavitation of tooth structure by a tacky/sticky sensation.

G. V. Black's Classification of Dental Caries and Restorations		
Class	Description	Pictorial View
I	Pits and fissures of anterior and posterior teeth.	
II	Proximal surface of posterior teeth. Commonly involves occlusal surface.	
III	Proximal surface of anterior teeth *not* involving the incisal edge.	
IV	Proximal surface of anterior teeth involving the incisal edge.	
V	Cervical (gingival) 1/3 of the facial or lingual surface.	
VI	Incisal edge of anterior teeth or cusp tips of posterior teeth.	

(b) Incipient: Beginning lesion; often not noticeable on radiographs; yellow to light tan in color, round or oval, slightly soft without cavitation

(c) Rampant: Rapidly progressing lesion; dark brown to black in color

(d) Recurrent: Occurs around an already present restoration; may need radiographs to detect; translucent gray to brown color beneath enamel

(4) Location of dental caries

(a) Pits and fissures located on occlusal surface of posterior teeth, facial and lingual pits/grooves of posterior teeth, and lingual pits of anterior teeth

     (b) Root surface develops on exposed cementum; yellow to dark brown or black in color

     (c) Smooth surface develops on facial, lingual, mesial, and distal surfaces

h. Attrition: Natural wearing of incisal biting surfaces; tooth-to-tooth wear; may be caused by malocclusion or bruxism—clenching or grinding of the teeth[5]

    (1) Typically noted on the chart in writing

    (2) May cause possible occlusal and supporting periodontal structure trauma

i. Abrasion: Mechanical wearing away of the tooth (e.g., by toothbrushing or by oral habits such as chewing on pens/pencils or pipe) (Figure 5–9)

    (1) Typically noted on the chart in writing

    (2) May cause occlusal trauma and increased susceptibility to decay

j. Abfraction: A noncarious lesion resembling cracks, notches, or lines around the cervical third of the tooth

    (1) Typically wedge-shaped cavity with sharp line angle

    (2) Primary causative factor of the lesion is tooth flexure; secondary factors are abrasion and acid erosion[7, 8]

k. Erosion: Loss of tooth structure as a result of chemical, not bacterial, action (e.g., complications caused by vomiting with bulimics, severe acid reflux)

    (1) Typically noted on the chart in writing

    (2) May evidence presence of systemic/mental disturbances, nutritional habits, and hypersensitive areas

l. Intrinsic staining of teeth, also known as *endogenous staining,*[10] includes stains within the tooth that cannot be removed

    (1) Typically noted on the chart in writing

    (2) May indicate presence of pulpal trauma

    (3) Observations

      (a) Gray indicates pulpal necrosis;[11] usually due to caries penetrating the pulp or the result of trauma to the tooth

      (b) Pink indicates trauma to the pulp, usually from internal resorption[10]

      (c) White flecks and/or white opaque and/or brown pits indicate presence of excess systemic fluoride during tooth development or hypoplasia

      (d) Shades of gray horizontal lines indicate exposure to tetracycline during tooth development; tooth will fluoresce when exposed to ultraviolet light[11]

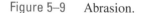

PRECLINICAL TIP

Assessing Your Knowledge: Along with assessing the medical history and dental tissues and conducting an examination of the head and neck, evaluation of erosion must also include assessment of salivary function.[9]

Figure 5–9   Abrasion.

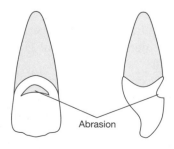

Abrasion

m. Extrinsic staining of teeth: Pigmented deposits that can be removed during instrumentation and polishing[5]
   (1) Typically noted on the chart in writing according to color, location, extent, and intensity
   (2) Aids in homecare instruction
   (3) Observations: Some colored stains are associated with chromogenic bacteria; remove as much extrinsic stain as possible with an instrument instead of a polishing agent to reduce the amount of tooth structure removed; it is possible for an extrinsic stain to become intrinsic if absorbed into the tooth structure
      (a) Brown is associated with poor oral hygiene and/or drinking colored beverages (e.g., coffee, tea, fruit juices, and wine)
      (b) Dark brown and black are associated with tobacco products
      (c) Yellow-brown and brown are associated with chlorhexidine gluconate or stannous fluoride; may be difficult to remove
      (d) Black usually occurs as thin lines on the facial and/or lingual surfaces near the cervical third of the tooth; found in healthy mouths; associated with iron and insoluble ferric sulfide
      (e) Green and yellow-green usually occur on the facial surface near the gingival half of anterior teeth; associated with poor oral hygiene
      (f) Orange commonly occurs on the facial and lingual of anterior teeth; associated with poor oral hygiene
n. Developmental malformations: Result during tooth germ initiation[2] (Note: listed below are just a few developmental malformations; for a more complete list, consult an oral pathology textbook)
   (1) Fluorosis: Ranges from white flecks to pitting to brown staining of the crown surface; caused from ingestion of too much fluoride during tooth development
   (2) Gemination: Two crowns joined together by a notched incisal area; usually has only one root; more frequently seen in the primary dentition;[4] confirmed by viewing radiographs
   (3) Fusion: Single large crown in place of two normal teeth; may have separate or fused roots;[10] confirmed by viewing radiographs
   (4) Talon cusp: Accessory cusp on a permanent incisor; located at the cingulum area[10]
D. Systematic method of charting: Develop a systematic method when charting the hard tissues to ensure that all components of the examination are performed.
E. Radiographic findings
   1. Include a thorough evaluation of the radiographs in the assessment of the hard tissues (e.g., to note any anomalies); radiographs assist in
      a. Detecting caries
      b. Identifying missing and unerupted teeth

c. Determining location of restorations and types of restorative materials

d. Noting pathology

e. Determining effect of malpositioned teeth on the periodontium

2. Determine frequency of radiographs, by need only, on an individual basis

III. Charting of the Soft Tissues (Periodontal Examination)

The purpose of charting soft tissues is to recognize and record areas of health, disease, and damage. It is also important to not only recognize these areas, but record the findings that may affect the health of the periodontium.

A. Gingiva[4, 5] (Figure 5–10)

1. Papillary (interdental) gingiva: Pointed gingiva located between the teeth

2. Col: Part of the papillary gingiva apical to the contact area connecting the facial and lingual gingiva ("valley between two mountain peaks"); non-keratinized and thus susceptible to disease

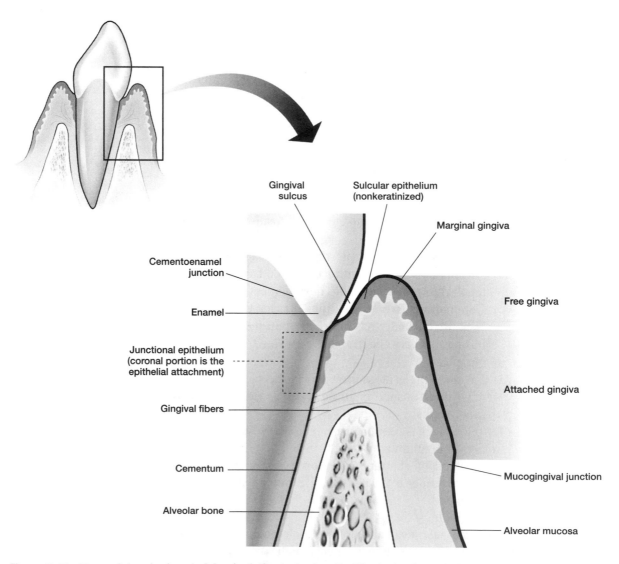

Figure 5–10   Parts of the gingiva. A. Marginal (free) gingiva; B. Gingival sulcus; C. Sulcular epithelium (nonkeritinized); D. Junctional epithelium (coronal portion of the epithelial attachment); E. Attached gingiva

3. Marginal (free) gingiva: Most coronal portion of the gingiva; entrance to the gingival sulcus
4. Gingival sulcus (gingival pocket): Space between the tooth and internal portion of the free gingiva
5. Sulcular epithelium: Extends from the marginal gingiva inside the gingival pocket; directly opposite the tooth structure
6. Junctional epithelium (attachment epithelium): Located at the bottom of the gingival sulcus
7. Attached gingiva: Extends from the free gingival groove to the alveolar mucosa

B. Descriptive terms (Table 5–1)
1. Color describes the color of the gingival tissue it most resembles; usually ranges from pink to red to hues of blue (bluish-pink to bluish-red); pigmented areas may be seen in health as well; factors affecting color include
   a. Vascular supply
   b. Thickness of keratinization of epithelium
   c. Presence of melanin pigmentation

Table 5–1   Gingival Descriptions: Health and Disease

		Characteristic in Healthy Tissue	Characteristics in Diseased Tissue
Color			
		Coral pink. Pigmented. Color associated with melanin. Usually limited to keratinized tissue.	Red. Dark pink to hues of blue. Pink—Fibrotic tissue.
Contour			
	Marginal gingiva	Flat against tooth. Knife-edged and scalloped.	Edematous—filled with fluid. Clefted—narrow slit in keratinized gingiva. Rolled—thickening of gingival margin, associated with edema.
	Papillary gingiva	Pyramid shape, fills interdental area. Note: May be flat if diastema is present.	Bulbous—balloon-like; usually result of severe edema. Cratered—scooped out, loss of interproximal tissue with facial and lingual gingiva remaining. Blunted—flat, loss of interproximal tissue.
Consistency			
	Marginal gingiva	Firm, resilient to pressure.	Edematous—fluid-filled due to loss of collagen and an accumulation of interstitial fluid. Shiny. Fibrotic, leather-like.
	Papillary gingiva	Firm.	Edematous. Shiny. Fibrotic—spongy, not resilient to compression.
	Attached gingiva	Firmly bound to bone. Stippled, orange peel appearance, may/may not be present.	Loss of stippling.

       d. Degree of gingival health

       e. Location of epithelium; attached, unattached, alveolar mucosa

  2. Contour denotes shape of the gingival tissue; how it lies around the tooth; factors affecting contour include

       a. Shape of teeth

       b. Alignment of teeth in arch

       c. Location and size of proximal contacts

       d. Degree of gingival health

  3. Consistency denotes resiliency of the gingival tissue; factors affecting consistency include

       a. Degree of health of the tissue

       b. Density of the tissue

       c. Firmness of the tissue

  4. Acute denotes sudden onset, sharp rise, and short course[12]

  5. Chronic means of long duration; frequent recurrence over a long time[12]

  6. Localized means confined to a definite location; specific number of teeth involved varies from person to person and school to school

  7. Generalized means spread throughout an area; specific number of teeth involved varies from person to person and school to school

C. Components

  1. Gingival assessment/description: Visual determination differentiating among normal, healthy tissues, and diseased tissues

       a. Healthy

          (1) Color—uniformly pink, coral pink, or pigmented

          (2) Contour—not enlarged; fits tightly around tooth

          (3) Consistency—firm; attached gingiva firmly bound to bone

       b. Diseased

          (1) Color

             (a) Acute disease—bright red

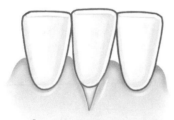

A V-shaped Stillman's cleft

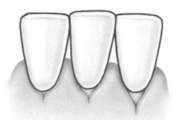

B Slit-like Stillman's cleft

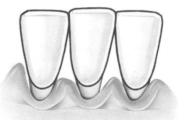

C Rolled "McCall's" festoons

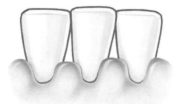

D Bulbous papilla

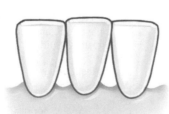

E Cratered papilla

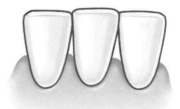

F Blunted papilla

Figure 5–11   Diseased gingiva.

(b) Chronic disease—dark pink to hues of blue (bluish-pink to bluish-red)

(2) Contour (Figure 5–11)

(a) Acute disease—edematous, enlarged, swollen, filled with fluid

(b) Chronic disease—clefted (i.e., Stillman's cleft), narrow V-shaped, or slit-like indentation in keratinized gingiva

(c) Rolled (McCall's festoon)—thickened gingival margin

(d) Bulbous—balloon-like papilla, usually result of severe edema; hyperplasia

(e) Cratered—scooped out interproximal papilla with facial and lingual gingiva remaining

(f) Blunted—loss of interproximal tissue

(3) Consistency

(a) Acute disease—edematous, soft, spongy, fluid filled

(b) Chronic disease—firm, hard, stippled, fibrotic, and leathery

D. Determine resiliency, sponginess, and presence of edema; use side of probe to gently press against tissue; observe reaction of tissue to probe

1. Probing depth (pocket depth): Distance between the junctional epithelium (base of pocket or sulcus) and gingival margin; does not detect disease activity or predict destruction of the periodontium[5]

   Note: The term *pocket* is commonly used when diseased periodontal tissues are present; sulcus is commonly used when healthy periodontal tissues are present—3mm or less is associated with health, 4mm or greater is associated with disease

   (Refer to probing technique in Chapter 8, "Instrumentation")

   a. Take and record probe readings at six aspects of each tooth—distolingual (DL), lingual (L), mesiolingual (ML), distofacial (DF), facial (F), mesiofacial (MF)

   b. Readings greater than 3mm may indicate attachment loss and periodontal disease or may indicate the presence of a pseudopocket; radiographs are necessary to differentiate periodontal pockets from gingival pseudopockets[5]

   c. Factors affecting probing depth[5]

   (1) Insertion force by the clinician—amount of pressure applied during procedure

   (2) Insertion point—some areas of the gingiva allow for easier insertion than others

   (3) Angulation of probe—excessive angulation can result in a false reading that is deeper than actual pocket, whereas insufficient angulation can result in a false reading that is shallower than the actual pocket

   (4) Degree of gingival inflammation—bleeding on probing may easily occur in inflamed areas, making it difficult to view the calibrations on the probe; fibrotic tissue can offer resistance to insertion of the probe

   (5) Presence of calculus—can impede downward progression of the probe into sulcus; requires operator to manipulate probe around deposit in order to get to base of sulcus

d. Types of pockets (Figure 5–12)
  (1) Gingival (pseudopocket): Gingival margin is coronal to cementoenamel junction (CEJ) because of inflammation of gingival tissues; reversible condition;[6] possible causes include
    (a) No loss of junctional epithelial attachment with presence of edema of gingival tissue
    (b) No apical migration of the junctional epithelium with presence of edema of gingival tissue
  (2) Periodontal pocket: Apical migration of the junctional epithelium resulting in an increased sulcus depth (pocket)
  (3) Total attachment loss: Add amount of recession from CEJ to gingival margin to probe reading

2. Bleeding on probing (BOP): Presence of bleeding during probing; elicited by the presence of bacterial plaque[13]
  a. One of the first cardinal signs of diseased/inflamed periodontal tissues
  b. Note areas of bleeding
    (1) Aids in educating patient about disease
    (2) Allows for evaluation of treatment at reevaluation and recall appointments
  c. Areas of chronic disease may not bleed, although active disease may be present
  d. After probe has been removed, observe sulcus for presence of bleeding (mild, moderate, heavy)
  e. Typically recorded on chart by specific tooth number

3. Exudate (suppuration, purulent exudate): Presence of pus in the periodontal pocket; color ranges vary from white to yellow
  a. Methods to determine presence of exudates include
    (1) Gently probe area and observe
    (2) Gently compress gingival tissue and observe
  b. Typically recorded on chart by specific tooth number

4. Mobility: Extent of movement of the tooth in either a horizontal and/or apical direction; indicates loss of supporting periodontal structure; most likely causes include occlusal trauma and bone loss from periodontal activity
  a. Technique for determining mobility
    (1) Use two single-ended blunt instruments: Place one on the facial aspect of the tooth and the other on the lingual aspect of the tooth
    (2) Gently rock the tooth in a facial-lingual direction while observing for movement of the tooth

PRECLINICAL TIP

Assessing Your Knowledge: Bleeding on probing may not be evident in cigarette smokers due to the effects of smoking on the health of the periodontium.[14]

Figure 5–12 Types of pockets: A. Healthy; B. Gingival C. Periodontal.

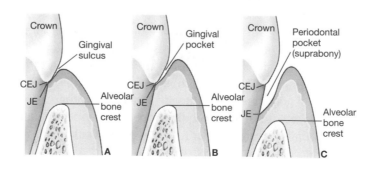

(3) Place one of the blunt-ended instruments on the occlusal surface or incisal edge to determine vertical movement

(4) Gently apply pressure in an apical direction while observing for movement of the tooth

b. Classification: Record on chart as N, 1, 2, 3, or I, II, or III

(1) N—normal, physiologic

(2) 1 or I—involves slight horizontal mobility, greater than normal

(3) 2 or II—involves moderate horizontal mobility, greater than a 1mm displacement; does not move vertically

(4) 3 or III—involves severe mobility and may move in both a horizontal and a vertical direction

5. Furcation involvement: Loss of bone and attachment between the furca of multirooted teeth[15]

a. Instrument used:—Furcation probe (e.g. Nabers)—designed to detect and measure the amount of attachment loss in the furca
Note: An explorer can also be used to assess furcation involvement, although the amount of attachment loss cannot be determined.

b. Classifications: Typically recorded schematically on chart (Figure 5–13)

(1) Class I—evidence of early bone loss in furca area; instrument can enter the depression leading to the furca

(2) Class II—evidence of moderate bone loss in furcation area; instrument can enter furca but cannot pass between roots

(3) Class III—evidence of severe bone loss in furcation area; instrument can pass between roots through entire furcation area

(4) Class IV—same as Class III with exposure resulting from gingival recession

c. Anatomic features

(1) Bifurcation—divergence of root trunk into two roots

(2) Trifurcation—divergence of root trunk into three roots

d. Technique for determining furcation involvement

(1) Maxillary first premolars—access locations are the mesial and distal aspect apical to contact area

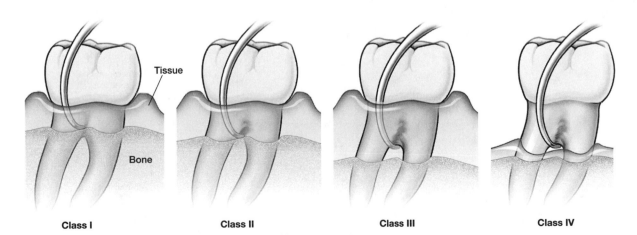

Class I   Class II   Class III   Class IV

Figure 5–13   Classification of furcation involvement.

        (2) Maxillary molars—access locations are the mesiolingual, buccal, and distolingual surfaces

        (3) Mandibular molars—access locations are the buccal and lingual surfaces

6. Recession: Apical migration of the marginal gingiva resulting in exposure of the root surface; loss of attachment (Figure 5–14)
   a. Distance between the CEJ and the marginal gingiva as measured with a periodontal probe
   b. Visual evidence of attachment loss
      (1) Visible recession—measured in millimeters from the CEJ to the gingival margin
      (2) Total (actual) recession—measured in millimeters from the CEJ to base of pocket

7. Open contacts: Nonexistent contacts between two adjacent teeth
   a. Commonly noted either schematically or in writing on chart
   b. Allow for food impaction, which may eventually cause periodontal problems
   c. Determine the presence of open contacts by visually examining contact area for open space or sliding floss through contact area

8. Periodontal screening and recording (PSR): Simplified system of assessing the status of periodontal health or disease utilizes a specially designed probe, with ball tip and colored calibrations at 3.5mm and 5.5mm; technique involves
   a. Dividing mouth into sextants
   b. Probing six sites per tooth, measuring pocket depth while assessing presence of overhangs, defective restorations, or bleeding
   c. Assigning each sextant a PSR code based on findings of the most periodontally involved tooth
   d. Documenting furcation involvement, mobility, mucogingival problems, and recession

Figure 5–14 Gingival recession: A. visible—measured from CEJ to gingival margin; B. actual—measured from CEJ to base of pocket.

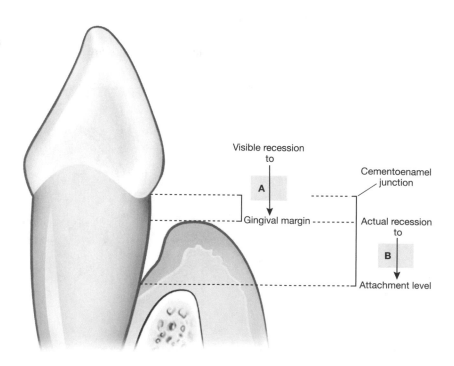

e. Determining if full-mouth periodontal examination charting is necessary if
(1) Two or more sextants scored Code 3
(2) One sextant scored Code 3 and Code[*]
(3) One sextant scored Code 4

Code	Description
Code 0	Colored area of probe remains completely visible in the deepest crevice of the sextant. • No calculus or defective margins are detected. • Gingival tissues are healthy, with no bleeding on probing.
Code 1	Colored area of probe remains completely visible in the deepest crevice of the sextant. • No calculus or defective margins are detected. • There is bleeding on probing.
Code 2	Colored area of probe remains completely visible in the deepest crevice of the sextant; supra or subgingival calculus is detected or defective margins are detected.
Code 3	Colored area of the probe remains partly visible in the deepest probe depth in the sextant.
Code 4	Colored area of the probe completely disappears, indicating probing depth greater than 5.5mm.
Code [*]	The symbol [*] is added to the sextant score whenever findings indicate clinical abnormalities such as • furcation invasion • mobility • mucogingival problems • recession extending to the colored area of the probe (3.5mm or greater)

9. Systematic method of assessment is imperative to develop when assessing the soft tissues to ensure a comprehensive and complete examination
10. Radiographic assessment: Thorough evaluation of the radiographs must be included in the assessment of the soft tissues; all radiographs should be accompanied by a documented interpretation of the patient's current periodontal health status; common radiographs include
    a. Horizontal bitewings: Accurately represent bone height in non-periodontally involved patients
    b. Vertical bitewings: Accurately represent bone height in patients with moderate to advanced periodontal disease
    c. Periapical films: Accurately represent periodontal status surrounding apex of tooth

Examination of the hard and soft tissues is an involved process that should be performed with attention to detail, and the findings should be documented. Initially, each component of this assessment procedure will be time consuming for the dental hygiene student. With exposure to a variety of conditions, the dental hygiene student should recognize and chart the findings with more efficiency, while maintaining the awareness of the importance of the exam.

QUESTIONS

1. Which of the following occlusal classifications is present when the buccal groove of the permanent mandibular first molar is mesial to the mesiobuccal cusp of the permanent maxillary first molar by at least the width of a premolar?
   a. Class II
   b. Tendency towards a Class II
   c. Class III
   d. Tendency towards a Class III

2. The MOST common crown fabricated in dentistry today is
   a. gold.
   b. temporary.
   c. veneer.
   d. porcelain fused-to-metal.

3. Dentures may be full or partial. They may also be fixed or removable.
   a. Both statements are TRUE.
   b. Both statements are FALSE.
   c. The first statement is TRUE. The second statement is FALSE.
   d. The first statement is FALSE. The second statement is TRUE.

4. Which of the following carious lesions is often *not* noticeable on radiographs but is still evident clinically as yellow to light tan in color?
   a. Arrested
   b. Incipient
   c. Rampant
   d. Recurrent

5. A patient states he grinds his teeth while sleeping. Clinical examination reveals wearing of incisal surfaces of the anterior teeth. This condition is called
   a. attrition.
   b. abrasion.
   c. erosion.
   d. abfraction.

6. All of the following methods are used to detect carious lesions EXCEPT one. Which one is the EXCEPTION?
   a. Radiographic
   b. Visual
   c. Tactile
   d. Percussion

7. According to G. V. Black's classification of dental caries and restorations, which of the statements accurately describes a Class II category?
   a. Pits and fissures of posterior teeth
   b. Proximal surfaces of posterior teeth
   c. Cervical third of posterior teeth
   d. Cusp tip of posterior teeth

8. The gingival structure that is the entrance to the sulcus is called
   a. papillary gingiva.
   b. col.
   c. marginal gingiva.
   d. gingival pocket.

9. When describing gingival conditions, which of the following terms would describe a long duration or a frequent occurrence over a long period of time?
   a. Acute
   b. Chronic
   c. Localized
   d. Generalized

10. Each of the following terms is used when describing the health or disease of the gingiva EXCEPT one. Which one is the EXCEPTION?
    a. Color
    b. Contour
    c. Consistency
    d. Connected

11. Several factors affect the probing depths achieved when completing a periodontal chart. One of the factors is excessive angulation, which can result in a reading shallower than the actual pocket.
    a. Both statements are TRUE.
    b. Both statements are FALSE.
    c. The first statement is TRUE. The second statement is FALSE.
    d. The first statement is FALSE. The second statement is TRUE.

12. All of the following factors affect the color of gingiva EXCEPT one. Which one is the EXCEPTION?
    a. Alignment of the teeth in the arch
    b. Presence of melanin
    c. Degree of gingival health
    d. Vascular supply

13. A loss of tooth structure as a result of a chemical means rather than bacterial is known as
    a. caries.
    b. attrition.
    c. abrasion.
    d. erosion.

14. When noting tooth surfaces, those located toward the midline are referred to as the
    a. mesials.
    b. distals.
    c. cervicals.
    d. incisals/occlusals.

15. An overbite measures the
    a. alignment of the maxillary central incisors to those of the mandibular incisors.
    b. movement of teeth out of the alveolar bone beyond occlusion.
    c. vertical overlap of the maxillary anterior teeth to the mandibular anterior teeth.
    d. horizontal overlap of the maxillary anterior teeth to the mandibular anterior teeth.

16. Which of the following statements describes prognathic occlusion?
    a. The maxilla and mandible appear to be in the same relation to each other.
    b. The mandible appears to be retruded in relation to the maxilla.
    c. The relationship is a Class II occlusion.
    d. The relationship is a Class III occlusion.

17. Which of the following classifications describes caries on the mesiobuccal cusp tip on tooth #14?
    a. II
    b. III
    c. IV
    d. V
    e. VI

18. Recession describes the apical migration of the marginal gingiva. It is measured with a periodontal probe between the CEJ and marginal gingiva.
    a. Both statements are TRUE.
    b. Both statements are FALSE.
    c. The first statement is TRUE. The second statement is FALSE.
    d. The first statement is FALSE. The second statement is TRUE.

19. Which of the following types of dental caries occurs adjacent to an already existing restoration?
    a. Arrested
    b. Incipient
    c. Rampant
    d. Recurrent

20. All of the following describe the col of the gingiva EXCEPT one. Which one is the EXCEPTION?
    a. Non-keratinized tissue
    b. Susceptible to disease
    c. Connects the facial and lingual gingiva
    d. Located at the bottom of the gingival sulcus

REFERENCES

1. Dofka, *Dental Terminology.* Albany, NY: Delmar Thomson Learning, 2000.

2. Jaroski-Graf, J. *Dental Charting, A Standard Approach.* Albany, NY: Delmar Thomson Learning, 2000.

3. Garvey, M. T., H. J. Barry, & M. Blake. Supernumerary Teeth: An Overview of Classification, Diagnosis, and Management. *Journal of the Canadian Dental Association* 65: 612–6, 1998.

4. Brand, R. and D. Isselhard. *Anatomy of Orofacial Structures,* 6th ed. St. Louis: Mosby, 1998.

5. Perry, D., P. Beemsterboer, & E. Taggart. *Periodontology for the Dental Hygienist,* 2nd ed. Philadelphia: Saunders, 2001.

6. Wilson, T. & K. Kornman. *Fundamentals of Periodontics.* Chicago: Quintessence, 1996.

7. Maneenut, C. Abfraction: A Non-Carious Cervical Lesion. *The Journal of the Dental Association of Thailand* 1997; 47: 310–319.

8. Tooth Abfraction Lesions. http://www.intelihealth.com, Harvard Medical School's Consumer Health Information, Reviewed by the faculty of The University of Pennsylvania School of Dental Medicine.

9. Gandara, B. K. & E. L. Truelove. Diagnosis and Management of Dental Erosion. *Journal of Contemporary Dental Practice,* 1(1), Fall 1999.

10. Ibsen, O. & J. Phelan. Oral Pathology for the Dental Hygienist, 3rd ed. Philadelphia: Saunders, 2000.

11. Merck Manual, Section 9, Chapter 106.

12. Merriam Webster Medical Dictionary.

13. Joss, A., R. Adler, & N. P. Lang. Bleeding on Probing, A Parameter for Monitoring Periodontal Conditions in Clinical Practice. *Journal of Clinical Periodontology,* 21(4), 402–08, 1994.

14. Machuca, G., I. Rosales, J. R. Lacalle, C. Machuca & P. Bullon. Effect of Cigarette Smoking on Periodontal Status of Health Young Adults; *Journal of Periodontology,* 71(1), 73–8, January 2000.

15. Al-Shammari, K. F., & C. E. Kazor & H. L. Wang, Molar Root Anatomy and Management of Furcation Defects; *Journal of Clinical Periodontology,* 28(8), 730–40, August 2001.

Chapter 6

Preventive Dentistry

Mary D. Cooper, RDH, MSEd, and Lauri Wiechmann, RDH, MPA

MediaLink

A companion CD-ROM, included free with each new copy of this book, supplements the procedures presented in each chapter. Insert the CD-ROM to watch video clips and view a large collection of color images that is also included. This multimedia library is designed to help you add a new dimension to your learning.

KEY TERMS

acquired pellicle. Organic layer of selective proteins that adheres to the hydroxyapaptite crystals of the tooth surface of a cleaned tooth surface when exposed to saliva.

attached bacterial plaque. Bacteria firmly attached to acquired pellicle, other bacteria, and tooth surfaces.

biofilm. A well-organized, cooperating community of microorganisms.

dental calculus. A hardened deposit resulting from the addition of mineral elements, such as calcium and phosphorus, to bacterial plaque.

disclosing agents. Selective dye in a solution, tablet, or lozenge form used to identify bacterial plaque on surfaces of teeth.

humectant. Ingredient that helps retain moisture and prevents toothpaste from drying.

intermicrobial matrix. Woven collection of different types of bacteria closely adhered to the tooth structure.

plaque. A dense, organized bacterial system embedded in an intermicrobial matrix that adheres closely to teeth, calculus, and other structures in the oral cavity.

therapeutic. Reduces a disease.

unattached (surface) bacterial plaque. Loose bacteria; washed away by saliva during swallowing.

LEARNING OBJECTIVES

After reading this chapter, the student will be able to:

- differentiate between primary, secondary, and tertiary services and the dental hygienists' involvement in each;
- discuss Maslow's hierarchy and recognize the need level at which a patient is from a given description;
- identify methods of motivation;
- diagram the learning ladder, listing each step of the ladder and describing what occurs at each step;
- define bacterial plaque;
- explain what occurs during each stage of the life cycle of plaque;
- differentiate between Gram-positive and Gram-negative bacteria based on the arrival to the bacterial plaque colony and the effects to the surrounding tissues;
- differentiate between an aerobic organism and an anaerobic organism, examining its relationship with oxygen and its arrival to the bacterial plaque colony;
- compare and contrast supragingival and subgingival plaque, emphasizing the type of bacteria present, origin, distribution, retention, and nutritional source;

- compare and contrast supragingival and subgingival calculus, emphasizing the appearance, nutritional source, and distribution;
- discuss the role of disclosing solution in oral hygiene instructions;
- describe the parts of the toothbrush;
- compare manual to power-assisted toothbrushes;
- name and describe the various toothbrushing methods;
- explain the functions for the following ingredients in dentifrices: humectants, foaming agents, flavoring agents, sweetening agents, coloring agents, and thickening agents;
- identify agents found in dentifrices and/or mouth rinses that either prevent caries, calculus formation, periodontal disease, or dental hypersensitivity;
- state reasons interdental care is essential to complement toothbrushing;
- state the purposes, indications, contraindications, and techniques for the following interdental cleaning aids: dental floss, dental floss holder, floss threader, knitting

yarn, pipe cleaner, gauze strip, interdental tip stimulator, wedge stimulator, toothpick holder, and interdental brush;

- demonstrate how to properly clean the tongue with a tongue cleaner or toothbrush;

- name the types of antimicrobial mouth rinses and state the specific purpose of each.

I. **Introduction**

Preventive dentistry includes the management of behaviors to prevent oral disease, the coordination and delivery of primary preventive oral hygiene services, the provision of secondary preventive intervention to prevent further disease, and the facilitation of the patient's access to care and implementation of oral care goals.

II. **Plaque consists of a dense, organized bacterial system embedded in an intermicrobial matrix that adheres closely to teeth, calculus, and other structures within the oral cavity**

A. Characteristics

1. Consist of white and soft material that are easily removed from the tooth surface
2. Over 500 bacterial species can be found in dental plaque[1]
3. Intermicrobial matrix involves glucan, a sticky substance secreted by certain bacteria that promotes adherence of the bacteria

B. Bacterial composition varies based on site, salivary components, duration at site, and oral hygiene practices of the patient

1. Directly involved with diseases of both the hard (teeth and bone) and soft (gingiva) tissues of the oral cavity
2. Immunological response to the bacteria depends on the susceptibility of the host, virulence of the bacteria, and specific types of bacteria present[2]

C. Development of plaque

The development, or life cycle, of plaque begins with the acquired pellicle stage, continues through bacterial colonization, and can terminate in mineralization

1. Acquired pellicle

a. Consists of an organic layer of selective proteins that adheres to the hydroxyapaptite crystals of a cleaned tooth surface when exposed to saliva[3, 4, 5, 6]

b. Includes four stages of formation

(1) Bathing of tooth by salivary fluids containing protein constituents
(2) Selective absorption of certain negatively and positively charged glycoproteins
(3) Loss of solubility of absorbed proteins
(4) Alteration of glycoproteins by enzymes from bacteria and oral secretions

c. Chemical composition of the acquired pellicle changes as it remains on the tooth; amino acid profiles differ when examined at 15 minutes and 1 hour

2. Bacterial colonization is comprised of complex, well-organized accumulation of bacterial flora commonly described as a biofilm

a. Biofilm is a well-organized, cooperating community of various types of microorganisms working together; properties of biofilm include[6]

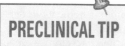

PRECLINICAL TIP

Protecting Your Knowledge: Gram staining is a method used to stain bacteria using a violet stain. It assists in classifying bacteria. Gram-positive bacteria absorb or retain the violet stain, whereas Gram-negative bacteria do not stain or are decolorized by alcohol used during the staining process.

(1) Microcolonies, composed of similar types of microorganisms; within microcolonies is a communication network

(2) Protective matrix, which surrounds these microcolonies; within the protective matrix, microcolonies are composed of differing environments

(3) Resistant to many anti-infective agents

b. Bacteria may grow as an independent resident or in coaggregated microcolonies; growing together allows the organisms to grow in an area where neither could survive independently[7]

c. Initial plaque formation—early plaque colonizers, Gram-positive cocci (round or spherical in shape) and rods, adhere to the acquired pellicle initiating bacterial colonization[8]

(1) Gram-positive bacteria are nondamaging to the periodontal tissues

(2) Organisms that coaggregate may benefit from the mutual bonding, as they may be retained during initial plaque formation[7]

(3) If the bacteria are not removed, the environment in the gingival sulcus becomes a mixture of Gram-positive and Gram-negative organisms

(4) Within three days of no oral hygiene, Gram-negative cocci are the predominant bacteria, followed by Gram-negative rods, Gram-positive cocci, and Gram-positive rods respectively[9]

d. Secondary plaque colonizers, Gram-negative spirochetes (spiral shaped), and vibrios (rod-like shaped) follow to continue the bacterial colonization; results in a thickness of bacteria;[8] Gram-negative bacteria are damaging to the periodontal tissues due to their motility, which allows penetration into the sulcus, therefore damaging the area

e. Timeline of colonization (Table 6–1)

(1) Days 1 to 2—made up primarily of aerobic Gram-positive cocci: *Streptococcus mutans* and *Streptococcus sanguis*

(2) Days 2 to 4—includes predominantly cocci, increasing numbers of Gram-positive filamentous (long, thick rods) forms, and slender rods

(3) Days 4 to 7—includes an increase in filaments and more mixed flora with rods, filamentous forms, and fusobacteria; plaque located near gingival margin begins to develop a more mature flora: Gram-negative spirochetes and vibrios

(4) Days 7 to 14—contains predominately spirochetes and vibrios, with an increase in white blood cells; more Gram-negative and anaerobic organisms are found

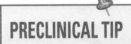

PRECLINICAL TIP

Protecting Your Knowledge: Aerobic organisms need oxygen to survive. Anaerobic organisms do not need oxygen to survive.

PRECLINICAL TIP

Protecting Your Knowledge: The presence of white blood cells indicates the immune system is helping defeat the bacteria.

Table 6–1   Timeline of Colonization of Bacteria

Days	Bacteria
1–2	Primarily aerobic Gram-positive cocci
2–4	Cocci, increased Gram-positive filamentous forms, and slender rods
4–7	Filamentous and fusobacteria; Gram-negative spirochetes and vibrios near gingival margin
7–14	Spirochetes and vibrios; increase in WBCs and more Gram-negative and anaerobic organisms

PRECLINICAL TIP

Protecting Your Knowledge: *Obligate aerobe* microorganisms cannot live or grow without oxygen. *Facultative anaerobic* microorganisms do not require oxygen to live, but they can survive in the presence of oxygen.

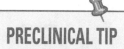

PRECLINICAL TIP

Protecting Your Knowledge: Saliva is the medium for suspension of bacteria. It serves as a means of transportation for the bacteria and carries chemical messengers.[11]

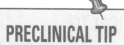

PRECLINICAL TIP

Protecting Your Knowledge: Subgingival instrumentation can remove retention structures other than tissue.

(5) Days 14 to 21—includes a continual increase of spirochetes and vibrios, white blood cells, and Gram-negative and anaerobic organisms

f. Location of bacteria

(1) Supragingival bacteria, located coronal to the gingival margin; consists of newly formed deposits (various Gram-positive, obligate aerobe species) and mature plaque (facultative anaerobic microorganisms)

(a) Plaque matures (acquires more bacteria) when it is not disturbed; it not only thickens in mass, but also migrates apically into the gingival sulcus

(b) Mature plaque contains more aggressive bacteria than does newly formed plaque

(c) Origin: Salivary microorganisms are selectively attracted to glycoproteins from acquired pellicle

(d) Distribution: Begins on proximal surfaces and other protected areas, which include any specific area where it is difficult to disturb bacteria such as rotated teeth and overhanging restorations

(e) Adhesion: Bacteria remain in close proximity
  • Attached bacterial plaque firmly attach to acquired pellicle, other bacteria, and tooth surfaces
  • Unattached (loose) bacterial plaque are washed away by saliva or during swallowing

(f) Retention: Retain on rough surfaces of teeth or restorations, malpositioned teeth, and carious lesions

(g) Nutritional source: Provided by saliva; enzymatic activity of salivary alpha-amylase may facilitate the breakdown of dietary starch to provide additional glucose for use by the bacteria in the near proximity[10]

(2) Subgingival plaque, located apical to the marginal gingiva; contains predominately motile, Gram-negative anaerobic rods and spirochetes[12]

(a) Origin: Apical growth of bacteria from supragingival plaque

(b) Distribution: Undisturbed area in mouth; if left undisturbed, distribution of the bacteria continues to progress apically, perforating the junctional epithelium and causing permanent, irreversible damage
  • Colonizing bacteria in shallow pockets are predominantly streptococci
  • Colonizing bacteria in deeper pockets are predominantly spirochetes and Gram-negative species[13]

(c) Adhesion: Different types of bacteria are localized throughout the subgingival plaque[14]
  • Attached bacterial plaque—includes tooth surface, subgingival pellicle, and calculus
  • Unattached (loose) bacterial plaque—floats between adherent plaque on tooth and pocket epithelium
  • Epithelium-associated plaque—includes invasive bacteria located in the gingival tissues of the periodontium

(d) Retention: Pocket holds plaque against tooth; other structures, such as calculus and overhanging margins, can also hold plaque within the sulcus

(e) Nutritional sources: Include gingival crevicular fluid, inflammatory exudate, and leukocytes

D. Identification methods

1. Disclosing agents: Selective dye in a solution, tablet, or lozenge form used to identify bacterial plaque on tooth surfaces

   a. Dye absorbs into soft dental plaque; available in single or multicolor forms; multicolor form distinguishes between new and old plaque

   b. Used during oral hygiene instructions to show patient areas of plaque and for self-examination of toothbrushing technique utilized at home

2. Direct vision: Plaque may be stained with beverages, food, or other pigmented agents, making it easier to see; thick plaque may appear dull, with a fur-like appearance

3. Tactile: Plaque may feel slimy or slippery

III. Calculus formation (bacterial mineralization) includes addition of mineral elements, such as calcium and phosphorus, to bacterial plaque; results in a hardened deposit[15, 16]

A. Process involves interactions between the bacterial plaque and the components of oral fluids—salivary proteins may be the catalyst to mineralizing the soft bacterial plaque into hardened calculus deposits[16]

B. Types

1. Supragingival calculus, located coronal to gingival margin

   a. Nutrient source: Saliva[17]

   b. Color: Includes white, creamy yellow, or gray; may be stained with food and/or beverages, tobacco, and other pigmenting agents

   c. Distribution: Most commonly found near opening of salivary gland ducts—facial surfaces of maxillary molars and lingual surfaces of mandibular anterior teeth;[17] presence has little impact on the surrounding gingival tissues, since toothbrushing can keep deposit plaque-free[17]

2. Subgingival calculus, located apical to gingival margin

   a. Nutrient source: Gingival crevicular fluid and inflammatory exudate[18]

   b. Color: Includes light to dark brown, dark green, or black; may appear as spicules (spurs) on proximal surfaces, ledges, rings, or grainy on all surfaces

     (1) Results from components in gingival crevicular fluid and inflammatory exudate, not food and beverage sources

     (2) Often gives gingiva appearance of cyanotic tissue due to dark color of calculus diffusing through tissue

   c. Distributions: Heaviest amount is located on proximal surfaces, lightest on facial surfaces; occurs with or without associated supragingival calculus deposits

   d. Detection

     (1) Most commonly detected with an explorer and may feel rough (like sandpaper) or provide slight resistance, causing vibrations of the explorer shank

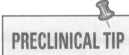

PRECLINICAL TIP

Protecting Your Knowledge: The porous composition of calculus allows for food and/or beverages, tobacco, and other pigmenting agents to permanently stain the deposit.

PRECLINICAL TIP

Protecting Your Knowledge: Smoking cigarettes increases the occurrence and severity of supragingival calculus.[18]

(2) Radiographs provide a valuable assessment tool when the deposits are large and dense

C. Identification methods

1. Visual examination

a. If supragingival calculus is not stained, it may be necessary to utilize compressed air to "dehydrate" it to view; deflect gingival margin for observation subgingivally

b. Dehydrating the calculus results in a chalky white appearance—a good self-evaluation tool to use during debridement; accomplish by using short blasts of air directed at the tooth—avoid directing into gingival sulcus when deflecting tissue to view subgingival calculus

c. Diseased gingival margin does not adapt closely to tooth surface where calculus is present; calculus is a physical irritant to the adjacent gingival tissue

d. Transillumination of anterior teeth depicts supragingival calculus as a dark, opaque, shadow-like area on proximal surface

2. Tactile: Utilize an explorer to detect supragingival and/or subgingival calculus deposits;[19] use a light lateral pressure with a light grasp to provide best tactile sensitivity

IV. **Prevention**

As health professionals, our main goal is to prevent diseases. Not only will treatment be minimized through preventive means, but cost will also be minimized for the patient—the more extensive the required treatment is, the more costly it will be for the patient. As dental hygienists, it is our responsibility to educate patients in order to help them prevent plaque diseases and keep their natural teeth for a lifetime. Preventive dentistry has three levels: primary, secondary, and tertiary prevention.

A. Primary prevention involves techniques and agents to forestall onset and reverse progression of disease, or arrest disease process before treatment becomes necessary; dental hygienists are at the forefront of primary preventive services; hygienists can provide

1. Patient education, health promotion, caries and nutrition counseling, and tobacco cessation education

2. Direct care—mechanical plaque removal, application of topical fluoride, and placement of pit and fissure sealants

B. Secondary prevention involves routine treatment methods to terminate a disease and/or restore tissues to as normal as possible

1. Dental hygienists can intercept the progression of periodontal disease and prevent advancement of disease by implementing periodontal debridement

2. Dentists can intercept the progression of diseases by

a. Placing restorations

b. Performing endodontics (root canal therapy)

c. Performing periodontal surgery

C. Tertiary prevention involves using measures necessary to replace lost tissues and rehabilitate patients so physical capabilities and/or mental attitudes are as near to normal as possible after secondary prevention has failed

1. Dental hygienists do not provide any tertiary services for the patient

2. Dentists restore areas, resulting in the return of function to the respective area; examples include prosthodontics (e.g., bridges, dentures, and implants) (Figure 6–1)

PRECLINICAL TIP

Protecting Your Knowledge: Subgingival calculus may be a direct contributing factor to periodontal inflammation.[17]

V. Principles of Learning and Motivation

In order to provide oral hygiene instruction to patients, the dental hygienist needs to understand some basic principles of learning and motivation. One-on-one care places the dental hygienist in a teaching position and the patient in a learning position. Understanding which needs are met allows the clinician to determine practical oral hygiene instruction and treatment.

A. Concepts

    1. Learning is more effective when an individual is physiologically and psychologically ready to learn

        a. Assess patient's readiness to learn about condition of oral cavity; question patient on importance of good oral health

        b. Address patient's main concern (e.g., bleeding gingiva, sensitive teeth, and halitosis)

    2. Motivation is essential for learning

        a. Forms of motivation include

            (1) Intrinsic motivation results from a patient's internal decision; patient wants oral health condition to improve

            (2) Extrinsic motivation involves outward influence; for example, dental hygienist may help the patient find a source of motivation to improve oral health; helps proceed to desired results at a faster rate

        b. Meeting patient needs involves inner forces that drive a person to action; lower needs, such as physiological and safety, must be met before the patient can concentrate on higher needs, such as love, ego, and self-fulfillment; as lower level needs are met, they become contained within the higher levels[20]

        c. Maslow's hierarchy of needs—developed by Abraham Maslow, humanistic psychologist; includes five levels of basic human needs: physiological, safety (security), love (social), self-esteem (ego), and self-actualization (self-fulfillment) (Figure 6–2)

            (1) Physiological needs—includes those necessary to maintain body homeostasis (e.g., food, water, oxygen, sleep); a patient who does not have this level met may only be concerned with the basics of toothbrushing

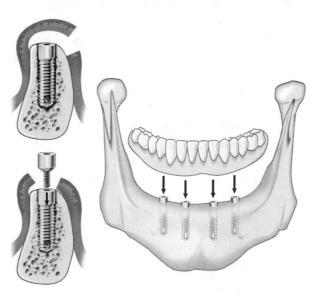

Figure 6–1   Endosseous dental implant.

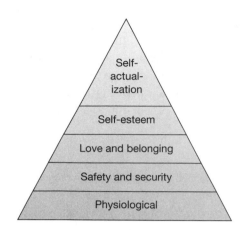

Figure 6–2   Maslow's hierachy of human needs.

    (2) Safety (security)—controls number of hazards that can cause physical and mental damage as well as guaranteeing a stable and predictable environment; meeting the needs on this level may find a patient expressing interest in methods to prevent decay

    (3) Love (social)—focuses on group acceptance, opportunity to give and receive friendship; needs met at this level may be evident when a patient inquires about tooth whitening methods (teeth have important cosmetic and social functions)

    (4) Self-esteem (ego)—involves feelings of self-worth, including achievement, confidence, competence, and status; patients at this level may smile frequently to express visual pride in their oral health

    (5) Self-actualization (self-fulfillment)—focuses on a positive tendency for development, growth, and self-enhancement; at this level, the patient may express satisfaction with the health of the oral cavity

3. Learner has to recognize and understand what is being taught and will learn only what is useful; it is important to consider what level of needs the patient has met before initiating oral hygiene instruction; individualize oral hygiene instructions to

    a. Allow learner the opportunity to understand health of oral cavity—requires dental hygienist to explain conditions of oral cavity thoroughly and at appropriate level

    b. Make information meaningful to the patient; utilizing a mirror and patient's chart delivers information in a visual manner that helps the patient get involved and accept condition

4. Learning takes place more rapidly when what is being taught has meaning; for example, associating location of disease in patient's mouth to information being presented allows the patient to "accept" the condition of the oral cavity

B. Learning ladder—designed to demonstrate how individuals learn in a sequential series of steps (Figure 6–3); a thorough assessment of the patient must be completed to help determine the patient's position on the learning ladder; once assessment is complete, the dental hygienist can implement individualized oral hygiene instructions that possess meaning to the patient

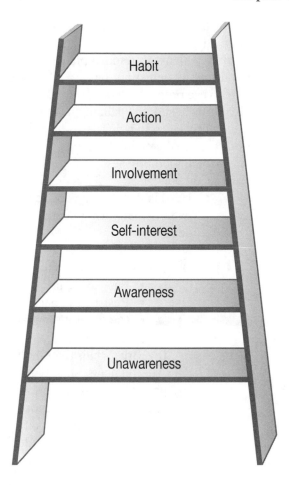

Figure 6–3   Learning ladder.

1. Unawareness involves possessing limited or inaccurate information; the patient may have a small amount of accurate information, but does not understand the entire concept, or the information the patient has is inaccurate; the dental hygienist must provide the patient with accurate information
2. Awareness involves obtaining correct information, but does not possess any personal meaning; getting the patient involved in the oral hygiene educational process helps the patient accept the condition and achieve the awareness level
3. Self-interest involves recognizing prospective objective with slight inclination to act; patient achieves awareness and shows interest in applying the information
4. Involvement—attitude is influenced and action is forthcoming; a desire to apply the knowledge and perform the correct skill is attained; patient begins to implement the knowledge and skills
5. Action—new concepts and practices are tested; actual application of the knowledge and skills is accomplished
6. Habit—commitment is reached in performing behavior; patient continues to implement the knowledge and skills incorporating them into the daily routine

VI. Mechanical Measures Used to Remove Bacterial Plaque

Removing dental plaque is an essential component in preventing and controlling several dental diseases. Compared to chemotherapeutic products,

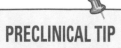

the toothbrush is a much more common means for reducing plaque and gingivitis.[21] The toothbrush is the most common and often the only device used by patients to remove plaque.[22] Therefore, it is the responsibility of the dental hygienist not only to recommend products and educate the patient to use proper techniques to accomplish thorough plaque removal, but also to make sure the patient understands what has been instructed. A way to confirm understanding is to have the patient demonstrate the instructions back to the dental hygienist.

A. Manual toothbrushes
  1. Components
    a. Head is the working end; consists of tufts of bristles in different patterns, lengths, and angles to aid even those with the poorest dexterity
      (1) Bristles
        (a) Nylon filaments
          • Easy to clean[23]
          • Resistant to bacteria and fungi[23]
          • Can tolerate multiple uses and temperatures without distortion[23]
        (b) Boar's hair (natural bristles)
      (2) All filaments should be soft, flexible, end-rounded, and polished finish to prevent gingival trauma and increase plaque and debris removal[23]
    b. Handle is the portion of toothbrush that is held; can be
      (1) Lengthened with a ruler, tongue depressor, or wooden spoon for those who may have difficulty raising their hand or arm[24]
      (2) Enlarged or be adjusted by shape and size for those with poor motor skills, grip problems, and spasticity[24]
    c. Shank is the section that connects head to handle
  2. Characteristics of an effective toothbrush include size, shape, and texture to conform to patient comfort
    a. Size: Selection should be based on size of patient's mouth—large enough to remove plaque effectively, yet small enough to access all areas of the mouth
    b. Shape
      (1) Handle: Modification may include angled, offset, angled and offset, small and narrow, large and wide, rounded, and squared; some allow patient to comfortably grasp toothbrush with little effort being placed on rotation and reaching posterior areas[23]
      (2) Head: May be designed in a diamond style or square; brushing plane may be flat, rippled, dome-shaped, or bilevel
    c. Bristles
      (1) Texture/firmness—indicates bristle resistance to pressure; composition involves tufted or multitufted and diameter of bristle; include
        (a) Tufted: Five or six tufts long and three tufts across
        (b) Multitufted: 10 or 12 tufts in three or four rows; positioned in close proximity, which allows for greater force during use

(c) Diameter: Usual range for adult toothbrush bristles is between 0.007 and 0.015 inches (filament size)

(2) Storage

(a) Keep toothbrush in a clean and open/aerated environment

(b) Should remain dry—therefore use multiple toothbrushes so every time a toothbrush is used, the bristles are as dry as possible

3. Types of manual toothbrushes

a. Adult toothbrushes: Patients should use soft-bristled toothbrushes, which provide a greater degree of flexibility to reach areas in the mouth as well as minimize the chance of tissue (hard and soft) trauma caused by harder bristled toothbrushes

(1) Soft toothbrush: Bristles 0.007 to 0.009 inches in diameter

(2) Medium toothbrush: Bristles 0.010 to 0.012 inches in diameter

(3) Hard toothbrush: Bristles 0.013 to 0.014 inches in diameter

(4) Extra hard toothbrush: Bristles 0.015 inches in diameter

b. Child toothbrush: Bristles are shorter and diameter is reduced to 0.005 inches

3. Replacement of toothbrushes

a. Reasons for replacement

(1) Decrease tissue trauma from bent, splayed, or matted bristles[25, 27, 28]

(2) Enhance effective plaque removal[25]

(3) Infection control—toothbrush can become contaminated by viruses,[29] so replace when ill

b. Timeframe for replacement varies depending on patient[27]—anytime between one to three months

c. Determination of wear: Visually examine brush;[25] check for worn bristles, splaying, matting, tapering, and/or bending of bristles

4. Toothbrushing

a. General objectives include

(1) Removing plaque and disturbing reformation

(2) Cleaning food, debris, and stain contained in plaque

(3) Stimulating gingival tissues

(4) Applying dentifrice or therapeutic agents

b. Methods include

(1) Horizontal: Position bristles perpendicular to crown of tooth; brush in a back-and-forth horizontal pattern

(2) Fones: Position bristles perpendicular to crown of tooth; brush in a circular (rotary) motion; similar to horizontal stroke with addition of rotary strokes (Figure 6–4)

(3) Leonard: Use up-and-down brushing motion over facial surfaces of closed posterior teeth

(4) Stillman: Position bristles at a 45-degree angle to apex of tooth, with part of brush resting on gingiva and other part on teeth; move brush using a vibratory motion while applying slight pressure; lift brush and repeat in next area (Figures 6–5 and 6–6a)

PRECLINICAL TIP

Protecting Your Knowledge: Up to the age of 11, children are unable to effectively remove plaque with a manual toothbrush.[26] Therefore, parental/guardian assistance is recommended.

PRECLINICAL TIP

Protecting Your Knowledge: Results of a study of dental practitioners stated that 95.6 percent felt that the dental hygienist should be the primary healthcare provider responsible for educating the patient about toothbrush replacement.[25]

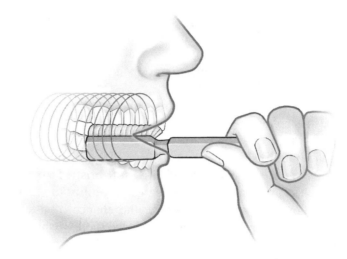

Figure 6–4   Fones method: Circular motion extending from maxillary to mandibular.

(5) Charters: Place brush at a 45-degree angle towards occlusal/incisal plane; move brush in several small rotary motions keeping bristles in contact with gingival margin (Figures 6–6b and 6–7)

(6) Bass: Place brush at a 45-degree angle to tooth apex; apply gentle pressure so bristles enter sulcus; use a vibratory motion (horizontal jiggle) to activate bristles (Figure 6–8)

(7) Roll: Position bristles parallel to and against attached gingiva; turn wrist to flex bristles first against gingiva and then facial/lingual surfaces; roll bristles coronally

c. Modified techniques

(1) Modified Stillman and Charters: Position bristles in same position as original method, then gently begin a vibratory motion; slowly press-roll bristles coronally, continuing vibratory motion during roll (Figure 6–9)

(2) Bass: Sulcular brushing is completed either before or after use of rolling method

d. General considerations when recommending a specific toothbrush/toothbrushing technique[25]

(1) Consider patient's oral health status: Number of teeth, alignment, mouth size, removable prostheses, orthodontic appliances, periodontal status, and gingival condition

Figure 6–5   Stillman method.

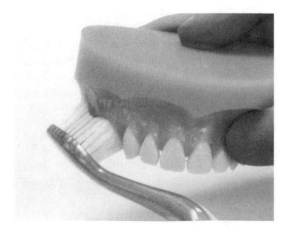

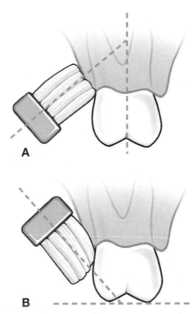

Figure 6–6   A. Stillman method;
B. Charters method.

(a) Horizontal: Most effective for children due to the bell-shaped anatomy of the primary dentition and ease of use
(b) Fones: Stimulates gingiva with rotary strokes; generally recommended to individuals needing an easier brushing technique due to physical and/or mental limitations
(c) Leonard: Generally used over the facial surfaces of the closed posterior dentition to provide both cleaning and stimulation of the gingiva
(d) Stillman: Generally recommended to clean the tooth and stimulate the gingiva
(e) Charters: Recommended to clean abutments, fixed bridges, around fixed orthodontic appliances, and when interproximal tissues are missing
(f) Bass: Recommended to remove plaque and debris from the gingival sulcus
(2) Review patient's systemic health status, muscular and joint diseases, and mental capabilities in case adaptations need

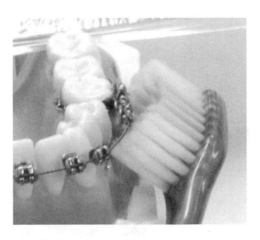

Figure 6–7   Charters method on orthodontics.

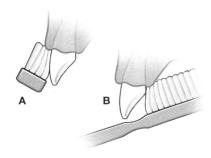

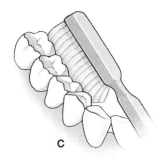

Figure 6–8   Bass (sulcular) method: Position bristles 45 degrees toward tooth apex; apply gentle pressure so bristles can enter sulcus.

to be made—can add bicycle grips and tennis balls to toothbrush handle

(3) Patient's age[30]

    (a) 4–24 months—primary dentition erupting; oral care should be performed by parent/guardian due to lack of manual dexterity

    (b) 2–4 years—primary dentition complete; some manual dexterity is developing, and children begin to learn how to brush, but parent/guardian should still assist with oral care

Figure 6–9   Modified Stillman method.

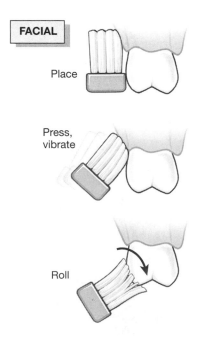

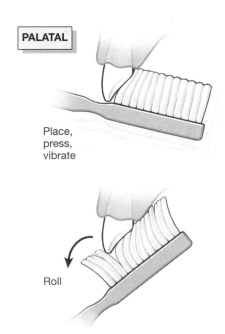

FACIAL

Place

Press, vibrate

Roll

PALATAL

Place, press, vibrate

Roll

(c) 5–7 years—primary teeth begin to shed and permanent teeth begin to erupt; manual dexterity continues to improve with parental/guardian involvement

(d) 8 years and up—mixed to permanent dentition; manual dexterity improved, but parental/guardian reinforcement is recommended

(4) Patient's interest and motivation

(5) Patient's manual dexterity—examples include

(a) Evaluating if patient can grasp toothbrush handle

(b) Determining if patient is capable of manipulating the toothbrush in a specified motion

(c) Determining if a caregiver needs to be present for oral hygiene instructions

(6) Ease and effectiveness in explaining and demonstrating toothbrushing technique

B. Power-assisted toothbrushes: Studies demonstrate that most power-assisted toothbrushes reduce plaque and gingivitis and remove stain more efficiently than manual toothbrushes[31]

1. Types[32]

a. Mechanical provides 300 to 8,000 strokes per minute

b. Sonic provides 15,000 to 31,000 strokes per minute

c. Combination of both

2. Components

a. Head—usually smaller than manual toothbrushes; removable to allow for replacement[33]

b. Mechanism of action (Figure 6–10)

(1) Reciprocating—back-and-forth or up-and-down motion

(2) Sonic—moves quickly

(3) Oscillating—swings back and forth with a steady, uninterrupted motion

(4) Rotational/counter-rotational—moves clockwise and then counterclockwise

c. Shank—connects into handle

d. Handle—contains power device (battery or electric current); portion of toothbrush that is held

3. Indications for use:[32, 33]

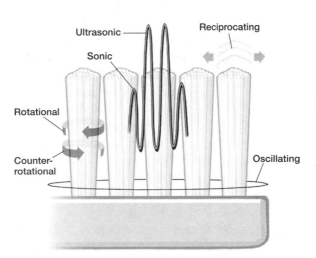

> **PRECLINICAL TIP**
>
> **Protecting Your Knowledge:** Evidence suggests that habits established during childhood and reinforced by dental professionals, parents, or guardians are likely to continue through adulthood.[30]

Figure 6–10 Movements of power-assisted toothbrushes: Include sonic, oscillating, reciprocation, and rotational/counter-rotational or a combination of these motions.

a. Children: May be more likely to brush all areas due to less effort involved and ease of use

b. Physically and mentally challenged: Provides the motion of the bristles requiring the patient minimal effort with placement

c. Elderly: Because elderly patients often suffer from arthritis or a decrease in dexterity, the handle of a power-assisted toothbrush may be easier to hold

d. Patients who require a larger handle due to arthritic and/or poor dexterity: Again, difficulty in grasping a smaller handle toothbrush may indicate use of a power-assisted toothbrush

e. Poorly motivated: Less motivated patients can benefit from the automatic motions provided from a power-assisted toothbrush

f. Implant care: Power-assisted toothbrushes provide effective, safe, and thorough plaque removal

4. Method of use—follow manufacturer's directions

C. Dental floss: Since toothbrushing cannot effectively clean the proximal areas, flossing is needed; regardless of effects made by dental healthcare professionals, data indicate that only 15 percent of patients floss regularly[23]

1. Types

a. Waxed—contains wax coating; broad and flat

(1) Indications for use—normal or without tight contact areas, irregular tooth surfaces, defective or overhanging restorations

(2) Precautions/contraindications—tight contact areas; use caution upon insertion to avoid causing "clefts" in the tissue

b. Unwaxed

(1) Indications for use—tight contact areas

(2) Precautions/contraindications—crowded teeth, heavy calculus deposits, defective or overhanging restorations

c. Tape—broad and flat waxed floss

(1) Indications for use—interdental space without tight contact areas

(2) Precautions/contraindications—none

d. Polytetrafluoroethylene—made of synthetic material

(1) Indications for use—tight contact areas and rough proximal tooth surfaces

(2) Contraindications—none

e. Tufted (SuperFloss manufactured by Oral B Laboratories)—contains a portion of waxed floss, followed by thicker tufted floss, and a portion of flexible plastic at the end

(1) Indications for use—under fixed bridges, through exposed furcations, between orthodontic bands and wires as well as implant abutments

(2) Precautions/contraindications—none

2. Method of use (spool method)

a. Use approximately 18 inches of floss

b. Wind bulk of floss around finger of one hand and remaining floss lightly around same finger of other hand

c. Secure floss with thumb and index finger of each hand leaving three-quarters to one inch of floss between digits

    d. Use thumb and index finger to guide floss between teeth using a see-saw motion

    e. Once past contact point, adapt floss to each interproximal surface by creating a C-shape (Figure 6–11)

    f. Move floss in an apical-coronal motion several times

    g. Repeat procedure on adjacent interproximal tooth with care to prevent damage to interproximal papilla

    h. Gently guide floss out of contact area using see-saw motion

    i. Obtain clean area of floss for next area

  3. Accomplishments achieved by using floss

    a. Removes plaque and debris that adhere to teeth, restorations, orthodontic appliances, fixed prostheses, interproximal gingiva, and implants

    b. Aids in identifying presence of subgingival calculus, overhanging restorations, and interproximal carious lesions

    c. Reduces gingival bleeding

    d. May use as a vehicle for applying polishing or chemotherapeutic agents to proximal or subgingival areas

D. Interdental brush: Small, spiral bristle brush; core of brush may be made of plastic, wire, or a nylon-coated wire (Figure 6–12); diameter of brush should be slightly larger than space being cleaned

  1. Indications for use

    a. Provide plaque removal at interproximal areas, in and around furcations, orthodontic bands, and fixed prostheses with large spaces present

    b. Provide gingival stimulation

    c. Apply chemotherapeutic agents

  2. Precautions/contraindications—avoid using when healthy interproximal papillae is present; also use caution to prevent damage to tooth, soft tissues, or implants with wire or plastic core

  3. Method of use

    a. Moisten brush with saliva, water, or chemotherapeutic agent

    b. Insert at an angle approximating normal gingival contour

    c. Activate by using an in-and-out motion

E. End-tuft brush: Single-tufted or group of small tufts (e.g., end-tuft and unituft) (Figure 6–13)

  1. Indications for use—to apply chemotherapeutic agents and use on areas not easily reached with other devices, such as

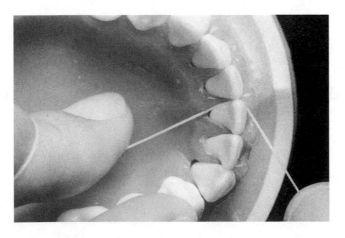

Figure 6–11   Creating a 'C' formation with dental floss.

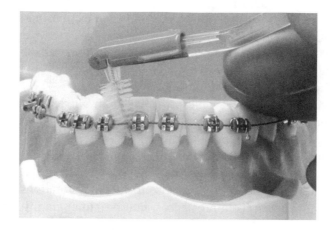

Figure 6–12   Application of interdental brush.

   a. Irregular gingival margins around migrated or malposed teeth
   b. Lingual and palatal tissues that elicit a gag reflex with a full-
      size toothbrush
   c. Distal areas of most posterior teeth
   d. Orthodontic appliances
   e. Pontics of fixed bridges
   f. Precision attachments associated with crown and bridge or im-
      plant abutments
   g. Proximal surfaces adjacent to edentulous spaces
   h. Furcations and open embrasures
2. Precautions/contraindications—avoid using when a normal contact
   area presents itself with interproximal papillae
3. Method of use
   a. Direct end of tuft into proximal area and along gingival margin
   b. Combine rotating motion with intermittent pressure
   c. Use sulcular brushing stroke
F. Toothpick holder: Utilized with a holder, the toothpick can be more
   effectively applied at a proper angle and access hard-to-reach areas
   (Figure 6–14)
   1. Indications for use
      a. Plaque removal at and just beneath gingival margin
      b. Interdental cleaning of concave proximal tooth surfaces
      c. Exposed furcation areas
      d. Orthodontic appliances

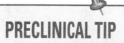

PRECLINICAL TIP

Protecting   Your   Knowledge:
When using a toothpick holder, interproximal areas can be cleaned in
a buccolingual direction.

Figure 6–13   Application of end-
tuft brush.

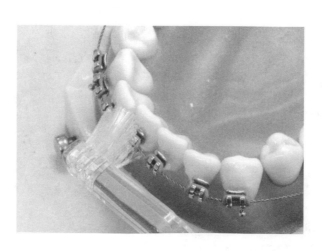

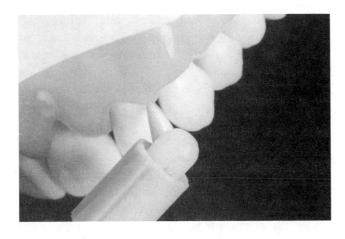

Figure 6–14 Application of tooth-pick holder.

    e. Application of chemotherapeutics
    f. Fixed prostheses
  2. Precautions/contraindications—avoid forceful subgingival insertion or vigorous proximal use to prevent gingival damage
  3. Method of use
    a. Moisten toothpick with saliva or water
    b. Apply toothpick perpendicular to gingival margin
    c. Use moderate pressure and trace around gingival margin of each tooth

G. Wedge stimulators: Plastic or wooden (balsa or birch) aids; triangular in cross section; use to remove plaque (Figure 6–15)
  1. Indications for use—use at interdental areas where tooth surfaces are exposed and interdental gingiva is missing: also use to massage underlying interdental papillae
  2. Precautions/contraindications—avoid using splayed wood—could force splinters into gingiva
  3. Method of use
    a. Soften wood by moistening in mouth
    b. Insert wedge from facial aspect with flat surface of triangular base resting on gingiva and tip of wedge angled coronally

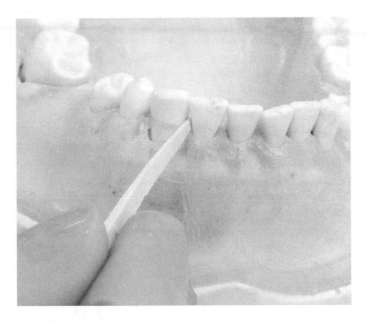

Figure 6–15 Application of wedge stimulator.

  c. Move wedge in and out (faciolingual direction) while applying moderate pressure

H. Gauze strips: Six-inch piece of gauze bandage (Figure 6–16)
  1. Indications for use—use on proximal surfaces of teeth adjacent to edentulous areas, teeth that are widely spaced, or implant abutments
  2. Precautions/contraindications—fold loose ends inwards to avoid gingival irritation
  3. Method of use
    a. Fold in half a one-inch wide, six-inch long gauze bandage—place fold toward gingiva
    b. Adapt gauze by wrapping it around the exposed proximal surface to the facial and lingual line angles
    c. Activate by using a "shoeshine" stroke from facial to lingual

I. Knitting yarn (Figure 6–17)
  1. Indications for use
    a. Proximal cleaning in areas where interdental papillae have receded
    b. Abutments of fixed prostheses
    c. Isolated teeth
    d. Teeth separated by diastemas
    e. Distal surface of most posterior teeth
  2. Precautions/contraindications—avoid using wool yarn where interdental gingiva is present
  3. Method of use in wide open embrasures
    a. Fold yarn in half using approximately eight inches
    b. Loop yarn through dental floss
    c. Insert floss through contact area and draw yarn into embrasure
    d. Clean tooth surface with a facial-lingual stroke

J. Pipe cleaner (Figure 6–18)
  1. Indications for use
    a. Proximal surfaces where interdental gingiva is missing
    b. Open furcation areas
    c. Separated teeth
  2. Precautions/contraindications—use caution: Sharp wire center can scratch cementum, gingiva, and implants

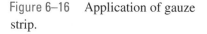
Figure 6–16   Application of gauze strip.

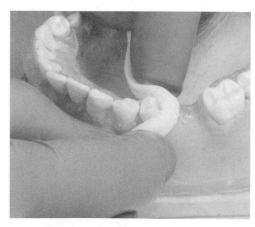

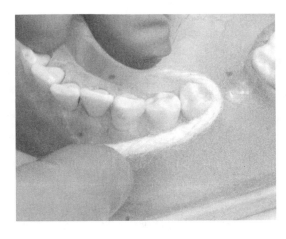

Figure 6–17   Application of knitting yarn.

3. Method of use
  a. Use one-third of a regular pipe cleaner
  b. Work end of cleaner through space
  c. Activate using an in-and-out motion
K. Interdental tip stimulator: Designed with a conical or pyramidal flexible rubber or plastic tip attached to a handle or to end of toothbrush (Figure 6–19)
1. Indications for use
  a. Cleans debris from interdental area
  b. Removes plaque at and just below gingival margin
2. Precautions/contraindications—use caution when inserting tip subgingivally to prevent damage to soft tissues
3. Method of use
  a. Place tip at 90-degree angle to long axis of tooth
  b. Utilize moderate pressure and trace along gingival margin or use a buccolingual (in-and-out) motion in open embrasure area
L. Floss holder: Y- or C-shaped yokes with handle allowing patient to manipulate floss (Figure 6–20); helpful for patients with limited dexterity
1. Indications for use are patients who[24]
  a. Have large hands
  b. Are physically challenged
  c. Lack normal dexterity
  d. Have caregivers providing oral care
  e. Prefer not to put hands in mouth

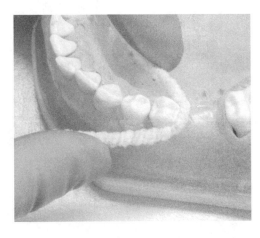

Figure 6–18   Application of pipe cleaner.

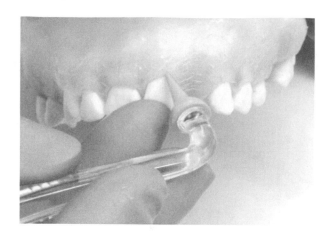

Figure 6–19   Application of interdental tip stimulator.

2. Precautions/contraindications—difficult to maintain tension of floss between prongs
3. Method of use
   a. Tightly secure floss between two prongs of yoke
   b. Use same technique as described for flossing
M. Floss (bridge) threader: Blunt-ended with a needle-like or loop device, where floss is inserted; made of a stiff, yet flexible plastic (Figure 6–21)
   1. Indications for use
      a. Through embrasure areas under contact points too tight for floss insertion
      b. Between proximal surface and gingiva of abutment teeth of fixed prostheses
      c. Under pontics
      d. Around orthodontic appliances
      e. Under splinting
   2. Precautions/contraindications—use caution when inserting point to avoid trauma to gingival tissues

Figure 6–20   Application of floss
holder.

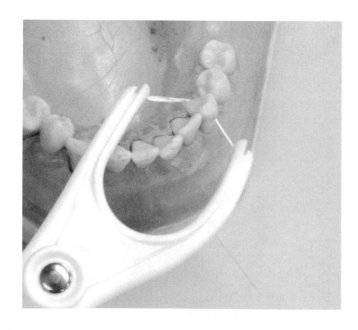

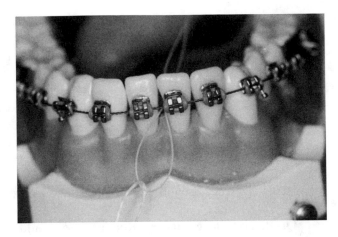

Figure 6–21 Application of floss threader.

3. Method of use
   a. Insert floss through threader
   b. Direct end of threader into target area
   c. Disengage floss from threader to adapt to tooth surface
   d. Utilize flossing technique previously described
N. Implant care (Figure 6–22): Several companies manufacture products especially for use on dental implants; use according to manufacturer's directions
O. Tongue Cleaners: Used to clean plaque from the dorsal (top) surface of the tongue
   1. Indications for use—indicated for those who smoke or who have fissured or elongated papillae (hairy tongue)
   2. Precautions/contraindications—none
   3. Method of use[34]
      a. Position tongue as far forward as possible
      b. Place tongue cleaner (can also use toothbrush) as far back as possible
      c. Apply gentle pressure and pull cleaner/brush forward
      d. Repeat procedure until entire dorsal surface of tongue is cleaned
P. Oral irrigator: Targeted application of a pulsated or steady stream of water or other irrigant used for cleansing and/or therapeutic purposes

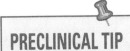

PRECLINICAL TIP

Protecting Your Knowledge: Implant care products are specifically manufactured from materials designed *not* to scratch the implant titanium material.

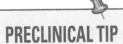

PRECLINICAL TIP

Protecting Your Knowledge: A study found that tongue coating and bleeding on probing (BOP) had a strong correlation to oral malodor in periodontal patients.[35]

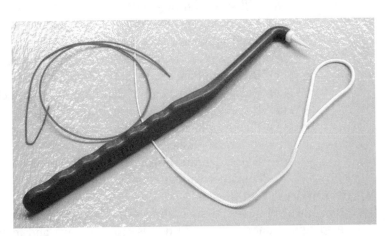

Figure 6–22 Implant care aids.

1. Indications for use—flush away loosely adherent microflora located coronal to gingival margin
2. Precautions/contraindications—avoid using on patients with a possible risk to subacute bacterial endocarditis
3. Method of use
   a. Direct jet tip toward interdental area holding tip at right angle to long axis of tooth
   b. Start on lowest pressure setting, increase slightly over time depending on condition of gingiva and tissue comfort
   c. Lean over sink
   d. Trace around each tooth, spending extra time at interproximal areas

Q. Removable appliances: Routine care should be taken to clean not only removable appliances, but also the underlying tissues
   1. Indications for use
      a. Prevent denture stomatitis
      b. Encourage regular oral self-examinations to observe changes of tissues
      c. Enhance oral cleanliness
   2. Precautions/contraindications—avoid alcohol or essential oils found in commercial mouth rinses—not compatible with denture acrylic
   3. Method of cleaning
      a. At home, use according to manufacturer's instructions
         (1) Immersion cleaners include
             (a) Hypochlorite solutions (contain alcohol)
             (b) Alkaline peroxide
         (2) Brushing
         (3) Combination of immersion cleaners and brushing
      b. In office
         (1) Wear gloves to handle appliances
         (2) Place 1 inch of water in the bottom of a beaker
         (3) Line beaker with plastic baggie
         (4) Place appliance in baggie
         (5) Add manufacturer tartar and stain remover to cover appliance
         (6) Place beaker in ultrasonic cleaner
         (7) Set timer for 10 minutes
         (8) Fill sink with two to three inches of water
         (9) Remove appliance from solution and rinse thoroughly
         (10) Hold appliance securely in palm without squeezing while brushing
         (11) Brush appliance with sterile denture brush
         (12) Use appropriate end of denture brush for each surface
         (13) Inspect appliance for remaining debris, calculus, and stain
         (14) Place appliance in cup with mouth rinse/water mixture
         (15) Return appliance to patient
         (16) Rinse denture brush thoroughly and place in cold sterile container with gluteraldehyde solution

VII. Dentifrices (Toothpastes)
Substance applied with a toothbrush or other applicator to remove bacterial plaque, materia alba, and debris from gingiva and teeth for cosmetic

purposes, and for applying specific agents to tooth surfaces for therapeutic purposes; available in gels and pastes, and contain active and inactive ingredients.

A. Active ingredients (therapeutic): Perform a specific preventive or treatment action; approximately 1 to 2 percent of dentifrices contain an active ingredient[36]

1. Fluoride
   a. Fluoride-containing dentifrice—contains up to 260 mg of fluoride; safe and effective fluoride content for over-the-counter dentifrice is 0.22 percent for sodium (NaF), 0.76 percent for monofluorophosphate (MFP), and 0.4 percent for stannous (SnF_2)
   b. Baking soda-peroxide-fluoride dentifrice (e.g., Mentadent)—combination of 0.75 percent stable peroxide gel, baking soda, and 1,100 ppm sodium fluoride

2. Antimicrobial dentifrices—chemical compounds used to supplement usual brushing and flossing in mechanical plaque control
   a. Stannous salts have reported activity against caries, plaque, and gingivitis
      (1) Marketed in United States as Crest Gum Care
      (2) Has shown superior efficacy in antimicrobial, plaque acidogenicity, gingivitis or gingival bleeding, and tartar control
   b. Triclosan—broad-spectrum antibacterial agent effective against wide variety of bacteria
      (1) Marketed in United States as Colgate Total
      (2) Approved by FDA in 1997 as the first dentifrice to help prevent gingivitis, plaque, and caries[36]
      (3) Received ADA's Seal of Acceptance for its benefit in reducing gingivitis, plaque, and caries
   c. Antitartar—active ingredients include
      (1) Tetrasodium phosphate and disodium dihydrogen pyrophosphate (e.g., Crest Tartar Control)—also inhibits some bacterial growth[36]
      (2) Zinc citrate trihydrate—tartar control versions for Aim and Close-Up—also inhibits growth of bacteria[36]
   d. Antihypersensitivity—used to treat dentinal hypersensitivity; active agents include potassium nitrate, strontium chloride, and sodium citrate

B. Inactive ingredients: Provide structure, texture, cleansing activity, color(s), flavor(s), and preserve toothpaste[36]

1. Humectants—retain moisture and prevent drying of dentifrice once exposed to air; examples include glycerin and sorbitol
2. Preservatives—prevent bacterial growth; help prolong shelf life; examples include alcohols and benzoates
3. Flavoring agents—impart pleasant flavor for patient acceptance; example includes menthol
4. Foaming agents—create a foaming effect; example includes sodium lauryl sulfate, which may cause canker sores
5. Coloring agents—enhance appearance; example includes vegetable dyes
6. Thickening agents—prevent separation of liquid and solid agents; example includes alginates

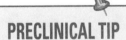

PRECLINICAL TIP

Protecting Your Knowledge: American Dental Association (ADA) seal of approval has not been rewarded to anticalculus products because the ADA recognizes calculus inhibition as a cosmetic effect. The seal is awarded due to anticaries effects of these products.

VIII.   **Mouth Rinses**

Mouth rinses are available in liquid form and serve as a delivery system for cosmetic and therapeutic agents.

A. Types
   1. Cosmetic—improve appearance of oral cavity (e.g., reduce oral malodor)
   2. Therapeutic—reduce some disease in mouth (e.g., dental caries, bacterial plaque, gingivitis); does not kill all bacteria in mouth, but reduces the number

B. Ingredients
   1. Oxygenating agents[37, 38]
      a. Purpose—use short-term to reduce symptoms of pericoronitis and necrotizing ulcerative gingivitis (NUG)
      b. Mechanism of action—cleanses by effervescent action; short-lasting antimicrobial effect—only as long as oxygen is released
      c. Adverse effects—long-term use results in overgrowth of bacteria, causing black hairy tongue
      d. Additional information—common ingredients include hydrogen peroxide, sodium perborate, and urea peroxide
   2. Chlorhexidine gluconate—0.12 percent prescription plaque control rinse;[37, 38] effective agent used to disinfect the oral mucosa as well as substantially reduce gingivitis occurrence, severity, and bleeding
      a. Purpose—inhibits and reduces development of plaque
      b. Mechanism of action—alters integrity of bacterial cell membrane and therefore damages the cytoplasm
         (1) Absorbed into teeth and pellicle
         (2) Time-released over 12 to 24 hours (substantivity), prolonging bactericidal effect
         (3) Lysis cell wall consisting of Gram-positive and Gram-negative microorganisms and fungi
      c. Adverse effects include
         (1) Temporary loss of taste
         (2) Bitter taste
         (3) Dryness, soreness, and burning sensation of mucosa
         (4) Epithelial desquamation—sloughing of oral mucosa
         (5) Discoloration (usually brown) of teeth, tongue, and restorations
         (6) Slight increase in supragingival calculus formation due to death of bacterial plaque and not being removed before mineralization occurs
      d. Additional information
         (1) Contains alcohol (11.6%), therefore contraindicated for alcohol-sensitive patients
         (2) Available in some countries as 0.2 percent solution
         (3) Use as a preprocedural rinse to lower oral bacterial count
         (4) Decreases supragingival bacterial plaque formation and inhibits development of gingivitis
         (5) Use for short-term adjunctive therapy after surgical treatment that limits mechanical plaque control
         (6) Use on selective patients to control inflammation with NUG
         (7) Use to encourage and motivate patients when oral hygiene has been neglected for a period of time

(8) Suppresses growth of *Streptococcus mutans,* which are involved in the dissolution of tooth structure

(9) Avoid using immediately before or after regular toothbrushing, as it is inactivated by most dentifrice surfactants

(10) Use as a 30-second rinse, twice daily, with 1 oz. of solution

(11) Common names include Peridex and Perioguard

3. Phenolic-related essential oils[37, 38]

   a. Purpose—reduces both plaque accumulation and severity of gingivitis by up to 34 percent

   b. Mechanism of action—disrupts cell walls and inhibits bacterial enzymes

   c. Adverse effects—has a bitter taste and may cause burning sensation to tissues

   d. Additional information

      (1) Active ingredients include thymol and eucalyptol, mixed with menthol and methylsalicylate

      (2) Original formula contains 26.9 percent alcohol; other variety contains 21.6 percent alcohol, therefore contraindicated for alcohol-sensitive patients

      (3) Common product name is Listerine

4. Quaternary ammonia compounds[37, 38]

   a. Purpose—recommended to control halitosis; reduces plaque and gingivitis

   b. Mechanism of action—decreases bacterial cell wall permeability and metabolism (bind to oral tissues through their strong positive charge)

   c. Adverse reactions include

      (1) Staining

      (2) Enhanced supragingival calculus formation

      (3) Burning sensation

      (4) Occasional tissue desquamation

   d. Additional information

      (1) Possesses no substantivity

      (2) Contains alcohol, therefore contraindicated for alcohol-sensitive patients

      (3) Common products include Cepacol and Scope

5. Sanguinarine[37, 38]

   a. Purpose—anti-gingivitis

   b. Mechanism of action—alters bacterial cell wall structure and may inhibit bacterial adhesion

   c. Side effect—occasional burning sensation

   d. Additional information

      (1) Contains 11.5 percent alcohol, therefore contraindicated for alcohol-sensitive patients

      (2) Common product name is Viadent

6. Fluoride (Stannous)[37]

   a. Purpose—may possess antiplaque properties for a short duration

   b. Mechanism of action—may alter bacterial cell metabolism or cell adhesion properties

   c. Additional information

      (1) Contains no alcohol

      (2) Available in paste or rinse form (0.4%)

      (3) May cause some staining

QUESTIONS

1. Which of the following is the proper order of the life cycle of plaque?
   a. Bacterial colonization, acquired pellicle, bacterial mineralization
   b. Bacterial mineralization, bacterial colonization, acquired pellicle
   c. Acquired pellicle, bacterial mineralization, bacterial colonization
   d. Acquired pellicle, bacterial colonization, bacterial mineralization

2. Which level of preventive dental services involves a dental hygienist intervening and stopping the progression of a disease?
   a. Primary preventive
   b. Secondary preventive
   c. Tertiary preventive

3. Using Maslow's hierarchy of needs, at which level would a person be who states he or she is "living month to month and trying to keep food on the table for the kids"?
   a. Physiological needs
   b. Safety
   c. Love
   d. Security

4. During oral hygiene instructions, you discuss the condition of the oral cavity with the patient. This patient is involved in the educational session and mentions that she would like to improve the condition of her gums and teeth. She is going to be a bridesmaid in her sister's upcoming wedding and she wants to feel good about her appearance. What type of motivation is this patient utilizing to improve her oral condition?
   a. Rewarding
   b. Praising
   c. Internal
   d. External

5. A mother is in the clinic with her 3-year-old child. You question the mother about the child's toothbrushing habits. The mother states that she brushes her daughter's teeth once a day with toothpaste, and the daughter brushes her own teeth once a day with toothpaste. You further question her on the toothpaste used, how much is placed on the brush, and whether the daughter expectorates after brushing. The mother states "I know it is not good for her, but I let her use enough toothpaste to cover the bristles. She says

it tastes good and that is the only way I can get her to brush." Where on the learning ladder is the mother with regards to toothpaste consumption?
   a. Unawareness
   b. Awareness
   c. Self-interest
   d. Involvement

6. Which of the following bacteria are predominant during early plaque formation?
   a. Gram-positive cocci
   b. Gram-negative cocci
   c. Spirochetes
   d. Vibrios

7. All of the following statements are true about the colonization of bacteria EXCEPT one. Which one is the EXCEPTION?
   a. As plaque matures, it thickens in mass and migrates subgingivally.
   b. Mature plaque contains more aggressive bacteria than early plaque.
   c. If left undisturbed long enough, white blood cells will colonize the bacterial matrix.
   d. The aerobic microorganisms penetrate to the base of the sulcus as plaque matures.

8. The nutritional source for both subgingival plaque and calculus is gingival crevicular fluid and inflammatory exudate. The bacteria involved with these deposits may be the causative agents in inflammation of the gingiva.
   a. Both statements are TRUE.
   b. Both statements are FALSE.
   c. The first statement is TRUE. The second statement is FALSE.
   d. The first statement is FALSE. The second statement is TRUE.

9. Which of the following identification methods aids in detecting the presence of subgingival calculus?
   a. Transillumination
   b. Disclosing solution
   c. Explorer
   d. Presence of bleeding

10. Which of the following is a white soft substance that is easily removed with toothbrushing?
    a. Acquired pellicle
    b. Bacterial plaque
    c. Dental calculus
    d. Softened enamel

11. Replacing toothbrushes should be done at the first evidence of the bristles splaying. Splayed bristles can increase tissue trauma, decrease plaque removal, and become contaminated by viruses.
   a. Both statements are TRUE.
   b. Both statements are FALSE.
   c. The first statement is TRUE. The second statement is FALSE.
   d. The first statement is FALSE. The second statement is TRUE.

12. All of the following auxiliary aids are effective to use when cleaning around orthodontic appliances EXCEPT one. Which one is the EXCEPTION?
   a. Floss holder
   b. Bridge (floss) threader
   c. Interdental brush
   d. Powered oral irrigator

13. Which of the following ingredients helps retain moisture and prevent drying in a dentifrice?
   a. Flavoring agent
   b. Humectant
   c. Thickening agent
   d. Preservatives

14. It is recommended patients use soft-bristled toothbrushes. The diameter of the soft bristle is large—between 0.013 to 0.014 inches.
   a. Both statements are TRUE.
   b. Both statements are FALSE.
   c. The first statement is TRUE. The second statement is FALSE.
   d. The first statement is FALSE. The second statement is TRUE.

15. All of the following are active ingredients in desensitizing dentifrices EXCEPT one. Which one is the EXCEPTION?
   a. Potassium nitrate
   b. Strontium chloride
   c. Sodium citrate
   d. Disodium dihydrogen pyrophosphate

16. Studies indicate that most power-assisted toothbrushes reduce plaque and gingivitis more efficiently than manual toothbrushes. Indications for using a power-assisted toothbrush include those with poor dexterity and for implant care.
   a. Both statements are TRUE.
   b. Both statements are FALSE.
   c. The first statement is TRUE. The second statement is FALSE.
   d. The first statement is FALSE. The second statement is TRUE.

17. All of the following are possible side effects of chlorhexidine gluconate EXCEPT one. Which one is the EXCEPTION?
   a. Bitter taste
   b. Epithelial desquamation
   c. Brown staining of teeth
   d. Black hairy tongue

18. Which of the following toothbrushing instructions describe the Fones method?
   a. The bristles are positioned perpendicular to the crown, and the brush is moved in a circular motion.
   b. The bristles are placed at a 45-degree angle toward the apex of the tooth—part on the gingiva and part on the tooth.
   c. The bristles are placed at a 45-degree angle toward the occlusal/incisal plane.
   d. The bristles are placed in the sulcus at a 45-degree angle toward the apex of the tooth.

19. All of the following are methods used when properly flossing EXCEPT one. Which one is the EXCEPTION?
   a. Use approximately 18 inches of floss.
   b. Secure the floss between the index finger and thumb.
   c. Leave one-and-one-half to two inches of floss between digits.
   d. Adapt floss through contact and use a "C" formation at proximals.

20. Which of the following toothbrushing methods is recommended to clean orthodontic brackets?
   a. Bass
   b. Fones
   c. Stillman
   d. Charters

REFERENCES

1. Rosan, G., & R. J. Lamont. Dental Plaque Formation. *Microbes Infect,* 2(3), 1599–1607, November 2000.
2. Socransky, S. S. & A. D. Haffajee. The Bacterial Etiology of Destructive Periodontal Disease: Current Concepts. *Journal of Periodontology* 63(4 Suppl.), 322–31, April 1992.
3. Schupbach, P., F. G. Oppenheim, U. Lendenmann, M. S. Lamkin, Y., Yao & B. Guggenheim. Electron-Microscopic Demonstration of Proline-Rich Proteins, Statherin, and Histatins in Acquired Enamel Pellicles In Vitro. *European Journal of Oral Sciences,* 109(1), 60–68, February 2001.

4. Yao, Y., J. Grogan, M. Zehnder, U. Lendenmann, B. Nam, Z. Wu, C. E. Costello, & F. G. Oppenheim. Compositional Analysis of Human Acquired Enamel Pellicle by Mass Spectrometry. *Archives of Oral Biology* 46(4) 293–303, April 2001.

5. Skjorland, K. K., M. Rykke, & T. Sonju. Rate of Pellicle Formation In Vivo. *Acta Odontologica Scandinavica,* 53(6), 358–62, December 1995.

6. Overman, P. R. Biofilm: A New View of Plaque. *The Journal of Contemporary Dental Practice,* 1(3), Summer 2000.

7. Palmer, R. J. Jr., K. Kazmerzak, M. C. Hansen, & P. E. Kolenbrander. Mutualism versus Independence: Strategies of Mixed-Species Oral Biofilms In Vitro Using Saliva as the Sole Nutrient Source. *Infection and Immunity,* 69(9), 5794–5804, September 2001.

8. Marsh, P. D., & D. J. Bradshaw. Dental Plaque as a Biofilm. *Journal of Industrial Microbiology,* 15(3), 169–75, 1995.

9. Bacterial Morphotypes of 3 day old plaque: Kwan-yat Z., P. Kam-man L. Samaranayake, & Attstrom R; *Journal of Clinical Periodontology,* 23, 403–406, 1996.

10. Scannapieco, F. A., G. Torres, & M. J. Levine. Salivary Alpha-Amylase: Role in Dental Plaque and Caries Formation. *Critical reviews in oral biology and medicine: an official publication of the American Association of Oral Biologists* 4(3–4), 301–7, 1993.

11. Rudney, J. D., Saliva and Dental Plaque. *Advances in Dental Research* 14, 29–39, December 2000.

12. Vrahopoulos, Barber, & Newman. The Apical Border Plaque in Severe Periodontitis: An Ultrastructural Study. *Journal of Periodontology,* 113–124, February 1995.

13. Wecke, J., T. Kersten, K. Madela, A. Moter, U. B. Gobel, A. Friedmann, & J. Bernimoulin. A Novel Technique for Monitoring the Development of Bacterial Biofilms in Human Periodontal Pockets. *FEMS Microbiology Letters,* 191(1), 95–101, October 1, 2000.

14. Noiri, Y., L. Li, & S. Ebisu. The Localization of Periodontal-Disease-Associated Bacteria in Human Periodontal Pockets. *Journal of Dental Research* 80(10), 1930–1934, October 2001.

15. Wong, L. Plaque Mineralisation In Vitro. *The New Zealand Dental Journal,* 94(415), 15–18 March 1998.

16. Nancollas, G. H., & M. A. Johnsson. Calculus Formation and Inhibition, *Advances in Dental Research,* 8(2), 307–11, July 1994.

17. White, D. J. Dental Calculus: Recent Insights into Occurrence, Formation, Prevention, Removal and Oral Health Effects of Supragingival and Subgingival Deposits. *European Journal of Oral Sciences,* 105(5 Pt 2): 508–522, October 1997.

18. Bergstrom, J. Tobacco Smoking and Supragingival Dental Calculus. *Journal of Clinical Periodontology,* 26(8), 541–547, August 1999.

19. Clerehugh, V., R. Abdeia, P. S. Hull. The Effect of Subgingival Calculus on the Validity of Clinical Probing Measurements. *Journal of Dentistry,* 24(5), 329–33, September 1996.

20. Rowan, John. Ascent and Descent in Maslow's Theory. *Journal of Humanistic Psychology,* Summer 1999.

21. Mann, G. When the Bristles Wear Out Don't Be in Doubt: How to Teach Patients about Toothbrush Replacement. *Journal of Practical Hygiene,* 8(5), 36–37, 1999.

22. Jepsen, S. The Role of Manual Toothbrushes in Effective Plaque Control: Advantages and Limitations. In N. P. Lang, R. Attstrom, & H. Loe. (Eds.), *Proceedings of the European Workshop on the Mechanical Plaque Control: Status of the Art and Science of Dental Plaque.* Berlin, Germany: Quintessence, 1998, 121–137.

23. Bantá, C. Y. Manual Toothbrushes—Pretty as a Picture and Just as Smart. *Journal of Practical Hygiene,* 8(5), 40–41, 1999.

24. Spears, D. Self-Study Course Module II, Preventive Dentistry for Persons with Severe Disabilities. Burtner, NC: Southern Association of Institutional Dentists, 1994.

25. Abraham, N. J., Cirincione, U. K. & Glass, R. T.: Dentists' and Dental Hygienists' Attitudes Toward Toothbrush Replacement and Maintenance. *Clinical Preventive Dentistry,* 12(5), 28–33, 1990.

26. Quinlisk, J., M. Roberts, & M. Taveres. An Evaluation of Children's Toothbrushing Habits and Techniques [abstract]. *Journal of Dental Research,* 78: 414, 1999. Abstract 2458.

27. Glaze, P. M., & A. B. Wade. Toothbrush Age and Wear as It Relates to Plaque Control. *Journal of Clinical Periodontology,* 13(1), 52–56, 1986.

28. Cronin, M., W. Dembling, P. B. Warren, & D. W. King. A 3-Month Clinical Investigation Comparing the Safety and Efficacy of a Novel Toothbrush (Braun Oral-B Plaque Remover) with a Manual Toothbrush. *American Journal of Dentistry,* 11(Spec No), S17–S21, 1998.

29. Collier, C., M. G. Scaletta, J. Stephens, R. Kimbrough, J. D. Kettering, & S. Meier. An In Vitro Investigation of the Efficacy of CPC for Use in Toothbrush Decontamination. *Journal of Dental Hygiene,* 70(4), 161–165, 1996.

30. Skotowski, M. C., R. Widmer, J. Strate, M. Cugini, & A. Nowak. A Practice-Based Evaluation of a Range of Children's Toothbrushes: Safety and Acceptance. *Supplement to Compendium of Continuing Education in Dentistry,* 23(3), 17–24, 2000.

31. Saxer, U. P., & S. L. Yanell. Impact of Improved Toothbrushes on Dental Diseases II. *Quintessence International,* 28(9), 573–593, 1997.

32. Jahn, C. Review of Automated Plaque Removal Products. *Journal of Practical Hygiene,* 5(9), 48–52, 2000.

33. Ortblad, K. Action Mechanisms of Various Automated Toothbrushes. *Journal of Practical Hygiene,* 8(5), 44–45, 1999.

34. Jahn, C. A. Tongue Cleaners: A Key to Fresh Breath and Health. *Journal of Practical Hygiene,* 10(4), 36–37, 2001.

35. Morita, M., & H. L. Wang. Relationship Between Sulcular Sulfide Level and Oral Malodor in Subjects with Periodontal Disease. *Journal of Periodontology,* 72(1), 79–84, 2001.

36. Parrott, P. B. The Building Blocks of Dentifrices. *Journal of Practical Hygiene,* 8(5), 48–50, 1999.

37. Chemical Agents for Control of Plaque and Gingivitis. Committee on Research, Science and Therapy, 1–10, April 1994.

38. Lyle, D. M. The Role of Pharmaceuticals in the Reduction of Plaque and Gingivitis. *Journal of Practical Hygiene,* 9(6), 46–49, 2000.

FLOSSING PERFORMANCE TASK SHEET

Student _____
Date _____
Instructor _____
Patient _____

*Option #1 - Wrap floss around middle fingers; use index fingers as guides.
*Option #2 - Wrap floss around index fingers.

Re-evaluation
Instr: _____
Date _____

Instr: _____
Date _____

	S	U	Comments	S	U	Comments	S	U	Comments
1. Uses approximately 18-24 inches of floss									
2. *Wraps floss around middle fingers.									
3. Establishes and *maintains* a fulcrum. (MUST have AT LEAST one fulcrum in anterior and two in posterior)									
4. Uses index finger as a guide.									
5. Inserts floss at an oblique angle to the tooth.									
6. Passes floss through contact area with see-saw motion.									
7. Controls floss to prevent snapping.									
8. Maintains short length - 3/4" to 1" between index fingers.									
9. Presses floss against teeth.									
10. Creates and maintains a "C" formation.									
11. Slides floss up and down with *scraping motion.*									
12. Avoids injuring the interdental papillae.									
13. Removes floss and prevents snapping.									
14. Wraps up the used floss and unwraps clean floss.									
15. Has an established pattern of flossing.									
16. Irrigates oral cavity to remove loose deposits.									

Courtesy of Indiana University Purdue University Dental Hygiene Program.

171

CLEANING REMOVABLE APPLIANCES PERFORMANCE TASK SHEET

Student _____

Date _____

Instructor _____

	S	U	Comments	S	U	Comments	S	U	Comments
1. Wears gloves to handle appliance(s).									
2. Places 1" of water in bottom of beaker.									
3. Lines beaker with a plastic baggie.									
4. Places appliance into plastic baggie.									
5. Adds Tartar & Stain Remover into baggie and covers appliance.									
6. Places beaker in ultrasonic cleaner.									
7. Sets timer for 10 minutes.									
8. Fills sink with 2–3" of water.									
9. Removes appliance from solution and rinses thoroughly.									
10. Holds appliance securely while cleaning.									
11. Brushes appliance with sterile denture brush under running water.									
12. Uses appropriate end of denture brush to clean each area of appliance.									
13. Inspects appliance.									
14. Places appliance in cup with correct mixture of mouth rinse and water.									
15. Appropriately sterilizes denture brush in cold sterilization.									

Courtesy of Indiana University Purdue University Fort Wayne Dental Hygiene Program.

Chapter 7

Ergonomics

Anne Nugent Guignon, RDH, MPH

MediaLink

A companion CD-ROM, included free with each new copy of this book, supplements the procedures presented in each chapter. Insert the CD-ROM to watch video clips and view a large collection of color images that is also included. This multimedia library is designed to help you add a new dimension to your learning.

KEY TERMS

ambidextrous. Refers to the ability to perform a task properly with either hand. The term is also used for products that can be used by either hand in contrast to a product or device that can be used by either the right or left hand.

contra angled. Term used to describe an instrument that features a slight bend backwards, away from the long axis of the instrument body. Some polishing devices and hand instruments are designed with such a bend.

cumulative trauma disorders. Originate from repeated stresses to the muscles, tendons, nerves, and supporting body structures, and are generally a result of activities that involve forceful exertions, awkward postures or positioning, repetition, and static loading.

depth of field. Measured in inches, with a typical range of 4 to 5 inches. Adequate depth allows movement of the head to view different parts of the mouth, unlike the fixed position obtained with a reading prescription alone.

ergonomics. Science used in the workforce to design tasks that adapt to the worker. Ergonomic study includes an analysis of the physical work environment, objects used in the environment, psychological factors, and work organization factors.

extension. Bending forward from a neutral position.

flexion. Bending backwards away from a neutral position.

magnification loupes. Special glasses fitted with telescopes allowing a larger view of the working field without compromising body posture.

musculoskeletal disorders (MSD). Conditions that affect the muscles, nerves, tendons, and supporting structures of the body. A wide variety of conditions can be classified as MSDs, and these disorders can be short term and episodic in nature or in certain cases can result in permanent impairment or disability.

neutral body posture. Places the body in a position where muscles are relaxed and the body is not placed in any stressful or awkward position.

pinch grip. Refers to how a clinician holds an instrument or device using the thumb, index, and middle fingers. The smaller the diameter of the instrument, the greater the pinch posture required to obtain a satisfactory grip.

radial deviation. Bending the wrist toward the thumb in the direction of the radius.

repetitive-stress injuries. Another term for cumulative trauma disorders.

right angled. Term used to describe an instrument that features an exact right angle in the body of the design. The attachment of the polishing cup in most prophy angles features this type of design.

static loading. Placing the body in one position for prolonged periods of time, resulting in an increase in muscle fatigue.

ulnar deviation. Bending the wrist toward the little finger in the direction of the ulna.

width of depth. Refers to the size of area being viewed. The most popular magnification strengths, 2.0x, 2.5x, and 2.6x, allow view of the entire mouth at one time. Higher levels of magnification result in a smaller field of view.

work-related musculoskeletal disorders (WMSD). Type of MSD that is a result of a work-related task.

working range. Distance from the eye to the actual working field. An accurate measurement of working range is made with the operator sitting in a relaxed upright position with shoulders relaxed, arms close to the side, and the patient positioned at a height comfortable to the operator.

LEARNING OBJECTIVES

After reading this chapter and participating in learning activities, the student will be able to

- describe and demonstrate correct operator positioning;

- describe and demonstrate correct patient positioning;
- list characteristics of an operator chair essential for adequate support;

- differentiate between through-the-lens and flip-up magnification loupes;
- list, discuss, and demonstrate methods of keeping the body in an ergonomic position while providing patient services;
- identify the more ergonomic product when examining different dental equipment and supplies;
- compare and contrast the types of examination and surgical gloves available;
- evaluate characteristics of instruments that make them ergonomically best for use;
- know what causes work-related musculoskeletal disorders (WMSDs), also known as repetitive-stress injuries (RSIs) or cumulative trauma disorders (CTDs);
- list which positions to avoid while practicing clinical dental hygiene;
- discuss how to eliminate static loading;
- integrate lifestyle activities that keep the mind and body healthy.

I. Introduction

Years ago, little attention was placed on workplace safety. However, with increased interest in occupational health, ergonomic issues are now being considered in a wide variety of professions. Thousands of injuries occur every year that can be directly traced to on-the-job tasks. Many of these injuries result from performing repetitive tasks that require the use of force and place workers in awkward postural positions. These injuries are further compounded in job settings where workers have little direct control over their schedules and a limited chance for breaks throughout the work period. Dental hygienists work in environments that frequently exhibit all of these characteristics; therefore, it is critical that students have a comprehensive understanding of ergonomic issues and the options available to avoid workplace-related injuries or disorders.

II. Ergonomic Positioning

A. Operator positioning: Correct positioning in the operator's chair contributes to overall operator well-being and helps prevent undue muscular fatigue and muscular imbalances;[1, 2, 3, 4] to establish correct positioning, maintain the following criteria:

1. Operator chair (Figure 7–1)
   a. Distribute body weight evenly on chair seat

Figure 7–1   Correct seating position–distribute body weight evenly on chair seat.

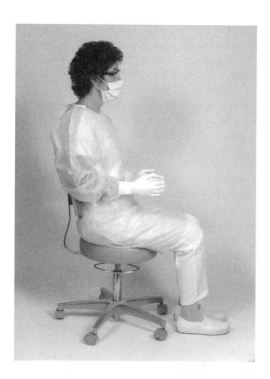

(1) Depth of seat: Space between edge of seat and knees should be one to three inches

(2) Width of seat: Should be minimum of two inches wider than buttocks

b. Position body so chair seat supports hips, thighs, upper and lower back, and behind the knees without impinging on the back of the legs (Figure 7–2)

c. Adjust back of chair to provide adequate support in the lumbar region of the back and support to hips and thighs

d. Elevate the chair so the hips are slightly higher than the knees; reduces strain on lower back

2. Posture: To prevent ergonomic injuries, practice proper posture positioning (Figure 7–3):

a. Sit up straight

b. Position head and neck directly over the shoulders: allows the upper body musculature to support the weight of the head (Figure 7–4)

c. Lean forward from the hips, keeping the back straight, and avoid rounding or hunching shoulders; shoulders should be relaxed and parallel to the floor

d. Place feet flat on the floor, shoulder-width apart, creating a tripod with the base of the operator's chair; avoid crossing ankles or knees, placing feet on chair rung, or balancing body weight on toes (Figures 7–5, 7–6, 7–7, and 7–8)

e. Position forearms parallel to the floor, keeping the wrists in a neutral position (Figure 7–9); avoid raising to a position where there is less than a 60-degree angle between the upper arms and forearms (Figure 7–10)

f. Keep arms close to the sides during instrumentation and avoid raising arms more than 20-degrees away from the body

g. Sit at 7:30, 9, 11, or 12 o'clock positions for right-handed clinicians (preferably 9:00 to 12:00) or 4:30, 3, 1, or 12 o'clock for left-handed clinicians (preferably 12:00 to 3:00)

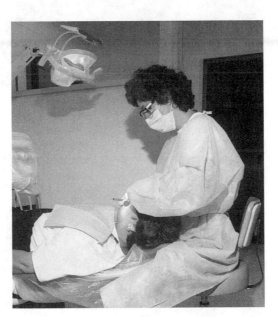

Figure 7–2   Position body so chair seat supports hips, thighs, back, and behind the knees without impinging on the back of the legs.

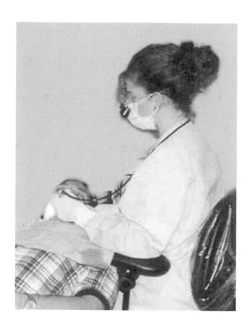

Figure 7–3   Sitting with proper body positioning.

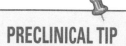

PRECLINICAL TIP

Positioning Your Knowledge: Exercise: Keeping the eyes level, reach arms straight out to the side and turn torso as far to one side as possible. Repeat on other side.[4]

      h. Straddle the patient chair to sit closer to the working field except when working at 5:30 or 7:30

B. Patient positioning: Dental chairs are generally made to accommodate large adult patients. However, operators are challenged to treat patients of all sizes. Therefore, consider the position and size of the patient in the dental chair during treatment to help reduce any unnecessary bending or twisting by the operator.[2, 4 5, 6] There are a number of ways clinicians can reduce unnecessary twisting and/or bending

Figure 7–4   Position head and neck directly over shoulders.

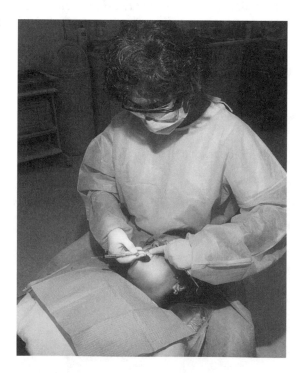

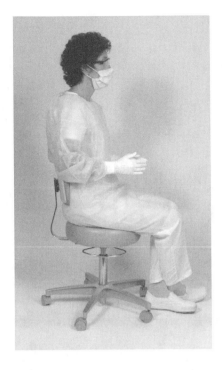

Figure 7–5   Avoid crossing ankles.

1. Position the patient's chair at a height where the operator can maintain neutral arm, shoulder, and wrist posture
2. Position patient's mouth parallel to the operator's elbow, approximately 18 inches from the operator's eyes
3. Utilize a mouth mirror for indirect vision
4. Ask the patient to turn the head toward or away from the operator to facilitate direct vision
5. Lift patient's chin (up) to improve access to the maxilla and tuck chin (down) to improve access to the mandible

Figure 7–6   Avoid crossing knees.

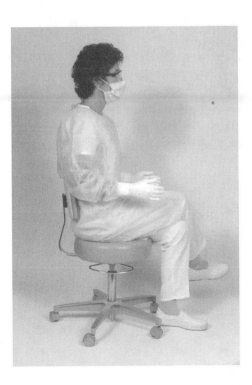

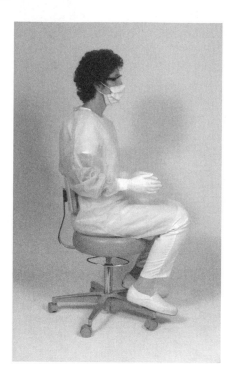

Figure 7–7   Avoid placing feet on chair rungs.

6. Position patient closer to the top of the chair to prevent from leaning over patient; use pillows, covered with barriers, or special children's seats to allow small children to sit closer to the top of the dental chair
7. Use supplemental head/neck/back supports for the elderly and patients with neck stiffness, osteoporosis, or other types of disabilities; cover all supports with infection control barriers such as plastic bags or headrest covers; supports include a variety of devices:

Figure 7–8   Avoid balancing weight on toes.

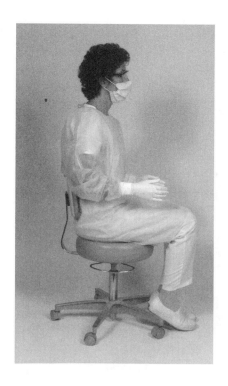

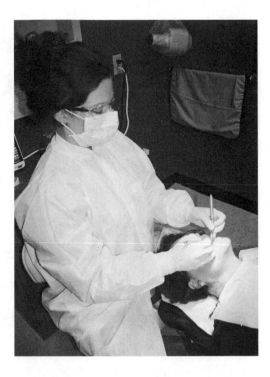

Figure 7–9   Maintain neutral arm and wrist position.

a. Special pillows that conform to individual's neck, filled with polystyrene beads, memory foam, or natural plant materials (Figure 7–11)
b. Small round, flat, or U-shaped air-filled or foam neck supports
c. Terrycloth towel rolled into the shape of a log or a roll of paper towels

C. Equipment placement: To access hand instruments, polishing devices, evacuation systems, power-driven scalers, and dental lights, position dental equipment to avoid any unnecessary bending and stretching;[1, 4, 6]

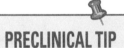

PRECLINICAL TIP

Positioning Your Knowledge: Exercise: While sitting, place hands on lower back with elbows bent. Pull back, bringing elbows together. Release and repeat.[4]

Figure 7–10   Avoid raising to a position with less than 60 degrees between the arms and forearms.

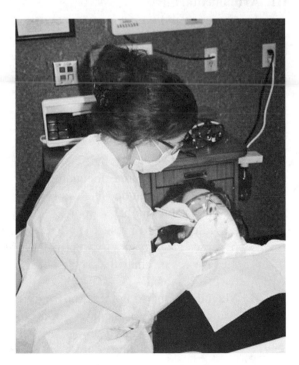

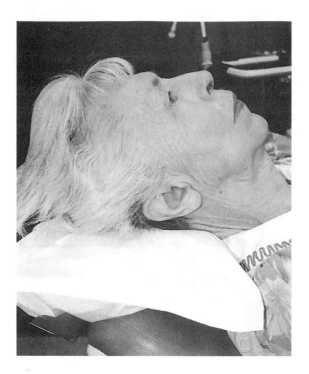

Figure 7–11   Use of a supplemental head support.

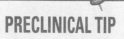
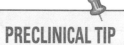
ways to reduce unnecessary bending, reaching, and stretching, and to maintain a neutral body posture include

1. Avoid flexion, extension, or deviation from a neutral position by properly positioning the neck, shoulders, elbows, and wrists
2. Place all frequently used instruments and equipment within an arm's length of reach, including dental light
3. Use side delivery, on the operator's dominant side, or over-the-patient delivery systems; avoid rear delivery systems
4. Adjust dental equipment height so it is compatible with the height of the operator

III. Armamentarium

The varieties and types of equipment used in the clinical setting can have a profound influence on the operator's overall well being, affecting comfort and reducing fatigue. Several categories of devices or equipment have a significant ergonomic effect and should be evaluated.

A. Operator chair: Dental clinicians spend the majority of their working day sitting. Select a chair that allows adequate body support for the back, legs and arms;[2, 4, 7, 8] operator chair should include the following characteristics

1. Adequate padding, sufficient to support body weight comfortably
2. Large seating area, adequate to provide good thigh support
3. Stable seat that does not rock
4. Adjustable lumbar support
5. Adjustable arm rests to give a relaxed rest area for the forearms
6. Low center of gravity to prevent chair from tilting
7. Five-caster chair that rotates freely and is not encumbered by debris (Figure 7–12)

B. Magnification: Magnification loupes are the most critical piece of equipment to help maintain good posture.[1, 3, 9] In addition, operators wearing magnification loupes are able to perform more precise, demanding clinical procedures.[10, 11, 12, 13, 14, 15] Reading glasses do not

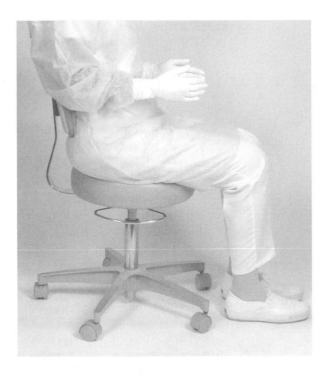

Figure 7–12   Use a five-caster chair that rotates freely.

provide operators with depth of field and therefore are not an appropriate substitute for magnification loupes. Also, wearing reading glasses with a higher diopter than an operator needs will only shorten the wearer's working distance, resulting in a more compromised posture. Magnification loupes offer the following benefits (Figure 7–13)

1. Improve posture by working in an upright position
2. Allow head movement within a five-inch range while still maintaining a clear view of the mouth
3. Decrease neck, shoulder, and back fatigue
4. Improve effectiveness for diagnosis and clinical treatment
5. Designed with the following features:

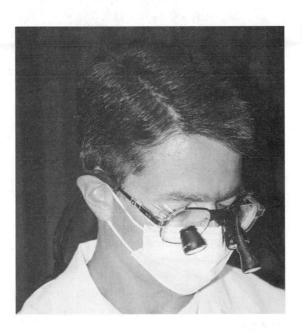

Figure 7–13   Magnification loupes.

a. Fabricated with the proper focal length for each operator
   (1) Through-the-lens (TTL) magnification loupes, fabricated by mounting loupes directly into a lens carrier
      (a) Provide greater width and depth of field than flip-up magnification loupes with the same power of magnification
      (b) Provide greater comfort for most because the magnification is mounted directly into the carrier lens
      (c) Custom-made according to each operator's specific measurements; therefore TTL's are not interchangeable between operators
   (2) Flip-up magnification loupes have binoculars mounted on a hinge attached to a frame
      (a) Must position the binoculars to correspond with individual needs
      (b) Not interchangeable with operators who have dissimilar working ranges
      (c) Prescription changes can be made by personal optician
b. Customized to accommodate individual vision requirements for distance, reading, or astigmatism corrections
c. Counterbalance weight by using an eyeglass support system, such as adjustable band behind the operator's head

C. Lighting: Clinical dental hygiene procedures require adequate illumination.[6] Factors that can affect the overall quality of light available to the dental hygienist include the following:
1. Dental unit light: Provides adequate use; drift free, and easily adjustable
   a. White, shadow-free light—aids in making precise clinical judgments
      (1) Lighting can alter the color of tissue
      (2) Insufficient or shadowy light can interfere with the overall ability to assess oral conditions
   b. Light covers—need to be kept clean from dust, smudges, and dirt, which can reduce available light
2. Mirrors: Types include
   a. Scratch-free mirrors—improve visibility
   b. Fog-free mirrors—maintain by wiping often with a gauze square moistened with mouthwash
   c. Lighted mirrors add site-specific illumination

D. Operator headlights: Although the dental unit light provides a source of illumination for operators, an auxiliary headlight can give a small two- to three-inch, specific bright beam of direct light to the working area.[11, 13] A wide selection of headlights are available, which attach either to magnification loupes or a headband apparatus. Auxiliary headlights can either provide additional illumination to the working field or allow the operator to perform clinical procedures independent of a traditional dental light. Headlights are particularly valuable in nontraditional clinical settings such as hospitals, schools, or extended care facilities.
1. Functions
   a. Provide constant illumination of working field
   b. Improve operator visibility

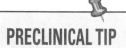

PRECLINICAL TIP

Positioning Your Knowledge:
Exercise: Position hands and arms straight above head. Stretch for 3 to 5 seconds. Release and repeat.[4]

2. Types
   a. Halogen lights
      (1) Do not provide as bright a light as fiber optic lights
      (2) One is available as battery-operated
      (3) Most must be plugged into a separate light generator
   b. Fiber optic lights
      (1) Lightweight
      (2) Provide a more precise beam with a greater light output
      (3) Must be plugged into a separate light generator
E. Gloves: A properly fitted glove is a key component for hand comfort (Figure 7–14).[1, 4, 16, 21, 32] It is imperative to select gloves that not only fit correctly, but are made of a non-irritating material.[17]
   1. Fit
      a. Should be adequate in the palm and wrist area (Figure 7–15)
         (1) Too tight—can cause constriction or irritation of delicate nerves and muscles
         (2) Too loose—decreases control and dexterity (Figure 7–16)
      b. Consider finger length as well
      c. Natural rubber latex gloves provide the most natural fit
      d. Recommend non-latex varieties to those concerned with potential allergic reactions to the plant proteins found in natural rubber latex
   2. Types of materials
      a. Two types are recommended for non-latex gloves
         (1) Nitrile rubber
            (a) Consists of a synthetic elastic material
            (b) Noted for its resistance to oil and many chemicals
            (c) More puncture resistant
         (2) Chloroprene
            (a) Consists of a synthetic rubber
            (b) Noted for its resistance to ozone, weathering, oil, and many chemicals
            (c) Adapts to hand sizes more comfortably than many nitrile products because of its softness and elasticity
      b. Powdered gloves are easier to don, but the powder can cause contact dermatitis in some wearers
         (1) Majority of gloves use cornstarch, which is less irritating than talc

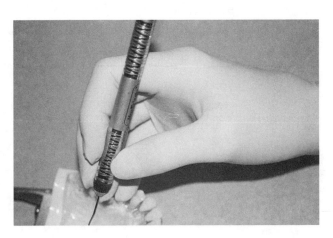

Figure 7–14   Wear properly fitting gloves.

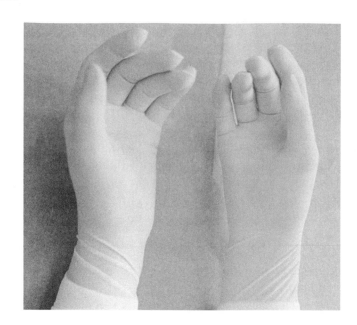

Figure 7–15   Incorrect glove size—tight palm with an incorrect finger length.

(2) Since the powder absorbs moisture, which reduces the discomfort from hand perspiration, dry skin can result

(3) Latex proteins can bind with the powder in latex gloves; this latex-contaminated powder may become aerosolized

c. Powder-free gloves—some have a special coating to make them easier to put on and take off

d. Textured gloves—surface provides traction for a better grip, even when wet, than gloves with a smooth finish

e. Right- and left-fitted gloves—fabricated so the thumb remains in a natural position relative to the palm (Figure 7–17); this is particularly beneficial in preventing hand fatigue, especially during lengthy procedures

f. Ambidextrous gloves—appropriate for all procedures but should be avoided by operators who experience thumb discomfort

F. Hand instruments: A wide variety of hand instruments are available today.[16, 18, 19] Operators should consider the following characteristics when selecting hand instruments:

Figure 7–16   Incorrect glove size—too large.

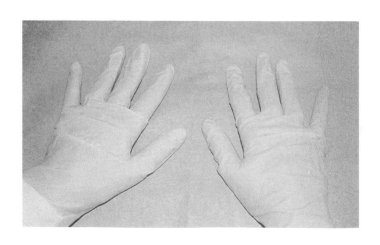

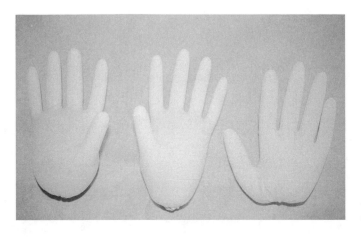

Figure 7–17 Types of gloves–right- and left-fitted gloves; ambidextrous gloves.

1. Handles
   a. Large diameter handles reduce pinch/grip on the shaft (Figures 7–18 and 7–19)
   b. Textured handles provide more traction and decrease pinch grip
   c. Padded handles reduce operator grip
   d. Autoclavable textured silicone grips can be added to existing instrument handles to increase diameter and reduce instrument pinch/grip (Figure 7–20)
   e. Disposable foam grips for mirror handles cushion the grip, which is especially beneficial when the mirror is used as a retraction tool
2. Double-ended instruments provide more balance than single-ended instruments
3. Sharp blades reduce overall pressure during instrumentation and increase effectiveness of calculus removal
4. Weights can vary by
   a. Material—instruments made with lightweight resin, hollow metal handles, or a combination of both are lighter in weight than all-metal varieties
   b. Balance—instruments designed so the weight is evenly balanced over the entire length of shaft
G. Polishing handpieces: Despite an increased emphasis on selective polishing, the slow-speed polishing handpiece still represents an important part of clinical appointments.[18, 19, 20, 21] The following factors should be considered in handpiece selection:

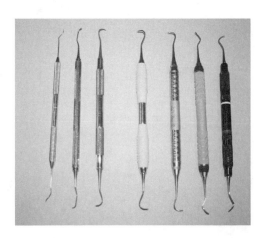

Figure 7–18 Small diameter instrument handles versus ergonomic shaft designs.

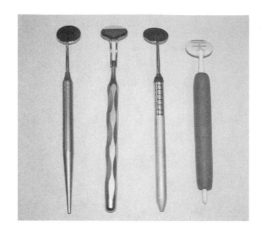

Figure 7–19   Large handled textured instruments—provide more traction and decrease pinch grip.

1. Weight
    a. Overall weight can vary from as little as 3 oz to more than 9 oz; heavier weight handpieces exhibit greater potential for hand fatigue and discomfort, so manufacturers have developed lighter weight polishing devices
    b. Balanced-weight handpieces are easier to hold; lightweight handpieces have been developed so the overall weight is evenly distributed over the length of the device rather than concentrated at the hose end, which causes unnecessary strain on the hand and wrist
2. Ability to swivel—non-swiveling handpieces can cause a deviated wrist position
    a. Use a polishing handpiece fabricated with a 360-degree swivel to reduce unnecessary torque on the hand or wrist
    b. Types of handpiece swivels
        (1) Fingertip swivel—allows altering the position of the prophy angle with a slight twist at the fingertips
        (2) Hose end swivel—allows for freely changing the angle of the polishing head
3. Larger diameter—allows grasping more loosely because less pinch grip is required to hold the handpiece shaft; larger handles allow operators to have a looser grip on the polishing device while still having control over the handpiece
4. Textured surface—improves grip

Figure 7–20   Adaptive silicone grips for instrument handles.

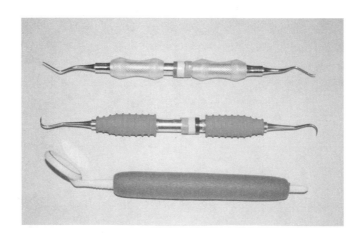

5. Locking mechanism—stabilizes polishing angle

6. Cordless polishing handpiece—eliminates air-hose weight and drag

H. Prophy polishing angles

1. Types

   a. Disposable plastic angles are lighter in weight than all-metal angles

     (1) Traditional configuration—designed to replicate all-metal angles and available in either contra- or right-angle designs

     (2) Extended straight attachment—elongated angle that replaces the metal shaft on some slow-speed polishing handpieces in addition to functioning as a polishing device

   b. All-metal angles—add weight to handpiece

2. Design

   a. Right-angle design requires flexion and extension of wrist in order to properly adapt the prophy cup to areas of the tooth surfaces

   b. Contra-angle design has a slight bend in the angle shaft, which facilitates a neutral wrist position during polishing procedures[20, 21]

3. Prophy cups

   a. Soft cups reduce polishing pressure, whereas firm cups increase fatigue

   b. Petite or junior-size cups are designed for areas with restricted access

I. Air hoses and hose positioning: Hoses that connect handpieces, air/water syringes, and suction systems can have a significant ergonomic impact on the wrist, forearm, and shoulder. Therefore, it is important to reduce any unnecessary weight, drag, or pull created by heavy, rigid, tightly-coiled, or short hose apparatus.[4, 18, 20, 21] It is also important to position all instruments that have hose or vacuum connections within easy reach.[1, 4, 6, 21]

1. Characteristics of hoses

   a. Tightly coiled versus smooth hose

     (1) Tightly coiled hoses—heavy, difficult to disinfect and maneuver; may increase resistance

     (2) Smooth hoses—reduce the overall drag and torque on the wrist and hand

   b. Rigid versus flexible hoses

     (1) Rigid hoses—limit the hand and wrist movements

     (2) Flexible hoses—easy to manipulate

   c. Short versus long hoses—short hoses cause unnecessary stress to the musculature of the hand

   d. Heavy versus lightweight hoses

     (1) Heavy hoses—require support of unnecessary weight as well as reduce tactile sensitivity

     (2) Lightweight hoses—easy to manipulate

2. Instruments with air or vacuum hose connections include

   a. Polishing handpiece

   b. Power-driven scaler

   c. Air/water syringe

   d. Saliva ejector

3. Handpiece positioning

a. Over-patient delivery—maintains neutral body postures
b. Raise bracket table—reduces overall weight of the handpiece cord
c. Extra long polishing hose—allows operator to drape the balance of the cord over the forearm

J. Suction devices: Saliva ejectors provide more flexibility than the heavier high-velocity (volume) evacuators. They are available in a variety of designs, ranging from a traditional plastic device to a curved design, which can be placed in either the buccal or lingual vestibule.

1. Certain curved configurations allow the saliva ejector to be placed in a stationary position in the patient's mouth, eliminating the need for the patient or operator to hold the device (Figure 7–21)
2. Evacuation devices available for polishing (Figure 7–22) include
   a. Padded saliva ejector or saliva ejector pillow—provides increased patient comfort and can be used as check retractors
   b. "Curly q" saliva ejector
   c. Mirror suction device—contains suction holes, can be attached to a vacuum hose, and allows for simultaneous evacuation and visibility
   d. Jet Shield—device that attaches to aid evacuation of aerosol produced by air polishers

IV. Occupational Risk Factors

The practice of dental hygiene presents a wide variety of occupational risk factors for musculoskeletal injuries.[22] WMSDs can result from a combination of clinical activities coupled with a variety of psychological risk factors;[1, 2, 7, 23, 24, 25, 26, 27] they can also be brought on by a single strain or trauma. Since these problems are frequently multifactorial, it is important to understand significant risk factors.[1, 2, 4, 6, 28, 29]

A. Cumulative trauma disorders

1. These disorders include a wide variety of physical injuries sustained by many types of workers
2. They are associated with jobs and tasks that involve repetitious movements over prolonged periods of time

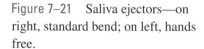

Figure 7–21   Saliva ejectors—on right, standard bend; on left, hands free.

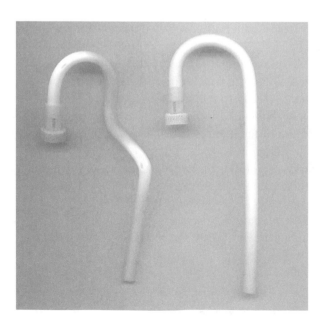

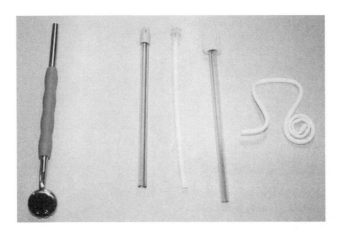

Figure 7–22   Types of suction devices (from left to right)—Mirror suction device, plastic-tipped saliva ejector, foam-tipped saliva ejector, padded saliva ejector, and a "curly q".

3. Most involve both muscles and nerves and can be short term and episodic in nature; in some cases can result in permanent impairment or disability[30]

B. Increase in musculoskeletal injuries among dental hygienists
1. The overall demographics of the dental hygiene profession have changed over the last four decades, just as the demographics of the entire workforce are not the same
2. More women are participating in the workforce for longer periods of time
3. Additional reasons for increased risk for injuries among dental hygienists include
   a. Longer professional careers
   b. Complex periodontal procedures that are more frequently scheduled
   c. Profession is more commonly full time than part time
   d. Increased emphasis on production in dental practices

C. Job and task risk factors
1. Forceful exertions: Tenacious deposits can be difficult to remove, often requiring significant force with hand scalers and curettes.[7, 21, 31] The application of force should *not* be applied to exploratory strokes, but rather reserved for the removal of deposits only. Advancements in power-driven scalers and the development of slimmer tips now allow for effective removal of deposits with reduced hand stress. Hand instrumentation can include hand movements, which result in the following actions:
   a. Sustained pinch grip—holding tightly to small diameter instruments with the thumb, index, and middle finger together
   b. Pulling motions—applied to hand instruments when removing deposits
   c. Mechanical stresses to digital nerves from sustained grasps—holding hand instruments for prolonged periods of time
2. Awkward clinician posture or position: Clinical dental hygiene procedures frequently place operators in compromising postural positions.[2, 6, 24] The negative effects of awkward positioning are magnified as these postures are maintained over a protracted period of time.[21, 23, 27, 33] Care must be taken to avoid positions that place unnecessary stress on the body's skeletal and neuromuscular apparatus. Positions to avoid include

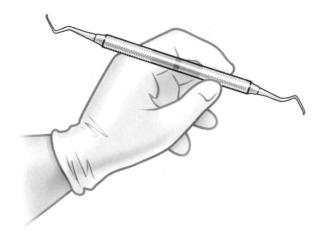

Figure 7–23   Wrist flexion.

     a. Deviating wrist from a neutral position, including flexion (Figure 7–23), extension (Figure 7–24), and radial and ulnar deviations

     b. Placing wrist or hand in awkward position

     c. Elevating elbow higher than 30-degrees (Figure 7–25)

     d. Bending forward from a sitting posture with hunched or rounded shoulders

     e. Raising one shoulder higher than the other (Figure 7–26)

     f. Bending head to one side; leaning head forward in an unsupported position by shoulder and neck

     g. Twisting the trunk of the body (Figure 7–27)

3. Repetition

     a. Majority of procedures performed in clinical dental hygiene, both manual and power-driven tasks, involve prolonged periods of repetition[16, 21, 24]

     b. High number of exertions or motions per unit of time involve

        (1) Hands, wrists, and/or arm movements

        (2) Vibration from both polishing and power-scaling devices

           (a) Generally these devices can be operated at lower speeds

Figure 7–24   Wrist extension.

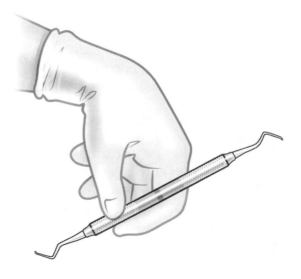

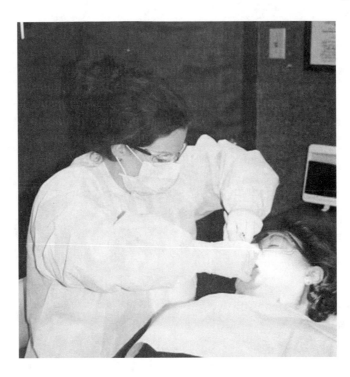

Figure 7–25 Avoid elevating elbows higher than 30 degrees.

     (b) Manually tuned power scalers can be adjusted to lower overall vibration, which reduces operator fatigue

4. Static loading: Dental hygienists often sit in static positions for long periods of time.[6, 23, 33] Static positions increase and accelerate muscle fatigue. Consider the following strategies to eliminate or reduce static loading:
  a. Take frequent breaks
  b. Work with feet on the floor
  c. Change sitting or standing position frequently

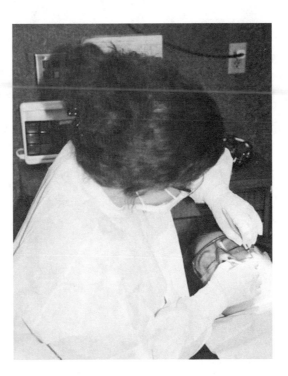

Figure 7–26 Avoid raising one shoulder higher than the other.

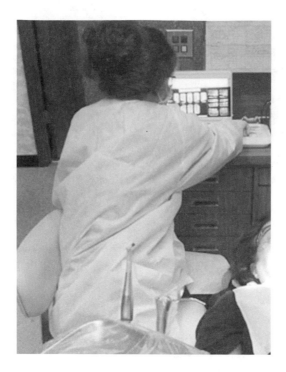

Figure 7–27   Avoid twisting trunk of body.

   d. Utilize backrest on operator chair
   e. Keep arms close to torso (Figure 7–28)
   f. Change instruments frequently
5. Localized contact stressors: A variety of other factors can increase physical risks for injury:
   a. Forcefully gripping small diameter tools
   b. Edge of chair seat cutting into back of thigh
   c. Resting wrists on sharp counter edge while writing

Figure 7–28   Work with arms comfortably close to torso.

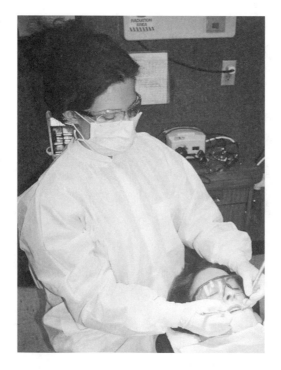

D. Psychosocial risk factors: Although psychosocial risk factors may be difficult to quantify and may vary in each work setting, they can have a significant modifying effect on the overall attitude of a worker.[35] It is important not to dismiss the impact of the common factors and concerns of practicing hygienists, which include

1. Performing repetitive work
2. Pressure to complete procedures in a specific timeframe
3. Feeling a lack of control over work pace
4. Lack of social support within the work setting
5. Too much or too little responsibility within a dental practice
6. Ability to cope with pain or minimize discomfort

E. Predisposing personal factors: Predisposing physical factors can exacerbate many injuries that are classified as RSIs.[24] WRMIs are much more likely to occur in workers who exhibit the following characteristics:

1. Poor general muscle tone
2. Abnormalities in size of carpal tunnel due to genetics or injury
3. Medical conditions such as arthritis and diabetes
4. Fluid retention
5. Pregnancy or taking oral contraceptives
6. Age—includes overall body strength and flexibility

F. Individual risk factors: The following factors may also increase the risk of occupational injuries. However, note that each can be modified by a lifestyle change.[6, 21, 33]

1. Leisure activities, such as knitting, gardening, and bike riding, place stress on small muscle groups
2. Lack of exercise or activity; obesity

G. Work organization factors: Since there will never be a standard dental hygiene practice day or patient load, it is important to consider the overall effect of the following factors and recognize that as the workload increases in intensity, difficulty, and number of days worked, the risk for injury will increase.[1, 21] Continuous dental hygiene practice, year after year, may also increase the potential for problems. Dental hygienists can negotiate a number of these factors in their employment settings.

1. Number of days worked per week
2. Total number of patients seen per day
3. Length of work shift
4. Number of back-to-back difficult cases
5. Number of rest breaks (laws in many states require rest breaks)
6. Environmental factors such as
   a. Noise—hard surfaces reflect sound; consider the overall effect from sources such as suction, handpiece, or power-driven scalers[20]
   b. Room temperature—cold room temperatures can aggravate some RSIs such as carpal tunnel syndrome[21]
   c. Lighting—insufficient lighting can create operator eyestrain[6]
   d. Physical layout of treatment facility—properly planned treatment rooms limit unnecessary operator bending and stretching; place frequently used items in easy-to-reach locations[1, 4, 5]

V. Personal Protection

Despite that dental hygiene practice can place enormous strain on the body, it is important to accept responsibility for good physical and mental

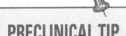

PRECLINICAL TIP

Positioning Your Knowledge: Since many dental hygienists work in environments where they are the only dental hygienist, many experience feelings of isolation. Therefore, it is important to make a concerted effort to remain in contact with other colleagues through activities such as professional meetings, study clubs, continuing education seminars, and dental hygiene Internet groups. Educational activities, networking, and reading professional journals help keep clinicians emotionally energized and refreshed.

health habits.[1] Operators who suffer from inadequate rest, insufficient exercise, chronic worry, high levels of stress, or poor nutrition cannot provide optimal dental hygiene services, and they place their bodies at higher risk for developing RSIs.[34, 35, 36, 37, 38] Activities and practices to try to incorporate on a regular basis include

A. Exercise, stretching, flexibility, and/or weight training—reduces stress and increases physical strength
B. Yoga or meditation—reduces stress and improves physical well-being
C. Good blood flow—necessary for soft tissue health
D. Massage therapy—promotes healthy soft tissue, improves circulation, and reduces muscular fatigue and tension
E. Chiropractic treatment—assures proper alignment of the body's skeletal, musculature, and nervous systems
F. Biofeedback training—promotes effective stress management
G. Personal hydration—supplies adequate fluid intake for the body
H. Vitamins/nutritional supplements—supply proper nutrients to help keep body healthy
I. Herbal teas or supplements—offer a calming effect and can aid in promoting rest
J. Adequate rest—allows the body to rejuvenate
K. Ergonomic pillow—designed to provide adequate support for the head and neck
L. Comfortable shoes—properly fitting shoes reduce leg and foot fatigue
M. Magnetic technology—some find that products designed with magnets reduce overall muscular pain

Dental hygiene can be a rewarding profession. However, it is physically taxing and mentally challenging, especially to those who practice daily over a period of several years. Since the foundation of dental hygiene practice is prevention, it is imperative to learn as many ergonomic preventive strategies as possible during the formal educational process. Dental hygienists, who take ownership of their careers and practice in an ergonomically safe manner from inception are less likely to develop workplace-related injuries and can look forward to a long and more comfortable career.

Once bad ergonomic habits develop, it can be time-consuming and difficult to learn new ways of working safely. While it is not possible to accurately predict who will develop a career-threatening injury or when a disability will occur, prevention is still the key to avoiding workplace-related musculoskeletal disorders. Countless hours of worry and physical discomfort can be avoided by adopting safe working habits. No amount of compensation will ever be sufficient to offset the devastating effects of a permanent disability or work-related injury.

Today, more and more dental hygienists are taking an active position in preventing injuries and reducing the risk of career burnout. For example, student and graduate hygienists are purchasing custom-made magnification loupes and larger diameter hand instruments and power scalers. Left-handed students are choosing to be right-handed operators, understanding that they will likely have to work in an area designed for the right-handed operator. Many operators are learning to understand the importance of realistic expectations rather than perfectionism, and they pace their clinical and personal lives accordingly. The emphasis on physical fitness in today's society further supports the goal of preventing injuries. Actions like these were unheard of decades ago, but they ensure a long, productive, and injury-free career.

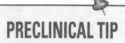

PRECLINICAL TIP

Positioning Your Knowledge: Dental hygienists should engage in activities that promote sound body and mind. These include hobbies or other activities that produce intellectual stimulation and/or relaxation and provide a sense of balance in life.

QUESTIONS

1. All of the following are proper posture techniques to be performed by the practicing clinical hygienist EXCEPT one. Which one is the EXCEPTION?
   a. Position head and neck directly over shoulders.
   b. Lean forward from the hips, keeping the back straight.
   c. Position arms more than 20 degrees away from the body.
   d. Keep arms as close to sides as possible.

2. In relationship to the operator's hips and knees, which of the following is the proper height of the operator's chair?
   a. The knees are slightly higher than the hips.
   b. The knees are parallel to the hips.
   c. The hips are slightly higher than the knees.
   d. There is no relationship between the hips and knees.

3. To maintain a neutral body posture, the operator should reduce unnecessary bending and stretching during the appointment. One way to do this is to place frequently used instruments an arm's length away from the seated position.
   a. The first statement is TRUE. The second statement is FALSE.
   b. The first statement is FALSE. The second statement is TRUE.
   c. Both statements are TRUE.
   d. Both statements are FALSE.

4. All of the following are positions operators should avoid EXCEPT one. Which one is the EXCEPTION?
   a. Keep wrist in neutral position
   b. Raise one shoulder higher than the other.
   c. Bend head to one side.
   d. Round the shoulders.

5. When selecting an operator chair, which of the following characteristics should the dental hygienist consider?
   a. The chair should have four casters.
   b. The seat should provide thin padding.
   c. The chair should provide a high center of gravity.
   d. The chair should have adjustable lumbar support.

6. All of the following strategies help eliminate or reduce static loading EXCEPT one. Which one is the EXCEPTION?

   a. Taking frequent breaks
   b. Keeping arms close to torso during instrumentation
   c. Working with feet elevated when possible
   d. Changing instruments frequently

7. Magnification loupes enable the operator to perform more precise clinical procedures. Flip-up magnification loupes provide a greater width and depth of field than through-the-lens magnification loupes.
   a. The first statement is TRUE. The second statement is FALSE.
   b. The first statement is FALSE. The second statement is TRUE.
   c. Both statements are TRUE.
   d. Both statements are FALSE.

8. While providing patient services, how should the operator be positioned on the operator's chair?
   a. Sit at the front edge of the seat with both feet planted firmly on the floor.
   b. Sit at the front edge of the seat with one foot on the base of the chair.
   c. Sit on the entire seat with one foot on the base of the chair.
   d. Sit on the entire seat with both feet planted firmly on the floor.

9. When evaluating dental equipment for ergonomic reasons, all of the following are acceptable features EXCEPT one. Which one is the EXCEPTION?
   a. Rigid hoses
   b. Swivel handpieces
   c. Long cord hoses
   d. Soft prophy cups

10. To help prevent unnecessary bending or twisting, the patient's chair should be positioned at a height where the operator can maintain a neutral body position. In addition, lifting the patient's chin to improve working on the mandibular arch and tucking the chin to work on the maxillary arch will also help the operator's body remain in a neutral position.
    a. Both statements are TRUE.
    b. Both statements are FALSE.
    c. The first statement is TRUE. The second statement is FALSE.
    d. The first statement is FALSE. The second statement is TRUE.

REFERENCES

1. Michalak-Turcotte, C., & M. Atwood-Sanders. Ergonomic Strategies for the Dental Hygienist, Part II. *Journal of Practical Hygiene,* 9(3), 35–38, 2000.

2. Nunn, P. J. Posture for Dental Hygiene Practice. In D. C. Murphy (Ed.), *Ergonomics and the Dental Care Worker.* Washington, D.C.: *American Public Health Association,* 1998, pp. 217–236.

3. Rucker, L. M., & M. A. Boyd. Optimizing Dental Operatory Working Environments. In D. C. Murphy (Ed.), *Ergonomics and the Dental Care Worker.* Washington, D.C.: *American Public Health Association,* 1998, pp. 301–318.

4. Tatro, D. E. Ergonomics for the Dental Hygienist. *Journal of Practical Hygiene,* 6(1), 35–39, 1997.

5. Oberg, T. Ergonomic Evaluation and Construction of a Reference Workplace in Dental Hygiene: A Case Study. *Journal of Dental Hygiene,* 67(5), 262–267, 1993.

6. Michalak-Turcotte, C. Controlling Dental Hygiene Work-Related Musculoskeletal Disorders: The Ergonomic Process. *Journal of Dental Hygiene,* 74(1), 41–48, 2000.

7. Milerad, E., & M. O. Ericson. Effects of Precision and Force Demands, Grip Diameter, and Arm Support During Manual Work: An Electromyographic Study. *Ergonomics,* 37(2), 255–64, 1994.

8. Parsell, D. E., M. D. Weber, B. C. Anderson, & G. W. Cobb, Jr. Evaluation of Ergonomic Dental Stools through Clinical Stimulation. *General Dentistry,* 48(4), 440–444, 2000.

9. Rucker, L. M., C. Beattie, C. McGregor, S. Sunell, & Y. Ito. Declination Angle and Its Role in Selecting Surgical Telescopes. *Journal of the American Dental Association,* 130(7), 1096–1100, 1999.

10. Rucker, L. M. Surgical Magnification: Posture Maker or Posture Breaker? In D. C. Murphy (Ed.), Ergonomics and the Dental Care Worker. Washington, D.C.: *American Public Health Association,* 1998, pp. 191–216.

11. Callen, C. What to Look for in Surgical Telescopes. *Dental Economics,* 91(6), 45,48, 2001.

12. Carter, J. Magnification in the Office. *Dental Equipment and Material,* 6(4), 10–11, 2001.

13. Morris, G. A., & M. I. Kokott. A Clear View No Longer Means a Stiff Neck. *Dental Economics,* 89(7), 82–4, 86, 1999.

14. Pencek, L. Benefits of Magnification in Dental Hygiene Practice. *Journal of Practical Hygiene,* 6(1), 13–15, 1997.

15. Syme, S. E., J. L. Fried, & H. E. Strassler. Enhanced Visualization Using Magnification Systems. *Journal of Dental Hygiene,* 71(5), 202–206, 1997.

16. Nunn, P. J., C. Hart, & F. Gaulden. "Perfect" Instrumentation Can be Hazardous to Your Health!—or Ergonomic Applications for the Prevention of Carpel Tunnel Syndrome. *Access,* 9(1), 37–43, 1995.

17. Powell, B. J., G. P. Winkley, J. O. Brown, & S. Etersque. Evaluations of the Fit of Ambidextrous and Fitted gloves: Implications for Hand Comfort, *Journal of the American Dental Association,* 125(9), 1235–1240, 1994.

18. Fredekind, R., & E. Cuny. Instruments Used in Dentistry. In D. C. Murphy (Ed.), *Ergonomics and the Dental Care Worker.* Washington D.C.: *American Public Health Association,* 1998, pp. 169–289.

19. Gomolka, K., & E. Cuny. Dental Ergonomics: Instrumental Ideas for Reducing Hand and Eye Strain. *Dental Products Report,* (3), 104–113, 2000.

20. Guignon, A. N. Handpiece. *Dental Economics,* 91(10), 96–100, 2001.

21. Gerwatowski, L. J., D. B. McFall, & D. J. Stach. Carpal Tunnel Syndrome—Risk Factors and Preventive Strategies for the Dental Hygienist. *Journal of Dental Hygiene,* 66(2), 89–94, 1992.

22. Liss, G., & E. Jesin. Musculoskeletal Problems Among Dental Hygienists: A Canadian Study. In D. C. Murphy (Ed.), *Ergonomics and the Dental Care Worker.* Washington, D.C.: *American Public Health Association,* 1998, pp. 143–168.

23. Finsen, L., H. Christensen, & M. Bakke. Musculoskeletal Disorders Among Dentists and Variation in Dental Work. *Applied Ergonomics,* 29(2), 119–25, 1998.

24. Hagberg, M. ABC of Work-Related Disorders: Neck and Arm Disorders. *British Medical Journal,* 313(7054), 419–22, 1996.

25. Horstman, S. W., B. C. Horstman, & V. Horstman. Ergonomic Risk Factors Associated with the Practice of Dental Hygiene: A Preliminary Study. *American Society of Safety Engineers,* 49–53, April 1997.

26. Mani, L., & F. Gerr. Work-Related Upper Extremity Musculoskeletal Disorders. *Primary Care,* 27(4), 845–64, 2000.

27. Oberg, T., A. Karznia, L. Sandsjo, & R. Kadefors. Workload, Fatigue and Pause Patterns in Clinical Dental Hygiene. *Journal of Dental Hygiene,* 89(5): 223–29, 1995.

28. Liskiewicz, S. T., & W. E. Kerschbaum. Cumulative Trauma Disorders: An Ergonomic Approach for Prevention. *Journal of Dental Hygiene,* 71(4), 162–67, 1997.

29. Poindexter, S. M. All the Right Moves: Ergonomics and the Dental Hygienist at Work. *Access,* 9(1), 19–28, 33, 1995.

30. Stitik, T. P., Conte, M., Foye, P. M., Schoen, D., Marini, J. S. An Analysis of Cumulative Trauma Disorders in Dental Hygienists. *Journal of Practical Hygiene,* 9(2), 19–25, 2000.

31. Nunn, P. J. Getting a Handle on Ergonomic Periodontal Instrument Design. *Access,* 11(3), 16–19, 1997.

32. Michalak-Turcotte, C., & M. Atwood-Sanders. Ergonomics Strategies for the Dental Hygienist, Part I. *Journal of Practical Hygiene,* 9(2), 39–42, 2000.

33. Bleeker, M. L. A Medical-Ergonomic Program for Prevention of Upper Extremity and Back Disorders in the Practice of Dentistry. In D. C. Murphy (Ed.), *Ergonomics and the Dental Care Worker.* Washington, D.C.: *American Public Health Association,* 1998, pp. 341–354.

34. Grace, E. Stress in the Practice of the Art and Science of Dentistry. In D. C. Murphy (Ed.), *Ergonomics and the Dental Care Worker.* Washington, D.C.: *American Public Health Association,* 1998, pp. 113–128.

35. Caravon, P., M. J. Smith, & M. C. Haims. Work Organization, Job Stress, and Work-Related Musculoskeletal Disorders. *Human Factors,* 41(4), 644–63, 1999.

36. Stevens, M. M. Harmony in Hygiene. *RDH,* 16(12), 27–29, 36, 1996.

37. Stevens, M. M. The Union of Mind and Body in Yoga Forges a Quiet and Relaxing Healing Process. *RDH,* 18(8), 44, 46–47, 1998.

38. Gorter, R. C., M. A. Eijkman, & J. Hoostraten. Burnout and Health Among Dutch Dentists. *European Journal of Oral Sciences,* 108(4), 261–67, 2000.

Chapter 8

Instrumentation

Nancy K. Mann, RDH, MSEd

 MediaLink

A companion CD-ROM, included free with each new copy of this book, supplements the procedures presented in each chapter. Insert the CD-ROM to watch video clips and view a large collection of color images that is also included. This multimedia library is designed to help you add a new dimension to your learning.

KEY TERMS

adaptation. Relationship between the working end (cutting edge) of the instrument and surface of the tooth when the terminal third of the working end is flush against the tooth.

angulation. Angle formed by the working end (cutting edge) of an instrument and the tooth surface.

channel scaling. Systematic overlapping pattern of strokes as wide as the toe/tip third of an instrument's cutting edge to help insure complete scaling of the tooth.

cross section. Section formed by a plane cutting through an object.

curette. Instrument with sharp cutting edges that meet at a rounded toe—forms a rounded back and has a spoon-shaped face; used for subgingival and supragingival scaling.

cutting edge. Line formed where the face and lateral edges of the working end meet at an angle.

dominant hand. Hand used for performing tasks that require control and precision; usually the writing hand.

exploration. Use of the tip of a dental instrument to evaluate a tooth or root surface.

face. Surface between the two lateral surfaces that converge to form a cutting edge; opposite the back of the instrument.

fulcrum. Point of stabilization for instrumentation with the ring finger.

handle. Part of the instrument that is held in the hand.

illumination (also called indirect illumination). Pool of light created from the dental light off the face of the mouth mirror.

indirect vision. Use of the mouth mirror for viewing intraoral structures.

insertion. Process of placing the instrument into the gingival sulcus.

lateral pressure. Pressure applied against the tooth surface with a scaling instrument when removing deposits during the working stroke.

lateral surface. Surface that meets the face to form two cutting edges.

line angle. Line formed by the junction of two tooth surfaces.

long axis. An imaginary dividing line that runs down the center of a tooth.

mirror-image. Double-ended instruments with paired working ends that complement each other; used for access to proximal surfaces.

modified pen grasp. Grasp used to hold most instruments; instrument is held between the pads of the thumb and the index finger, with the side of the middle finger supporting the shank or placed lower on the handle.

nondominant hand. Opposite hand from the writing hand.

palm grasp. All four of the fingers contact the handle in the palm of the hand; grasp used for the air/water syringe and mirror.

parallel lines. Equally distant lines that run in the same direction and never meet.

perpendicular lines. Lines that meet at right angles.

retraction. Moving an obstruction, such as the tongue or the cheek, away from the task area for better access and control.

scaler. Instrument with sharp cutting edges that meet in a point; used for supragingival calculus removal.

shank. Part of the instrument that connects the handle to the working end; it is either straight or has one or more bends.

stroke. Single unbroken movement of an instrument during the task it was designed to perform.

exploratory stroke. Instrument movement used with a light grasp to evaluate tooth/root surface for deposits or surface irregularities.

horizontal stroke (circumferential). Movement of the instrument using a pull stroke perpendicular to the long axis of the tooth.

oblique stroke. Movement of the instrument using a pull stroke in a diagonal direction across the long axis of the tooth.

pull stroke. Movement of the instrument toward the clinician.

push stroke. Movement of the instrument away from the clinician.

scaling stroke. Movement of the instrument to dislodge and/or remove supragingival and subgingival calculus.

vertical stroke. Movement of the instrument using a pull stroke parallel to the long axis of the tooth.

walking stroke. A combination push/pull stroke used with a light grasp during exploration of a tooth/root surface.

working stroke. Activation of the instrument to perform a stroke.

tactile sensitivity. Ability to detect, through vibration, the texture and characteristics of the tooth/root surfaces by touching; changes in the surface of the tooth or root are transmitted from the instrument tip to the fingertips through the shank of the instrument.

terminal shank. Portion of the shank closest to the working end and an important part of the instrument for determining the correct working end, angulation, and adaptation.

tip. Pointed one-third of the working end of an explorer, probe, or sickle scaler.

toe. Rounded one-third of the working end of a curette.

transillumination. Reflection of light through the teeth with the mirror from the lingual aspect while the teeth are viewed from the facial.

universal (instrument). Instrument that can be used on all surfaces of all teeth; for example, universal curette.

working end. Part of the instrument used for the task or procedure; connects the shank at the opposite end of the handle and can be a blade or wire-like.

LEARNING OBJECTIVES

Upon reading this chapter, the student will be able to:

- identify classification, design name, and design number of instruments in student kit;
- identify the instrument shank and working end;
- demonstrate the proper technique and form for a modified pen grasp;
- demonstrate correct principles of instrumentation in the preclinical setting;
- discuss the purpose of instrument adaptation;
- differentiate between exploratory and working strokes;
- indicate where the mirror should be placed in the oral cavity in relation to the working area;
- describe the correct probing technique;
- discuss the role of the explorer in caries detection;
- discuss the role of the explorer in periodontal therapy;
- describe the correct exploring technique;
- identify the design features of the sickle scaler;
- differentiate between anterior and posterior (universal) sickle scalers;
- describe the correct instrumentation technique used with the posterior sickle scaler;
- describe the correct instrumentation technique used with the anterior sickle scaler;
- identify the design features of the universal curette;
- differentiate between the designs of the universal curette and sickle scaler;
- describe the correct instrumentation technique used with universal curette;
- identify the three types of strokes used during scaling;
- describe the use of lateral pressure when implementing scaling strokes;
- describe two methods used to determine instrument sharpness;
- discuss the primary objective of sharpening;
- describe the correct technique used to sharpen sickle scalers;
- differentiate between flat and curved sickle scalers and demonstrate how to sharpen each correctly;
- list the disadvantages of using a dull instrument during scaling;
- list and describe the different types of sharpening stones;
- describe the correct technique used to sharpen universal curettes.

I. Introduction

As reviewed in Chapter 7, proper positioning of the body and equipment are essential to help maintain a long, comfortable, and healthy career in dental hygiene. In addition, mastering sound principles of instrumentation, from the beginning of your career, will help develop skills that will make you an excellent clinician.

A. Seating positions

To determine appropriate seating positions for instrumentation in the mouth, use the small hand on the face of a clock as a guide. Clock seating positions enable the operator to sit and maneuver around the patient so access in the oral cavity is accomplished comfortably and efficiently.

1. Right-handed operator—utilize clock positions beginning at 7:30; work zone is through 11:30 to 12:00

2. Left-handed operator—utilize clock positions beginning at 4:30; work zone is through 12:00 to 12:30

B. Dental light position: To properly position the dental light, shine light onto patient's bib and slowly adjust into position on patient's dentition; avoid shining light in patient's eyes

1. Maxillary arch (Figure 8–1)—position light over the patient's chest and angle toward the maxillary teeth; adjust patient's chair nearly parallel with the floor with the patient's feet positioned slightly higher than the head

2. Mandibular arch (Figure 8–2)—direct light over the oral cavity toward the mandibular teeth (directly overhead); position patient's chair back at a 20-degree angle with the floor[1]

II. Instrument Characteristics and Design

Include three basic parts: handle, shank, and working end.

A. Handle: Portion of the instrument that is held

1. Sizes vary; common sizes include 3/8″, 5/16″, 1/4″, and 3/16″

a. Smaller handle may increase operator fatigue, since it is more difficult to grasp

b. Larger handle may decrease operator fatigue, since it is easier to grasp[2]

2. Composition

a. Hollow (empty in middle)

(1) Conducts vibrations with greater accuracy and amplification than a solid handle

(2) Provides good tactile sensitivity

(3) Eases handling due to lighter weight, producing less operator fatigue

b. Solid (filled with metal in the middle)—heavier to hold; decreases tactile responsiveness

c. Discussion of metals

(1) Stainless steel

PRECLINICAL TIP

Adapting Your Knowledge: Regardless of which clock seating position the operator chooses, the most important concept is to maintain a neutral body position.

PRECLINICAL TIP

Adapting Your Knowledge: Autoclaving does *not* change the hardness of an instrument, because the temperature required to temper or make a molecular change in steel tips is higher than 400° F.[4]

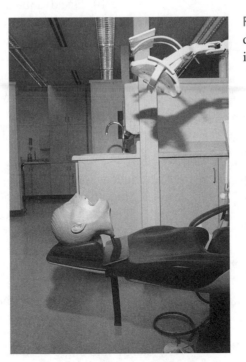

Figure 8–1 Properly positioned dental light when working on maxillary arch.

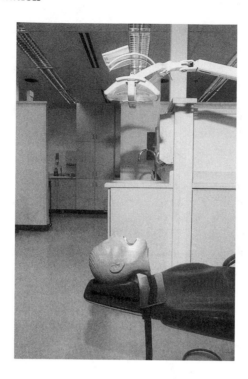

Figure 8–2   Properly positioned dental light when working on mandibular arch.

      (a) Advantages
- Resists corrosion
- Easy to maintain
- Lightweight

      (b) No disadvantages

  (2) Carbon steel

      (a) Advantages
- Holds a cutting edge for greater length of time
- More rigid

      (b) Disadvantages—more brittle, so more likely to fracture; corrodes easily
- Requires additional steps in sterilization and instrument processing, such as separating carbon from noncarbon instruments in the ultrasonic bath and sterilization, or there is a risk of cross corrosion
- Some manufacturers recommend a milk bath (special solution) for carbon steel items prior to sterilization; in addition, chemical vapor or dry heat is recommended over a steam autoclave

3. Surface texture (Figure 8–3)
  a. Smooth—difficult to hold (grasp) due to smooth texture
  b. Scored or serrated—easier to maintain grasp due to positive gripping surface[2, 3]
  c. Ribbed or knurled—easier to maintain grasp; can help increase tactile sensitivity and rotational control[4]
  d. Resin (medical grade resin overlaid on stainless steel)—provides a cushion grip that is less likely to slip and therefore provides comfort to the operator

B. Shank: Joins handle and working end; tapered and thinner than handle
1. Length and angle of shanks

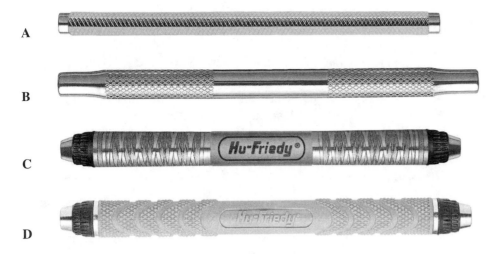

A

B

C

D

Figure 8–3   Types of surface textures on instruments. A. Smooth B. Scored or serrated C. Ribbed or knurled D. Resin. (Photo-Courtesy of Hu-Friedy Manufacturing Company)

    a. Length of shank—a longer shank is needed when instrumenting a longer crown length and greater/deeper pocket depth

    b. Angle of shank in relation to area of application

        (1) Anterior teeth—in general, the straighter the shank on an instrument, the more anterior its area of use; however, when using a universal scaler with an angled shank, both anterior and posterior teeth can be instrumented (e.g., IUFW 204); shank continues in a straight line with the handle

        (2) Posterior teeth—the longer and more curved the shank on an instrument, the more posterior its area of use; sometimes referred to as contra-angled, or offset; bend in shank removes it from the same plane as the handle

  2. Types of shanks

    a. Functional shank—portion of instrument between handle and working end (Figure 8–4)

    b. Terminal or lower shank—located nearest to working end and adjacent to blade; can be used as a visual guide to help determine correct end for instrumentation

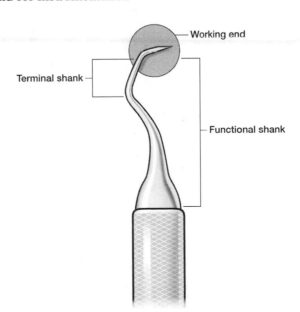

Working end

Terminal shank

Functional shank

Figure 8–4   The functional shank is the portion of the instrument between the handle and working end. The terminal shank is adjacent to the blade.

c. Flexible versus rigid—selection is based on the objective of the procedure to be performed, such as removing fine versus heavy calculus deposits
  (1) Flexible
    (a) Fluctuates slightly when encountering object
    (b) Use to detect subgingival calculus and/or remove fine calculus deposits
    (c) Provides the best tactile sensation to the operator's fingers through the shank and handle (e.g., explorers and curettes)[4]
  (2) Rigid
    (a) Enables instrument to withstand force of lateral pressure without flexing[5]
    (b) Decreases tactile sensitivity, but improves the ability to remove heavy calculus deposits (e.g., sickle scalers and rigid curettes)

C. Working end: Part of the instrument that determines its purpose and function
  1. Use and classification of instrument
    a. Single-ended—designed with only one working end
    b. Double-ended—designed with two different working ends; double-ended mirror-image working ends are paired for working in interproximal surfaces
    c. Cone socket handle—accepts a threaded insert containing the shank and working end of an instrument
    Note: A disadvantage of the cone socket tip is that it can become loose or torque while in use, and the thread pattern frequently does not allow for correct tip alignment and balance when fully secured.[6]
  2. Blade—the working end (cutting edge) of a sharp instrument; parts include (Figure 8–5a and 8–5b)
    a. Cutting edge—line where the lateral surface and face of blade meet
    b. Back—place where the lateral surfaces meet or are continuous to its formation
    c. Face—surface between the two lateral surfaces that converge to form a cutting edge, opposite the back of the instrument
    d. Tip—pointed end of a sickle scaler, explorer, or probe
    e. Toe—rounded end of a curette

> **PRECLINICAL TIP**
>
> **Adapting Your Knowledge:** While whole instruments are most commonly used, some regions of the country use cone socket instruments.

> **PRECLINICAL TIP**
>
> **Adapting Your Knowledge:** Some instruments have thinner blades, which allow access around tighter, healthy tissue or areas of restricted anatomy.

Figure 8–5A   Parts of the sickle scaler blade. Sickle scalers are triangular in cross section. Working ends are straight or curved.

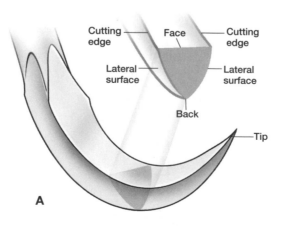

A

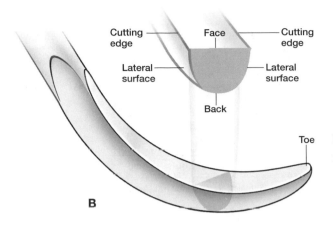

Cutting edge — Face — Cutting edge

Lateral surface — Lateral surface

Back

Toe

B

Figure 8–5B   Parts of the curette blade. Curette scalers are half-moon shaped in cross section.

D. Instrument balance: Occurs when working end of the instrument is in line with the center of the handle; an unbalanced instrument is more difficult to use due to increased stress on the muscles of the arm and hand[3] (Figure 8–6)

III. **Instrument Classifications**

Determined by instrument use, such as assessment or diagnostic, and scaling. Since the main focus of this textbook is for preclinical instruction, advanced instruments are not presented.

The following is an overview of instrument classifications. Each instrument is further described individually in detail by design, function, and use.

A. Periodontal probe: Assessment instrument used in periodontal charting and in measuring oral lesions or deviations, such as overjet or midline deviation

B. Explorer: Assessment instrument used for the detection of calculus, caries, and/or tooth or root surface irregularities, depending on design

C. Curette: Removes deposits and stain (see Table 8–1 for areas of application and usage)

D. Sickle scaler: Removes deposits and stain (see Table 8–1 for areas of application and usage)

E. Design name and number (Figure 8–7): States name of the instrument; often bears the name of the school or individual responsible for its development; instrument markings are labeled along the length or around the instrument handle

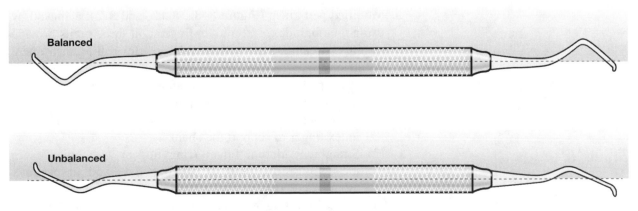

Balanced

Unbalanced

Figure 8–6   Instrument balance. Balance results when the working end of the instrument is in line with the center of the handle.

Table 8–1   Scaling Instrument Selection Guide

	Application	Working Ends	Shank	Purpose and Use
Anterior Sickle	Anterior sextants Supragingival	One or two, single or paired	Straight or slightly curved	Facial and linguals Interproximal calculus and stain removal
Posterior Sickle	Posterior sextants Supragingival	One or two, single or paired	Modified or contra-angled	Facial and linguals Interproximal calculus and stain removal
Universal Curette	Anterior sextants Supra- and subgingival	Two, paired	Flexible or rigid Straight	Circumferential of all tooth surfaces Light calculus deposit removal apical to gingival margin
	Posterior sextants Supra- and subgingival		Flexible or rigid Contra-angled	

This table has been adapted with permission from Colleen R. Schmidt, RDH, MS, "Task Analysis of the Nevi 1 and Nevi 2 Periodontal Instruments." *Journal of Practical Hygiene,* 11(3) 15–19, 2002.

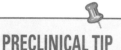

PRECLINICAL TIP

Adapting Your Knowledge: A left-handed operator may choose to instrument with the right hand, because many dental operatories in private practice are designed for right-handed operators.

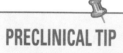

PRECLINICAL TIP

Adapting Your Knowledge: When fingertips are blanched, the grasp is too tight.

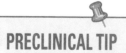

PRECLINICAL TIP

Adapting Your Knowledge: Place the shank of the instrument against the pad of the middle finger.

1. If labeled along the length of the handle, then each working end is identified by the number closest to it
2. If labeled around the handle, then the first number on the left identifies the working end at the top of the handle, and the second number identifies the working end at the bottom

F. Manufacturer's name: The name of the company that manufactures the instrument; many of the same types of instruments are manufactured by different companies

IV. **Principles of Instrumentation**

  A. Hands: For instrumentation, use the
   1. Dominant hand—the hand used to write
   2. Nondominant hand—use to hold mirror and retract in some areas

  B. Grasp
   1. How the clinician holds and controls movement of the instrument and maintains a firm finger rest in a controlled manner[7]
   2. Purposes
      a. Increases tactile sensitivity in the fingertips when using a light grasp
      b. Decreases trauma to hard and soft tissues, therefore reducing discomfort to the patient during the examination and scaling procedures
      c. Decreases fatigue in operator's arm, hand, and fingers[5]
   3. Types of grasps
      a. Modified pen grasp (Figure 8–8a, 8–8b, and 8–c); achieved by using thumb, index, and middle fingers; all three digits provide stability, strength, and control, and allow for rolling instrument in fingers
         (1) Place pads of bent thumb and index finger near junction of handle and shank across from one another
         (2) Place side of middle finger pad lower than the thumb and index finger to support the shank
         (3) Straighten fulcrum finger (ring finger) with knuckles in locked position; used to stabilize the hand in patient's mouth; keep fingers stacked
         (4) Relax little finger—serves no function and should be held in a comfortable manner

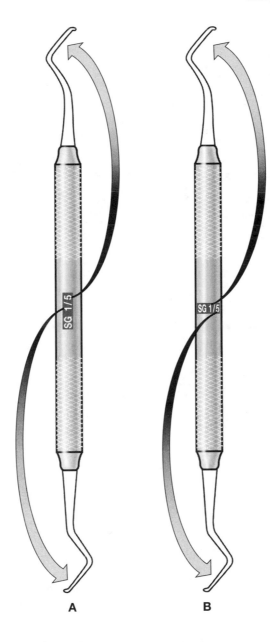

Figure 8–7 Design name and number. A. When the instrument markings are labeled along the length of the instrument handle, each working end is identified by the number closest to it. B. When the markings are labeled around the handle, the first number on the left identifies the working end at the top of the handle, and the second number identifies the working end at the bottom.

b. Palm grasp (Figure 8–9)
  (1) Provides little tactile sensitivity and flexibility
  (2) Utilize with
    (a) Air/water syringe; activate buttons with thumb pad
    (b) Mirror when *not* in use, such as in the anterior region when using index finger to retract lip
  (3) Placement
    (a) Place instrument handle in palm of hand
    (b) Cup the handle with palm and fingers
c. Pen grasp—using an instrument: (Figure 8–10a and 8–10b)
  (1) Place pads of bent thumb and index finger near junction of handle and shank across from one another
  (2) Place instrument *across* the pad of middle finger, which is lower than the thumb and index finger, to support the shank

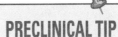

PRECLINICAL TIP

Adapting Your Knowledge: Some schools teach students to use the pen grasp when instrumenting the maxillary left lingual sextant.

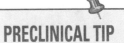

PRECLINICAL TIP

Adapting Your Knowledge: *Always* use a fulcrum with the dominant hand during instrumentation.

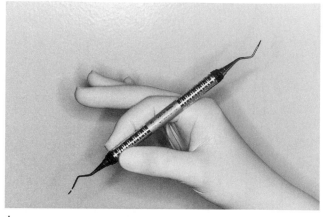

A

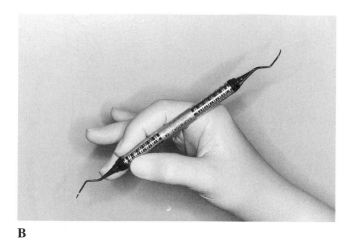

B

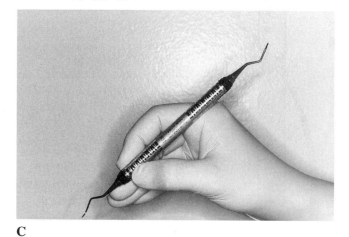

C

Figure 8–8   Forming the modified pen grasp. 8-8A. Place thumb and index finger pads across from one another near the junction of the handle. 8-8B. Place side of middle finger below the thumb and index finger. 8-8C. Modified pen grasp with straight fulcrum finger.

C. Instrument fulcrum
1. Support or finger on which the hand turns when moving an instrument; acts as a lever where hand pivots
2. Purposes
   a. Provides stability for the operator's grasp—fulcrum, or "finger rest," serves to stabilize the hand and instrument by providing a rest point when instrument is activated
   b. Helps prevent injury from uncontrolled pressure or movement
   c. Provides control of the instrument

PRECLINICAL TIP

Adapting Your Knowledge: When using the modified pen grasp, the fulcrum finger is the ring finger. It should remain in a straight and locked position.

Figure 8–9   Palm grasp.

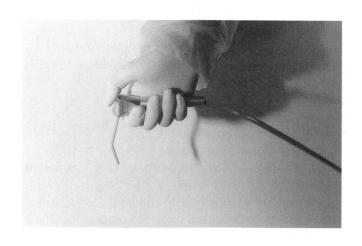

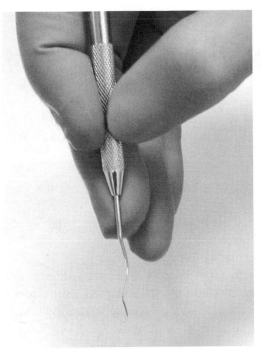
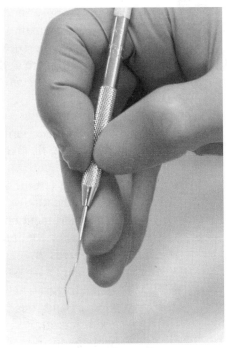

A   **B**

Figure 8–10   Instrument grasps. A. Modified pen grasp. B. Pen grasp is formed by placing instrument across the pad of the middle finger.

      d. Provides patient comfort by providing secure grasp of instrument

      e. Helps provide effective and efficient calculus removal—fulcrum becomes the pressure point to apply force for deposit removal

  3. Placement—intraoral fulcrum (Figure 8–11)

      a. Place fulcrum finger on tooth or teeth of same arch and as close as possible to working area—one to four teeth away; control of instrument is compromised when the fulcrum is positioned too far away

      b. Face palm toward occlusal or incisal plane

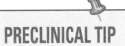

PRECLINICAL TIP

Adapting Your Knowledge: Instrumentation requires short fingernails! Not only can long fingernails cut the patient's soft tissue, but they can also interfere with a proper fulcrum and can harbor bacteria.

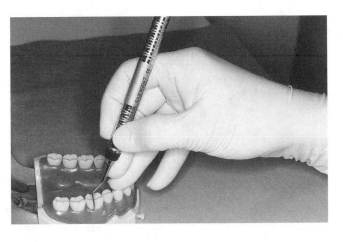

Figure 8–11   Intraoral fulcrum is established by placing fulcrum finger on tooth/teeth of same arch.

4. Pressure—apply moderate pressure on fulcrum finger to balance action of instrument
   a. Excessive pressure leads to decreased stability and tactile sensitivity and increased operator fatigue
   b. Light pressure can reduce effective deposit removal
D. Adaptation
   1. Relationship between the instrument and surface of the tooth or soft tissue; place terminal part of the working end, or lower one-third of blade, flush against the tooth
   2. Technique (Figure 8–12)
      a. Place the terminal shank of the instrument parallel to the long axis of the tooth
      b. Roll instrument between the thumb and index finger during activation for continued proper adaptation
   3. Difficult areas to maintain adaptation
      a. Line angles—instrument must be rolled between thumb and index finger to keep the end third of blade adapted against tooth
      b. Convex and rounded surfaces—due to unique anatomy of each tooth, carefully accommodate all concavities and convexities with the instrument
      c. Proximal root surface—cautiously place instrument far enough interproximally to get under contact
E. Insertion
   1. Place the instrument into the gingival sulcus
   2. Technique (Figure 8–13)
      a. Position terminal shank parallel to the long axis of tooth
      b. Use a short, oblique stroke and carefully insert the blade end third into the sulcus close to zero degree angulation (face of blade is closed and nearly flat against the surface) until resistance of the epithelial attachment is felt—soft and resilient like a rubber band
      c. Extend to the depth of the sulcus; utilize the periodontal chart to determine depth; avoid pushing down too forcefully, which could pierce the epithelial attachment
F. Angulation
   1. Angle formed with the tooth surface by the working end of an instrument

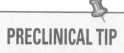

PRECLINICAL TIP

Adapting Your Knowledge: Maintain correct adaptation *and* angulation at all times. This assists with detection and removal of calculus.

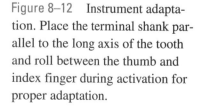

Figure 8–12   Instrument adaptation. Place the terminal shank parallel to the long axis of the tooth and roll between the thumb and index finger during activation for proper adaptation.

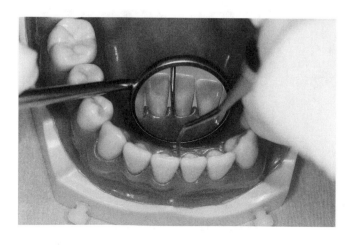

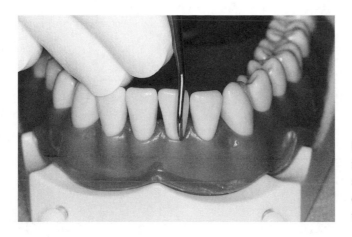

Figure 8–13   Proper instrument insertion. Using a short, oblique stroke, carefully insert the end third of the blade close to a zero angulation into the sulcus.

2. Angle can vary between 0 and 90 degrees depending on instrument and task
   a. Explorers—use to detect caries and explore supra- and subgingivally
      (1) Detecting caries—use 90-degree angle
      (2) Exploring supra- and subgingivally—use 5-degree angle or less during activation—angle is closed
   b. Scaler and curette—use to remove deposits and stain; use 45-degree to 90-degree angle during activation—blade angle is open (Figure 8–14)
G. Stroke
   1. A single unbroken movement made by an instrument
   2. Motions include
      a. Exploratory stroke to assess teeth
      b. Scaling stroke to remove deposits; directions include (Figure 8–15)
         (1) Vertical—stroke is parallel to long axis of tooth
         (2) Oblique or diagonal—stroke is diagonal to long axis of tooth
         (3) Horizontal—stroke is perpendicular to long axis of tooth

PRECLINICAL TIP

Adapting Your Knowledge: A light grasp enhances tactile sensitivity, allowing the operator to feel vibrations.

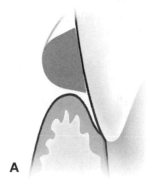
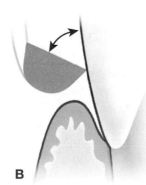
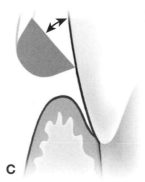
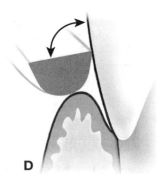

A   B   C   D

Figure 8–14   Blade angulation. A. Correct angulation for blade insertion—zero. B. Correct angulation for scaling—45 degrees to 90 degrees. C. Blade too closed for scaling—less than 45 degrees. D. Blade too open for scaling—more than 90 degrees.

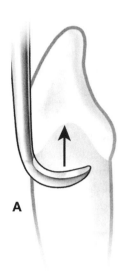
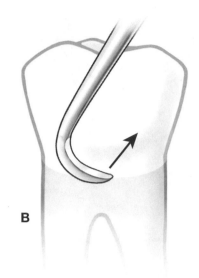
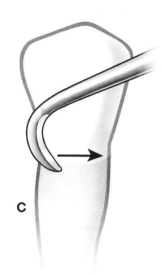

Figure 8–15   Basic stroke directions. A. Vertical B. Oblique C. Horizontal.

PRECLINICAL TIP

Adapting Your Knowledge: Follow correct and proper seating positions. Most errors made by beginning operators can be traced back to improper patient/operator positioning.

PRECLINICAL TIP

Adapting Your Knowledge: Caution: AVOID USING FINGER MOTIONS TO MAKE INSTRUMENT MOVE! This tires the fingers and produces ineffective strokes.

PRECLINICAL TIP

Adapting Your Knowledge: When properly using the wrist/forearm to rock, the handle of the instrument resembles a pendulum, swinging from side to side.

c. Push or insertion stroke allows access of instrument into gingival sulcus

3. Types of strokes
   a. Exploratory stroke—use a light, feeling stroke with explorers to assess area, detect calculus, and differentiate between smooth and rough sensations
      (1) Use a feather-light grasp and fulcrum to allow maximum tactile sensitivity
      (2) As the tip is drawn over the tooth surface, bumps, rough areas, and catches can be detected from the vibrations created through the shank of the instrument—imagine feeling concrete as opposed to a smooth tile floor
   b. Working/scaling stroke—use with scaler or curette to remove deposits
      (1) Use firm grasp (tighten up) with overlapping strokes
      (2) Place end third of blade just under the deposit
      (3) Apply pressure to the handle by tightening the grasp and fulcrum while using a pull stroke toward the crown of the tooth
      (4) Apply increased pressure on fulcrum by pressing down on the pad of the ring finger
      (5) Apply increased lateral pressure on handle with thumb; use power from the wrist and arm to engage the cutting edge of the instrument for calculus removal
      (6) Finish with exploratory strokes to check effectiveness of stroke

4. Activation—wrist rock
   a. With wrist in neutral position, position hand straight with arm—wrist should *never* be bent up or down, which can cause strain and injury to the joint

b. Synchronize hand and arm in one motion to move instrument (avoid finger motion!)
   (1) Pivot—allows movement at fulcrum point while keeping hand straight with arm
       (a) Pivot on pad of fulcrum finger, from side to side, allowing movement of the instrument across tooth surface
       (b) Keep fulcrum finger straight and rigid in a locked position
       (c) Use lateral or rocking movement of the wrist to activate the instrument; allows the sharp cutting edge to scale or debride the tooth surfaces
   (2) Roll—use thumb and index finger, and turn end third of blade (working end) toward tooth
       (a) Use to adapt the end third of working end across the interproximal surface to prevent tissue trauma
       (b) Simultaneously, rock the wrist laterally and activate vertical working strokes

V. **Operator Positions**
   Establish seating positions that allow optimum access to oral cavity with minimal strain on the operator. (see Table 8–2 and Table 8–3)

VI. **Instruments**
   Regardless of instrument being used, the basic fundamentals of instrumentation must be applied. (Note: Right-handed operator positions are noted first; left-handed operator positions are noted second, in parenthesis, for each respective instrument and instrumentation pattern section).
   A. Mirror (Figure 8–16)
      1. A key instrument that aids in the visual aspect of the examination and scaling procedures
      2. Purposes
         a. Retraction—prevents interference with cheeks, tongue, and lips
            (1) Cheek—gently retract by placing mirror face toward buccal mucosa or with back of mirror when face is needed for reflection/indirect vision (Figure 8–17)
            (2) Angle of mouth—adjust shank to help avoid pinching the tissue (Figure 8–18)
            (3) Tongue—retract and position mirror head between lateral and dorsal surfaces of tongue (Figure 8–19)
         b. Indirect vision—achieved by looking in the mirror to view image (Figure 8–20)
         c. Indirect illumination—achieved by pooling light from the mirror face (Figure 8–20)
         d. Transillumination—use to examine teeth for interproximal carious lesions on anterior teeth; achieved by reflecting light through the teeth—to examine facials, reflect from linguals
      3. Characteristics—consists of a handle and a cone socket; available in various handle diameters
      4. Types
         a. One-sided
         b. Two-sided—image can be seen from both sides
         c. Front surface—reflects image on the front of the surface, producing a clear image

PRECLINICAL TIP

Adapting Your Knowledge: Use a slow wrist rock during instrumentation. Using a nursery rhyme, such as Hickory Dickory Dock, ensures a slow rhythmic rock.

PRECLINICAL TIP

Adapting Your Knowledge: Keep thumb knuckle bent out to facilitate rolling of instrument in fingers. Practice this!

PRECLINICAL TIP

Adapting Your Knowledge: A range has been given for seating positions to offer flexibility. However, to determine the correct position for the operator, *always* keep wrist and body in neutral position.

Table 8–2   Positions for Right-Handed Operator

Sextant	Operator Position	Patient Head Position	Patient Chin Position	Light Position	Mirror	Instrument Fulcrum
1	Facial: 10:00 with arm at 9:00 Lingual: 10:00–10:30	Facial: Slightly away Lingual: Toward	Up	Over chest, angled up	Facial: Retract cheek; use indirect vision for molars, direct vision for premolars; avoid resting rim of mirror on gingiva or alveolar bone Lingual: Use indirect vision and illumination	As close as possible to working area without blocking light
2	11:00–11:30	Straight or slightly toward	Up	Over chest, angled up	Facial: Palmed; use direct vision, retract with nondominant index finger Lingual: Use indirect vision and illumination	As close as possible to working area without blocking light
3	Facial: 9:00–11:30 Lingual: Alternate A, 9:00 Alternate B 10:00–11:30	Facial: Toward Lingual: Alternate A, away Alternate B, toward	Up	Over chest, angled up	Facial: Retract cheek; use illumination, indirect vision for molars, direct vision for premolars Lingual: Use indirect vision	Facial and lingual: Alternate A, as close as possible to working area Lingual: Alternate B, maxillary anteriors
4	Facial: Distals at 9:00, mesials at 11:30 Lingual: 9:00	Facial: Toward Lingual: Away	Down	Over mouth	Facial: Retract cheek; use indirect vision for molars, direct vision for premolars Lingual: Retract tongue; use indirect vision for distal of molars, direct vision where possible	As close as possible to working area without blocking light
5	Facial: Surfaces toward—7:30–9:00; surfaces away—11:30 Lingual: Surfaces toward—7:30–9:00; surfaces away—11:30	Straight or slightly toward	Down	Over mouth	Facial: Palmed, use direct vision; retract with nondominant index finger Lingual: Use indirect vision, transillumination, illumination, and retract tongue	As close as possible to working area without blocking light
6	Facial—9:00 Lingual: Distals at 9:00, mesials at 11:00	Facial: Slightly away Lingual: Toward	Down	Over mouth	Facial: Retract cheek, use indirect vision for molars, direct vision for premolars Lingual: Retract tongue, use indirect vision and illumination	Incisal/occlusal of canine/premolar area

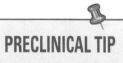

PRECLINICAL TIP

Adapting Your Knowledge: Of all the types of mirrors, the front surface mirror is preferred.

d. Plane or flat—reflects image on the back of the surface that can produce a double image
e. Concave—magnifies image but can also distort it
5. Grasp—use modified pen in nondominant hand (opposite hand from instrumentation) (Figure 8–21)
6. Fulcrum—place ring finger on tooth surface (see Figure 8–21 and note locked finger position)
7. Insertion—gently insert; avoid hitting the teeth during insertion, positioning, or movement
8. Adaptation—use sufficient pressure to maintain retraction—avoid pulling too hard and applying pressure on alveolar mucosa, floor of mouth, retromolar area, maxillary tuberosity, hard palate, or tongue

Table 8–3 Positions for Left-Handed Operator

Sextant	Operator Position	Patient Head Position	Patient Chin Position	Light Position	Mirror	Instrument Fulcrum
1	Facial: 2:00 with arm at 3:00	Facial: Toward	Up	Over chest, angled up	Facial: Retract cheek; use indirect vision for molars, direct vision for premolars	Facial and lingual: Alternate A, as close as possible to working area
	Lingual: Alternate A, 3:00 Alternate B, 12:30–1:00	Lingual: Alternate A, away Alternate B, toward			Lingual: Use indirect vision and illumination	Lingual: Alternate B, maxillary anteriors
2	12:30–1:00	Straight or slightly toward	Up	Over chest, angled up	Facial: Palmed; use direct vision; retract with non-dominant index finger Lingual: Use indirect vision, illumination, and trans-illumination	As close as possible to working area without blocking light
3	Facial: 2:00 with arm at 3:00	Facial: Away	Up	Over chest, angled up	Facial: Retract cheek; use indirect vision; avoid resting rim of mirror on gingiva or alveolar bone	As close as possible to working area without blocking light
	Lingual: 12:30–2:00	Lingual: Toward			Lingual: Use indirect vision and illumination	
4	Facial: 3:00	Facial: Away	Down	Over mouth	Facial: Retract; use indirect vision and illumination	Incisal/occlusal area of canine/premolar area
	Lingual: 3:00–4:30	Lingual: Toward			Lingual: Retract tongue; use indirect vision and illumination	
5	Facial: Surfaces toward—3:00–4:30; surfaces away—12:30	Straight or slightly toward	Down	Over mouth	Facial: Palmed; retract with nondominant index finger; use direct vision	As close as possible to working area without blocking light
	Lingual: Surfaces toward—3:00; surfaces away—12:30	Straight			Lingual: Use indirect vision, illumination, transillumination, and retract tongue	
6	Facial: 3:00	Facial: Toward	Down	Over mouth	Facial: Retract cheek; use indirect vision for molars, direct vision for premolars	
	Lingual: 3:00–4:30	Lingual: Away			Lingual: Retract tongue; use indirect vision	As close as possible to working area without blocking light

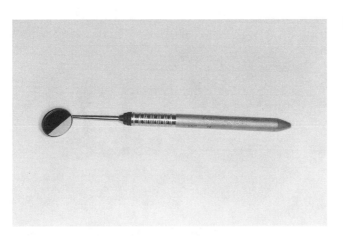

Figure 8–16 Dental mirror.

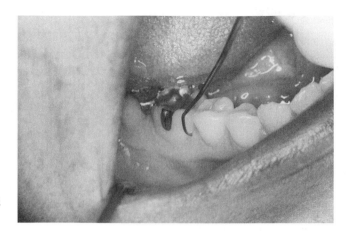

Figure 8–17   Retracting cheek with dental mirror.

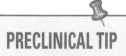

PRECLINICAL TIP

Adapting Your Knowledge: Much time is spent during instrumentation with the mirror in the non-dominant hand. Practice this skill!

9. Angulation—achieved by rolling mirror in the fingers of the non-dominant hand; rotate the view from mesial to distal where indirect vision is necessary (see Tables 8–2 and 8–3)
10. Maintain clear vision—can obtain by
    a. Warming the mirror (rubbing) along patient's buccal mucosa to coat with saliva
    b. Instructing patient to breathe through nose
    c. Dipping mirror head in commercial solution or mouthwash
11. Care of mirrors—avoid contact with polishing paste, which can scratch face of mirror; replace scratched mirror heads when indicated; if not using an autoclave cassette, wrap mirror head with a gauze square to protect face from being scratched by other instruments
    See Mirror Skill Sheet at end of chapter.
    The remaining instrument sections summarize each specific instrument introduced. A majority of the information is repeated from other instrument sections. This allows the student to learn about a specific instrument with all the information presented in a few pages. This format also instills that the same principles of instrumentation are to be implemented for all instruments.
B. Explorer
    1. Assessment and detection instrument used to examine the hard surfaces of the teeth and also to evaluate the tooth/root surfaces for the presence of deposits

Figure 8–18   Retracting angle of mouth with dental mirror.

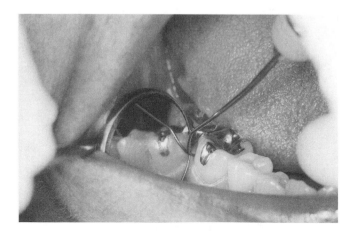

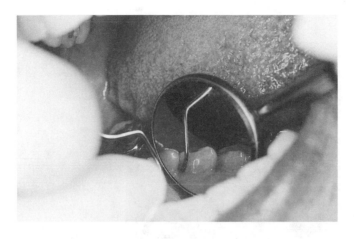

Figure 8–19   Retracting tongue with dental mirror.

2. Provides the greatest amount of tactile sensitivity of any dental instrument
3. Purposes
   a. Caries detection—shank of explorer is more rigid
      (1) Technique
         (a) Use straight explorer or Shepherd's hook (#23) explorer (Figure 8–22)
         (b) Keep point perpendicular to the surface being evaluated
         (c) Trace outline of restorations to detect defects or recurrent carious lesions; apply light-to-moderate pressure in all pits and fissures
      (2) Evaluation—area of decay will stick and feel soft or catch in the surface; operator will feel resistance upon removal
   b. Calculus detection and root surface evaluation—shank of explorer is more flexible, permitting vibrations to be easily felt; allows the operator to locate deposits, irregular tooth structures, and other anomalies[8]
4. Types of calculus-detecting explorers (Figure 8–23)
   a. 11/12 explorer
      (1) Design
         (a) Universal instrument
         (b) Double-ended with mirror-image working ends, fine metal tip, and rounded back to prevent tissue laceration
         (c) Long terminal shank

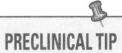

PRECLINICAL TIP

Adapting your Knowledge: The point of the explorer is the working end.

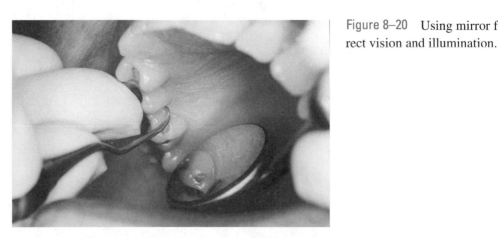

Figure 8–20   Using mirror for indirect vision and illumination.

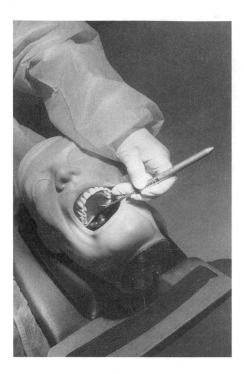

Figure 8–21   Using modified pen grasp with mirror.

        (2) Allows for adaptation into deeper pockets or areas of limited access[9]
    b. Pigtail explorer or cowhorn (3CH)
        (1) Design
            (a) Universal instrument
            (b) Double-ended with mirror-image working ends; fine metal tip with rounded back to prevent tissue laceration
        (2) Adapts to all surfaces; however, short curve limits use in deep pockets
    c. Orban-type explorer—single-ended instrument, yet can be paired easily with another explorer or probe (e.g., TU-17)
        (1) Possesses a long, wire-like, straight terminal shank with a tip bent at 90 degrees to the terminal shank
        (2) Use in narrow pockets, especially in the anterior and facial and lingual surfaces of posterior teeth
  5. Determination of correct working end for calculus detection (Figure 8–24)

Figure 8–22   Straight explorer or Shepherd's hook.

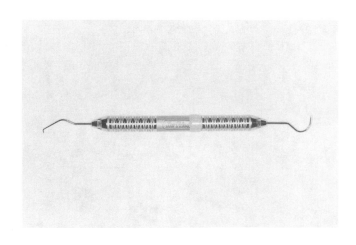

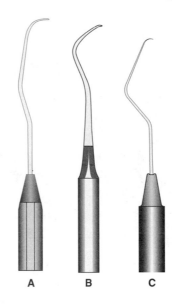

Figure 8–23 Types of calculus-detecting explorers. A. 11/12 B. Pigtailed or cowhorn C. Orban-type.

   a. Place terminal shank parallel to the long axis of the tooth—reduces trauma to the tissues and increases the probability of detecting deposits
   b. Place tip into interproximal and position handle toward opening of oral cavity
6. Grasp—use feather-light modified pen grasp
7. Instrument fulcrum—use intraorally and as close as possible to the working area
8. Insertion—place tip flush against tooth surface
9. Adaptation—place working end parallel to the long axis of the tooth with tip toward tooth (Figure 8–25); use one of the following options to keep tip adapted to tooth and to prevent tissue trauma
   a. Option 1—roll the explorer with thumb and support with index finger around line angles
   b. Option 2—stop and reposition at line angles
10. Angulation—use 5-degree angle
11. Activation
   a. Explore from gingival margin to base of sulcus
   b. Use short, overlapping, systematic strokes to feel each surface area

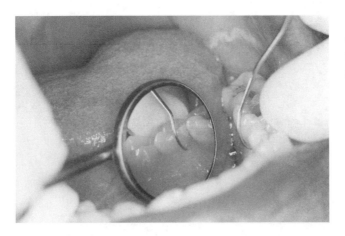

Figure 8–24 Correct working end determination of the explorer. Place terminal shank parallel to the long axis of the tooth.

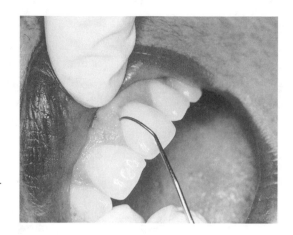

Figure 8–25   Proper explorer adaptation. Keep tip adapted to tooth at all times.

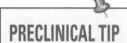

PRECLINICAL TIP

Adapting Your Knowledge: Roll instrument continuously to adapt tip of instrument to tooth surface.

   c. Slightly overlap strokes at line angles to avoid leaving gaps of unexplored tooth surface
12. Instrumentation pattern
   a. Sextant 1 (maxillary right)
      (1) Facial
         (a) Operator position—10:00 with arm at 9:00 (left-handed, 2:00 with arm at 3:00) (Figure 8–26)
         (b) Patient's head—position slightly away from operator
         (c) Patient's chin—position up
         (d) Light—position over chest, angle up
         (e) Mirror—use for retraction when face of mirror is toward cheek; use illumination when face of mirror is toward teeth—usually to view distal surfaces
         (f) Instrument fulcrum—position as close as possible to working area without blocking light
      (2) Lingual
         (a) Operator position—10:00 to 11:30 (left-handed, 2:00 to 12:30); avoid excessive bending and/or leaning to avoid blocking light (Figure 8–27)
         (b) Patient's head—position toward operator
         (c) Patient's chin—position up
         (d) Light—position over chest, angle up
         (e) Mirror—fulcrum on opposite maxillary premolar; use for indirect vision and illumination

Figure 8–26   Seating position for facial surfaces of Sextant 1 (maxillary right).

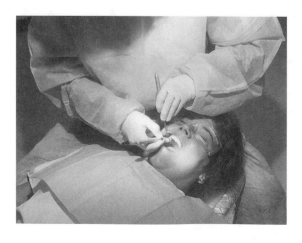

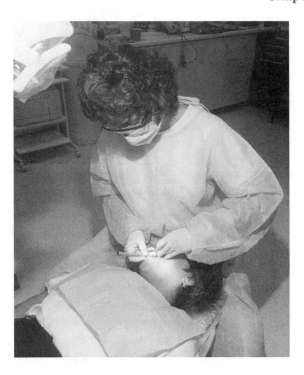

Figure 8–27   Seating position for lingual surfaces of Sextant 1.

  (f) Instrument fulcrum—position as close as possible to working area

(3) Application (facial and lingual) (Figure 8–28)

  (a) Insert tip at distal line angle

  (b) Activate vertical/oblique strokes toward distal, making sure to always keep tip against tooth

  (c) Roll tip around into proximal surface, finishing under contact

  (d) Turn tip toward mesial and reposition at distal line angle

  (e) Reinsert at distal line angle and use vertical/oblique strokes to move instrument toward mesial line angle

  (f) Stop at mesial line angle; use one of the following options to help keep tip adapted to tooth and to prevent tissue trauma

   • Option 1—roll the explorer with thumb and support with index finger around line angle

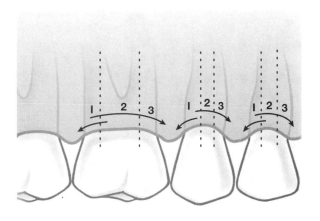

Figure 8–28   Application pattern of explorer. 1. Begin at the distal line angle and explore distal third. 2. Reposition instrument and explore cervical third. 3. Explore to mesial line angle and finish mesial third under contact.

- Option 2—stop and reposition at line angle
   (g) Proceed around line angle into proximal surface, finishing under contact

b. Sextant 2 (maxillary anteriors): Mentally divide each tooth down the center; surfaces from midline to interproximal toward operator are called *toward;* surfaces from midline to interproximal away from operator are called *away*

   (1) Facial (Figure 8–29)
      (a) Operator position—11:00 to 11:30 (left-handed, 1:00 to 12:30)
      (b) Patient's head—position straight or slightly toward the operator
      (c) Patient's chin—position up
      (d) Light—position over chest, angle up
      (e) Mirror—in nondominant hand, palm mirror and retract lip with index finger; use direct vision
      (f) Instrument fulcrum—position as close as possible to working area

   (2) Lingual (Figure 8–30)
      (a) Operator position—11:00 to 11:30 (left-handed, 1:00 to 12:30); avoid leaning and/or bending excessively over patient
      (b) Patient's head—position straight or slightly toward operator
      (c) Patient's chin—position up
      (d) Light—position over chest, angle up
      (e) Mirror—fulcrum on opposite maxillary premolars; use indirect vision, illumination, and transillumination

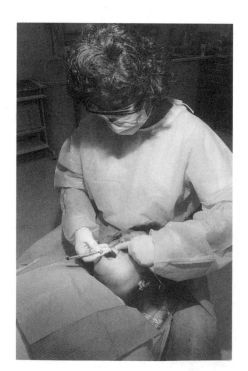

Figure 8–29   Seating position for facial surfaces of Sextant 2 (maxillary anterior).

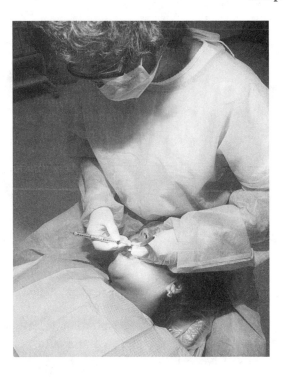

Figure 8–30   Seating position for lingual surfaces of Sextant 2.

(f) Instrument fulcrum—position as close as possible to working area

(3) Application (Figure 8–31a and 8–31b)

    (a) Facial

- Insert tip slightly past midline of tooth
- Activate vertical/oblique strokes toward operator, across cervical, making sure to always keep tip against tooth (Figure 8–32)
- Roll tip around line angle into proximal surface, finishing under contact; complete all surfaces toward operator
- Reposition tip at midline of tooth

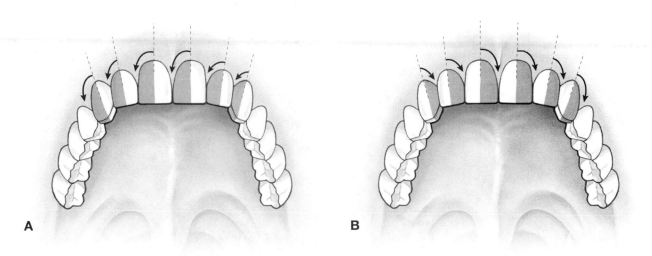

Figure 8–31A   Exploring facial surfaces toward operator.   8–31B Exploring facial surfaces away from operator.

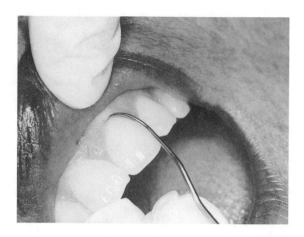

Figure 8–32   Exploring surfaces toward operator.

- Activate vertical/oblique strokes away from operator, across cervical, making sure to always keep tip against tooth (Figure 8–33)
- Roll tip around line angle into proximal surface, finishing under contact; complete all surfaces away from operator

(b) Lingual
- Insert tip slightly past midline of tooth
- Activate vertical/oblique strokes away from operator, across cervical, making sure to always keep tip against tooth
- Roll tip around line angle into proximal surface, finishing under contact; complete all surfaces away from operator
- Reposition tip at midline of tooth
- Activate vertical/oblique strokes toward operator, across cervical, making sure to always keep tip against tooth
- Roll tip around line angle into proximal surface, finishing under contact; complete all surfaces toward operator

c. Sextant 3 (maxillary left)
(1) Facial (Figure 8–34)
(a) Operator position—9:00 to 11:30 (left-handed, 3:00 to 12:30)

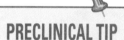

PRECLINICAL TIP

Adapting Your Knowledge: Refer to the enclosed CD-ROM to view alternative instrumentation methods for anterior teeth.

Figure 8–33   Exploring surfaces away from operator.

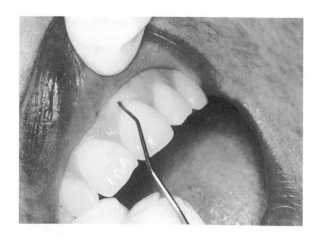

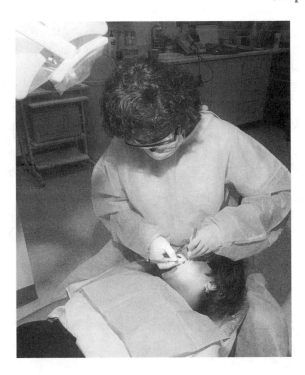

Figure 8–34   Seating position for facial surfaces of sextant 3 (maxillary left).

(b) Patient's head—position toward operator
(c) Patient's chin—position up
(d) Light—position over chest, angle up
(e) Mirror—retract cheek with mirror face toward teeth for indirect vision; use direct vision for premolars; avoid resting rim of mirror on gingiva or alveolar bone
(f) Instrument fulcrum—position as close as possible to working area without blocking light

(2) Lingual (Figure 8–35a)
　(a) Alternate Position A
　　• Operator position—9:00 (left-handed, 3:00)
　　• Patient's head—position up and away from operator
　　• Patient's chin—position up
　　• Light—position over chest, angle up
　　• Mirror—fulcrum on opposite maxillary premolars; use indirect vision and illumination
　　• Instrument fulcrum—position as close as possible to working area
　(b) Alternate Position B (Figure 8–35b)
　　• Operator position—10:00 to 11:30 (left-handed, 2:00 to 12:30)
　　• Patient's head—position toward operator
　　• Patient's chin—position up
　　• Light—position over chest, angle up
　　• Mirror—position on the opposite maxillary premolar area
　　　Tip: If the operator fulcrums on the facial surfaces of the opposite maxillary premolar teeth, it helps retract the lip, allowing for greater illumination.

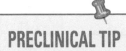

PRECLINICAL TIP

Adapting Your Knowledge: When working in areas with limited direct vision, keep face of mirror toward the teeth so distal surfaces can be viewed. Neutral body positions should always be maintained.

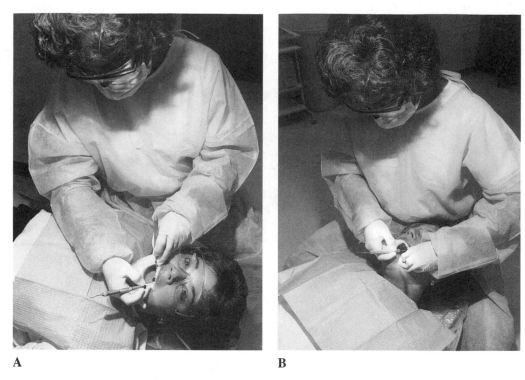

A   **B**

Figure 8–35A   Seating position for lingual surfaces of sextant 3—Alternate position A–9:00.
8-35B Seating position for lingual surfaces of sextant 3—Alternate position B–11:00.

- Instrument fulcrum—using the pen grasp, position on the maxillary anteriors, making sure to place grasp toward middle of handle

(3) Application (facial and lingual)
   (a) Insert tip at distal line angle
   (b) Activate vertical/oblique strokes toward distal, making sure to always keep tip against tooth
   (c) Roll tip around into proximal surface, finishing under contact
   (d) Turn tip toward mesial and reposition at distal line angle
   (e) Reinsert at distal line angle and use vertical/oblique strokes to move instrument toward mesial line angle
   (f) Stop at mesial line angle; use one of the following options to help keep tip adapted to tooth and to prevent tissue trauma
      - Option 1—roll the explorer with thumb and support with index finger around line angle
      - Option 2—stop and reposition at line angle
   (g) Proceed around line angle into proximal surface, finishing under contact

d. Sextant 4 (mandibular left)
   (1) Facial
      (a) Operator position
         - Distals—9:00 (left-handed, 3:00) (Figure 8–36a)

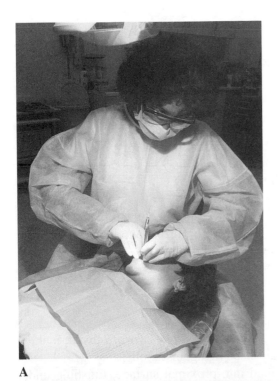

A

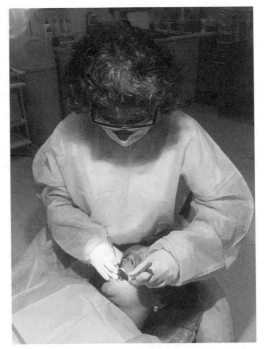

B

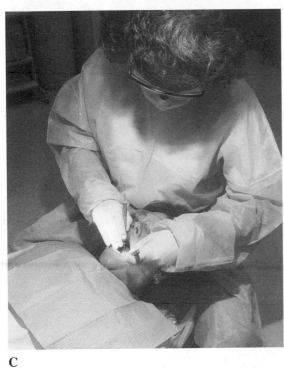

C

PRECLINICAL TIP

Adapting Your Knowledge: Note how changing operator's seating position in this sextant helps to keep hand straight with arm.

Figure 8–36 Seating position for facial surfaces of sextant 4. A. Distal third. B. Middle third. C. Mesial third.

- Middle—10:00 (left-handed, 2:00) (Figure 8–36b)
- Mesials—11:30 (left-handed, 12:30) (Figure 8–36c)
    (b) Patient's head—position toward operator
    (c) Patient's chin—position down
    (d) Light—position over mouth
    (e) Mirror—retract cheek with mirror face toward teeth for molars; retract for premolars using direct vision
    (f) Instrument fulcrum—position as close as possible to working area

(2) Lingual
    (a) Operator position—7:30 to 9:00 (left-handed, 4:30 to 3:00)
        • Position 1—7:30 (left-handed, 4:30); place knees together at side of chair facing 12:00 position (Figure 8–37a)
        • Position 2—9:00 (left-handed, 3:00); straddle chair with weight evenly distributed (Figure 8–37b)
    (b) Patient's head—position away from operator
    (c) Patient's chin—position down
    (d) Light—position over mouth
    (e) Mirror—fulcrum on opposite mandibular premolar area; retract tongue with mirror face toward teeth; use indirect vision and illumination
    (f) Instrument fulcrum—position as close as possible to working area

(3) Application (facial and lingual)
    (a) Insert tip at distal line angle
    (b) Activate vertical/oblique strokes *toward* distal, making sure to always keep tip against tooth
    (c) Roll tip around into proximal surface, finishing under contact
    (d) Turn tip toward mesial and reposition at distal line angle
    (e) Reinsert at distal line angle and use vertical/oblique strokes to move instrument toward mesial line angle
    (f) Stop at mesial line angle; use one of the following options to help keep tip adapted to tooth and to prevent tissue trauma

Figure 8–37A   Seating position for lingual surfaces of sextant 4—Position 2.

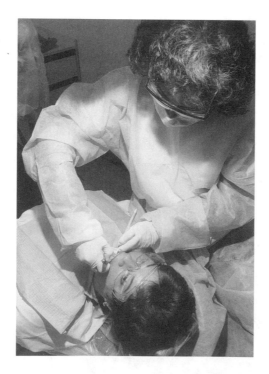

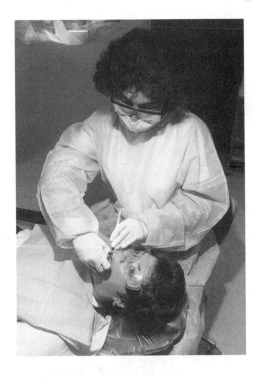

Figure 8–37B Seating position for lingual surfaces of sextant 4—Position 1.

- Option 1—roll the explorer with thumb and support with index finger around line angle
- Option 2—stop and reposition at line angle
  (g) Proceed around line angle into proximal surface, finishing under contact
e. Sextant 5 (mandibular anterior)
  (1) Facial and lingual (surfaces toward)
      (a) Operator position—7:30 to 9:00 (left-handed, 4:30 to 3:00) (Figure 8–38a)
      (b) Patient's head—position straight or slightly away

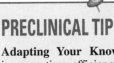

PRECLINICAL TIP

Adapting Your Knowledge: To increase time efficiency, complete all facial surfaces toward you, then complete all lingual surfaces toward you before instrumenting the surfaces away from you.

Figure 8–38A Seating position for sextant 5 (facial and lingual [surfaces toward]).

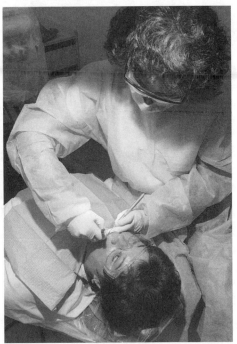

(c) Patient's chin—position down

(d) Light—position over mouth

(e) Mirror—use palm grasp and retract lip with index finger of nondominant hand for facial surfaces; use indirect vision for lingual surfaces

(f) Instrument fulcrum—position as close as possible to working area

(2) Facial and lingual (surfaces away) (Figure 8–38b)

(a) Operator position—11:30 (left-handed, 12:30)

(b) Patient's head—position straight or slightly toward

(c) Patient's chin—position down

(d) Light—position over mouth

(e) Mirror—use palm grasp and retract lip with index finger of nondominant hand for facial surfaces; use indirect vision for lingual surfaces

(f) Instrument fulcrum—position as close as possible to working area

(3) Application

(a) Surfaces toward operator (facial and lingual)

- Insert tip slightly past midline (Figure 8–39a)
- Activate vertical/oblique strokes toward operator, across cervical, making sure to always keep tip against tooth
- Roll tip around line angle into proximal surface, finishing under contact

(b) Surfaces away from operator (facial and lingual)

- Reposition tip at midline of tooth
- Activate vertical/oblique strokes away from operator, across cervical, making sure to always keep tip against tooth (Figure 8–39b)
- Roll tip around line angle into proximal surface, finishing under contact

Figure 8–38B   Seating position for sextant 5 (facial and lingual [surfaces away.])

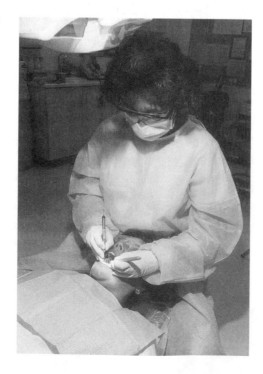

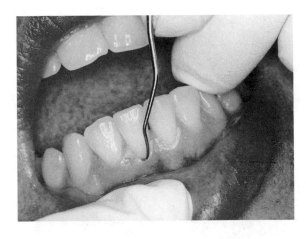

Figure 8–39A   Application of explorer on sextant 5—surfaces toward operator.

f. Sextant 6 (mandibular right)
  (1) Facial
    (a) Operator position—7:30 to 9:00; (left-handed, 4:30 to 3:00)
       • Position 1—7:30 (left-handed, 4:30); place knees together at side of chair facing 12:00 position (Figure 8–40)
       • Position 2—9:00 (left-handed, 3:00); straddle chair with weight evenly distributed
    (b) Patient's head—position slightly away
    (c) Patient's chin—position down
    (d) Light—position over mouth
    (e) Mirror—retract cheek; use indirect vision for molars, direct vision for premolars
    (f) Instrument fulcrum—position on incisal/occlusal of mandibular canine/premolar area
  (2) Lingual (Figure 8–41)
    (a) Operator position
       • Distals—9:00; (left-handed, 3:00)
       • Middle—10:00 (left-handed, 2:00)
       • Mesials—11:30 (left-handed, 12:30)
    (b) Patient's head—position toward operator
    (c) Patient's chin—position down
    (d) Light—position over mouth
    (e) Mirror—retract cheek with mirror face toward teeth for molars; retract for premolars using direct vision

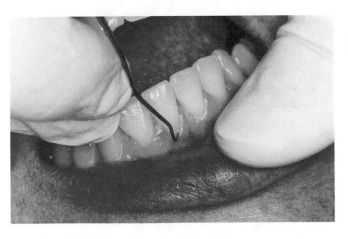

Figure 8–39B   Application of explorer on sextant 5—surfaces away from operator.

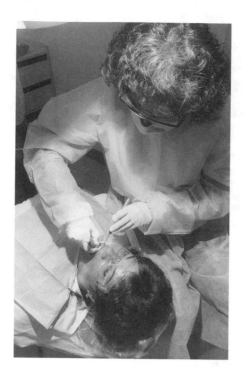

Figure 8–40   Seating position 1 for facial surfaces of sextant 6.

(f) Instrument fulcrum—position as close as possible to working area
(3) Application (facial and lingual)
  (a) Insert tip at distal line angle
  (b) Activate vertical/oblique strokes toward distal, making sure to always keep tip against tooth
  (c) Roll tip around into proximal surface, finishing under contact
  (d) Turn tip toward mesial and reposition at distal line angle

Figure 8–41   Seating position for lingual surfaces of sextant 6.

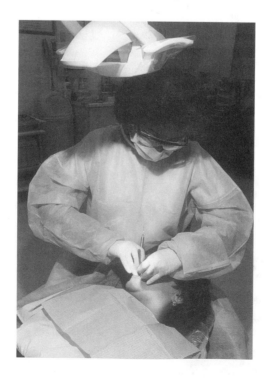

(e) Reinsert at distal line angle and use vertical/oblique strokes to move instrument toward mesial line angle (Figure 8–42)

(f) Stop at mesial line angle; use one of the following options to help keep tip adapted to tooth and to prevent tissue trauma
   - Option 1—roll the explorer with thumb and support with index finger around line angle
   - Option 2—stop and reposition at line angle

(g) Proceed around line angle into proximal surface, finishing under contact
   See Calculus-Detecting Explorer Skill Sheet at end of chapter.

C. Probe
1. A slim "measuring-stick" instrument used to assess periodontal health and measure oral lesions or deviations
2. Used to complete the periodontal exam and assess the periodontal health of patients
3. Characteristics: Working-end shape is cylindrical or flat rod with a measuring stick; calibrated into millimeters to measure gingival sulcus or pocket depth
4. Types and working ends: Single- or double-ended with a variety of marking combinations; can be paired with an explorer (Figure 8–43)
   a. PSR probe—round shape; color-coded with 0.5 mm ball on end; sextants are assigned a code based on findings during assessment
   b. Marquis probe—round shape with alternating colored increments 3 millimeters apart; goes up to 12 millimeters (black and silver are a popular combination)
   c. UNC probe—round shape with markings at every millimeter, 1 to 12, but color-coded at 5, 10, and 12 millimeters
   d. Novatech—round shape, right-angled for posteriors, with markings at 3, 6, 9, and 12 millimeters
   e. Michigan O probe—round in shape with markings at 3, 6, and 8 millimeters
   f. Williams probe—round in shape with markings at 1, 2, 3, 5, 7, 8, 9, and 10 millimeters

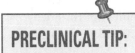

PRECLINICAL TIP:

Adapting Your Knowledge: Although examples of flat-rod probes are not shown, they are available.

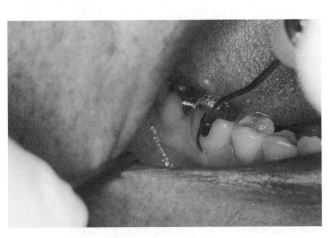

Figure 8–42   Application of explorer on sextant 6.

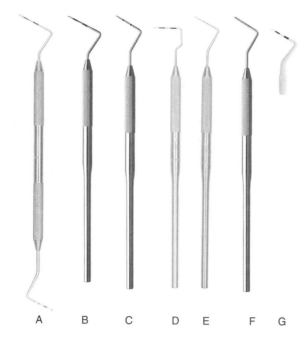

Figure 8–43   Types of Periodontal Probes. Courtesy of Hu-Friedy Manufacturing Company A. PSR (lower end) B. Marquis C. UNC D. Novatech. E. Michigan O F. Williams G. PCV12PT. (Colorvue)

A   B   C   D   E   F   G

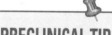

PRECLINICAL TIP

Adapting Your Knowledge: Twenty-five grams of force is necessary to indent the pad of the thumb about 1 to 2 mm.

   g. Plastic probe—round shape; used to assess implants; since implants are made of titanium, a metal instrument will scratch the implant; an example is the PCV12PT Colorvue probe by Hu-Friedy with alternating yellow/black markings at 3, 6, 9, and 12 millimeters

5. Grasp—use modified pen
6. Instrumentation fulcrum—position as close as possible to working area
7. Insertion—gently insert blunted tip into sulcus with 20 to 25 grams of force until the rubberband-like epithelial attachment is felt[10] (Figure 8–44)
8. Adaptation—always maintain the sides of the probe on the tooth
9. Angulation
   a. Place probe parallel to long axis of tooth on direct facial or lingual surfaces (Figure 8–45)
   b. Avoid tilting the probe sideways or away from the tooth, except in the interproximal where the probe must be directed beneath the contact point
   c. Angle into sulcus following curvature of root, especially in the col area; avoid overangling probe—results in a false measure-

Figure 8–44   Proper insertion and adaptation of probe.

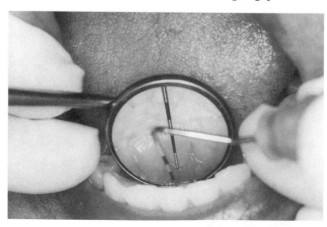

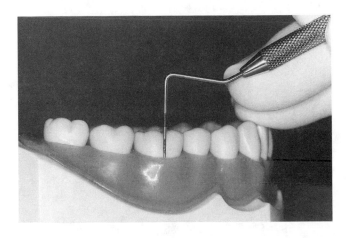

Figure 8–45   Place probe parallel to long axis of tooth.

ment; use one of the following options to keep tip adapted to tooth and to prevent tissue trauma

(1) Option 1—roll the probe with thumb and index finger around line angles

(2) Option 2—stop and reposition at line angles

10. Activation—use a walking stroke

a. Move up and down, or "bob," along the epithelial attachment around the tooth, with each movement only 1 to 2 mm apart; keep instrument in the sulcus making contact with the junctional epithelium (Figure 8–46)

b. Two-point contact—maintain contact between the tooth and probe at two sites on the instrument: the shank and tip (Figure 8–47)

11. Reading and recording measurements—depths are measured from the base of the pocket or junctional epithelium to the margin of the free gingiva; record the deepest reading in each of the following six locations on each tooth (Figure 8–48)

a. Distofacial—measure from distofacial line angle to distal interproximal col area

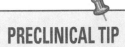

PRECLINICAL TIP

Adapting Your Knowledge: Avoid dragging the probe along the epithelial attachment to insure thorough assessment of the sulcus and to avoid rupturing the junctional epithelium.

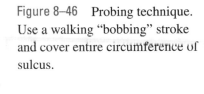

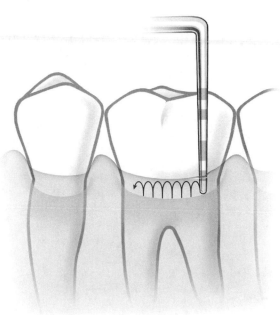

Figure 8–46   Probing technique. Use a walking "bobbing" stroke and cover entire circumference of sulcus.

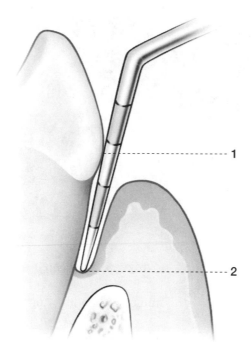

Figure 8–47   Two-point contact with the probe. Maintain contact between the tooth and probe at 2 sites—the shank and tip.

b. Facial—measure between distofacial and mesiofacial line angle
c. Mesiofacial—measure from mesiofacial line angle to mesial interproximal col area
d. Distolingual—measure from distolingual line angle to distal interproximal col area
e. Lingual—measure between distolingual line angle and mesiolingual line angle
f. Mesiolingual—measure from mesiolingual line angle and mesial interproximal col area

12. Record keeping—it is imperative to record accurate and neat probing depths in record of treatment
   a. Patient record—provides a legal document; periodontal chart could be subpoenaed in a court of law
   b. Aids in determining status of periodontal disease
   c. Allows for evaluation/reevaluation of treatment

13. Challenges of probing include

Figure 8–48   Reading and recording measurements. There are six areas from which probe readings are obtained. DL=distolingual; L=lingual; ML=mesiolingual; DF=distofacial; F=facial; MF=mesiofacial.

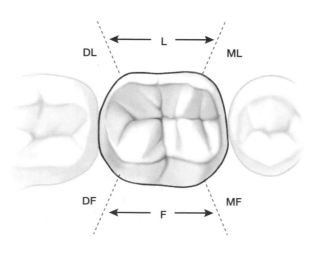

a. Keeping tip parallel to long axis of tooth, except in interproximals where tip needs to be angled under the contact

b. Angling into col area without overangling or underangling (Figure 8–49)

    (1) Overangling occurs when the probe is too hyperextended; results in a false high reading

    (2) Underangling results in a false shallow reading

c. Encountering obstacles, such as calculus, tooth-margin discrepancies, caries, and pontics, instead of base of epithelial attachment

d. Having visibility obstructed due to hemorrhage or excess soft deposits

14. Instrumentation pattern

  a. Sextant 1 (maxillary right)

    (1) Facial

      (a) Operator position—10:00 with arm at 9:00 (left-handed, 2:00 with arm at 3:00)

      (b) Patient's head—position slightly away from operator

      (c) Patient's chin—position up

      (d) Light—position over chest, angle up

      (e) Mirror—use for retraction when face of mirror is toward cheek; use illumination when face of mirror is toward teeth—usually to view distal surfaces

      (f) Instrument fulcrum—position as close as possible to working area without blocking light

    (2) Lingual

      (a) Operator position—10:00 to 11:30 (left-handed, 2:00 to 12:30); avoid excessive bending and/or leaning to avoid blocking light

      (b) Patient's head—position toward operator

      (c) Patient's chin—position up

      (d) Light—position over chest, angle up

      (e) Mirror—fulcrum on opposite maxillary premolar; use indirect vision and illumination

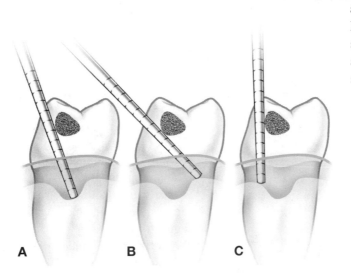

Figure 8–49   Probing the contact area. A. Correct angulation. B. Overangling at the contact results in high readings. C. Underangling at the contact results in shallow readings.

A   B   C

(f) Instrument fulcrum—position as close as possible to working area

(3) Application (facial and lingual)

(a) Insert tip at distal line angle

(b) Activate walking strokes toward distal, making sure to always keep tip against tooth

(c) Walk tip into proximal surface, finishing under contact

(d) Reposition and reinsert tip at distal line angle

(e) Reactivate walking strokes to move instrument across cervical toward mesial line angle

(f) Stop at mesial line angle

(g) Reposition and proceed with walking strokes around line angle into proximal surface, finishing under contact

b. Sextant 2 (maxillary anteriors)

(1) Facial

(a) Operator position—11:00 to 11:30 (left-handed, 1:00 to 12:30)

(b) Patient's head—position straight or slightly toward operator

(c) Patient's chin—position up

(d) Light—position over chest, angle up

(e) Mirror—in nondominant hand, palm mirror and retract lip with index finger; use direct vision

(f) Instrument fulcrum—position as close as possible to working area

(2) Lingual

(a) Operator position—11:00 to 11:30 (left-handed, 1:00 to 12:30); avoid leaning and/or bending excessively over patient

(b) Patient's head—position straight or slightly toward operator

(c) Patient's chin—position up

(d) Light—position over chest, angle up

(e) Mirror—fulcrum on opposite maxillary premolars; use indirect vision, illumination, and transillumination

(f) Instrument fulcrum—position as close as possible to working area

(3) Application

(a) Facial

• Insert tip at line angle closest to operator

• Activate walking strokes toward the interproximal with tip heading toward operator, making sure to always keep tip against tooth

• Walk tip around line angle into proximal surface, finishing under contact

• Reposition tip at same line angle

• Reactivate walking strokes away from operator, across cervical, making sure to always keep tip against tooth

• Walk tip around line angle into proximal surface, finishing under contact

---

PRECLINICAL TIP

Adapting Your Knowledge: When completing a periodontal charting, establish a pattern that is best for the operator to follow.

(b) Lingual
  - Insert tip at line angle away from operator
  - Activate walking strokes toward the interproximal with tip heading away from operator, making sure to always keep tip against tooth
  - Walk tip around line angle into proximal surface, finishing under contact
  - Reposition tip at same line angle
  - Reactivate walking strokes toward operator, across cervical, to line angle closest to operator
  - Walk tip around line angle into proximal surface, finishing under contact

c. Sextant 3 (maxillary left)
  (1) Facial
    (a) Operator position—9:00 to 11:30 (left-handed, 3:00 to 12:30)
    (b) Patient's head—position toward operator
    (c) Patient's chin—position up
    (d) Light—position over chest, angle up
    (e) Mirror—retract cheek with mirror face toward teeth for indirect vision; use direct vision for premolars; avoid resting rim of mirror on gingiva or alveolar bone
    (f) Instrument fulcrum—position as close as possible to working area without blocking light
  (2) Lingual
    (a) Alternate position A
      - Operator position—9:00 (left-handed, 3:00)
      - Patient's head—position up and away from operator
      - Patient's chin—position up
      - Light—position over chest, angle up
      - Mirror—fulcrum on opposite maxillary premolars; use indirect vision and illumination
      - Instrument fulcrum—position as close as possible to working area
    (b) Alternate position B
      - Operator position—10:00 to 11:30 (left-handed, 2:00 to 12:30)
      - Patient's head—position toward operator
      - Patient's chin—position up
      - Light—position over chest, angle up
      - Mirror—position on the opposite maxillary premolar area

        Tip: If the operator fulcrums on the facial surfaces of the opposite maxillary premolar teeth, it helps retract the lip, allowing for greater illumination.
      - Instrument fulcrum—using the pen grasp, position on the maxillary anteriors, making sure to place grasp toward middle of handle
  (3) Application (facial and lingual)
    (a) Insert tip at distal line angle
    (b) Activate walking strokes toward distal, making sure to always keep tip against tooth

    (c) Walk tip into proximal surface, finishing under contact

    (d) Reposition and reinsert tip at distal line angle

    (e) Reactivate walking strokes to move instrument across cervical toward mesial line angle

    (f) Stop at mesial line angle

    (g) Reposition and proceed with walking strokes around line angle into proximal surface, finishing under contact

d. Sextant 4 (mandibular left)

  (1) Facial

    (a) Operator position
- Distals—9:00 (left-handed, 3:00)
- Mesials—11:30 (left-handed, 12:30)

    (b) Patient's head—position toward operator

    (c) Patient's chin—position down

    (d) Light—position over mouth

    (e) Mirror—retract cheek with mirror face toward teeth for molars; retract for premolars using direct vision

    (f) Instrument fulcrum—position as close as possible to working area

  (2) Lingual

    (a) Operator position—7:30 to 9:00 (left-handed, 4:30 to 3:00)
- Position 1—7:30 (left-handed, 4:30)—place knees together at side of chair facing 12:00 position
- Position 2—9:00 (left-handed, 3:00)—straddle chair with weight evenly distributed

    (b) Patient's head—position away from operator

    (c) Patient's chin—position down

    (d) Light—position over mouth

    (e) Mirror—fulcrum on opposite mandibular premolar area; retract tongue with mirror face toward teeth; use indirect vision and illumination

    (f) Instrument fulcrum—position as close as possible to working area

  (3) Application (facial and lingual)

    (a) Insert tip at distal line angle

    (b) Activate walking strokes toward distal, making sure to always keep tip against tooth

    (c) Walk tip into proximal surface, finishing under contact

    (d) Reposition and reinsert tip at distal line angle

    (e) Reactivate walking strokes to move instrument across cervical toward mesial line angle

    (f) Stop at mesial line angle

    (g) Reposition and proceed with walking strokes around line angle into proximal surface, finishing under contact

e. Sextant 5 (mandibular anterior)

  (1) Facial and lingual

    (a) Operator position—7:30 to 9:00 (left-handed, 4:30 to 3:00)

    (b) Patient's head—position straight or slightly away

    (c) Patient's chin—position down

    (d) Light—position over mouth

    (e) Mirror—use palm grasp and retract lip with index finger of nondominant hand for facial surfaces; use indirect vision for lingual surfaces

    (f) Instrument fulcrum—position as close as possible to working area

  (2) Application

    (a) Facial

- Insert tip at line angle closest to operator
- Activate walking strokes toward the interproximal with tip heading toward operator, making sure to always keep tip against tooth
- Walk tip into proximal surface, finishing under contact
- Reposition and reinsert tip at same line angle
- Reactivate walking strokes away from operator, across cervical, making sure to always keep tip against tooth
- Reposition and proceed with walking strokes around line angle into proximal surface, finishing under contact

    (b) Lingual

- Insert tip at line angle away from operator
- Activate walking strokes toward the interproximal with tip heading away from the operator, making sure to always keep tip against tooth
- Walk tip into proximal surface, finishing under contact
- Reposition and reinsert tip at same line angle
- Reactivate walking strokes across the cervical, toward operator
- Stop at line angle
- Reposition and proceed with walking strokes around line angle into proximal surface, finishing under contact

f. Sextant 6 (mandibular right)

  (1) Facial

    (a) Operator position—7:30 to 9:00 (left-handed, 4:30 to 3:00)

- Position 1—7:30 (left-handed, 4:30)—place knees together at side of chair facing 12:00 position
- Position 2—9:00 (left-handed, 3:00)—straddle chair with weight evenly distributed

    (b) Patient's head—position slightly away

    (c) Patient's chin—position down

    (d) Light—position over mouth

    (e) Mirror—retract cheek; use indirect vision for molars, direct vision for premolars

    (f) Instrument fulcrum—position on incisal/occlusal of mandibular canine/premolar area

  (2) Lingual

    (a) Operator position

- Distals—9:00 (left-handed, 3:00)
- Mesials—11:30 (left-handed, 12:30)

(b) Patient's head—position toward operator
(c) Patient's chin—position down
(d) Light—position over mouth
(e) Mirror—retract cheek with mirror face toward teeth for molars; retract for premolars using direct vision
(f) Instrument fulcrum—position as close as possible to working area

(3) Application (facial and lingual) (Figure 8–50)

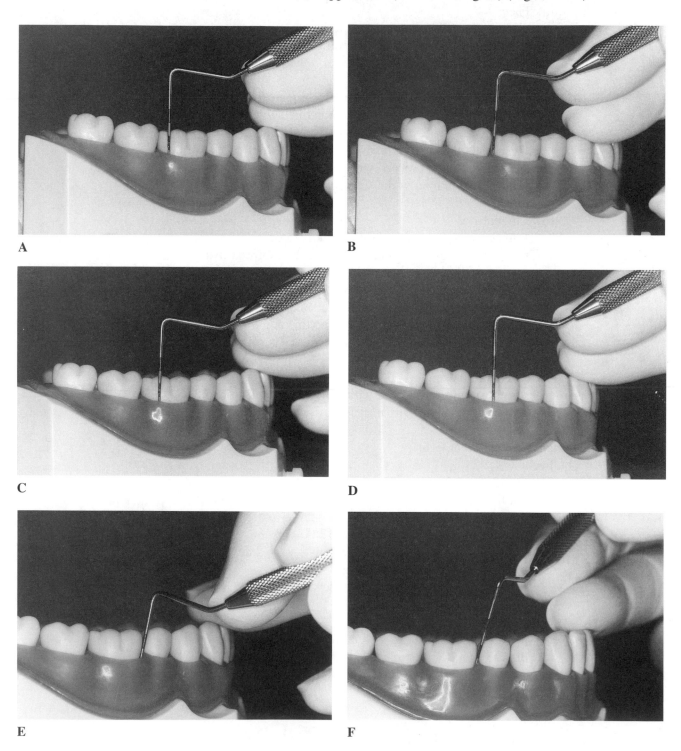

A

B

C

D

E

F

Figure 8–50   Probing technique.

  (a) Insert tip at distal line angle

  (b) Activate walking strokes toward distal, making sure to always keep tip against tooth

  (c) Walk tip into proximal surface, finishing under contact

  (d) Reposition and reinsert tip at distal line angle

  (e) Reactivate walking strokes to move instrument across cervical toward mesial line angle

  (f) Stop at mesial line angle

  (g) Reposition and proceed with walking strokes around line angle into proximal surface, finishing under contact

   See Probe Skill Sheet at end of chapter.

D. Scaler

 1. A scaling instrument with two cutting edges that meet at a point

 2. Use to remove supragingival calculus, stain, and light-to-moderate subgingival calculus if deposit is an extension of a supragingival deposit

 3. Characteristics

  a. Working end has two cutting edges and is triangular in cross section (refer to Figure 8–5)

  b. Two lateral surfaces meet to form a sharp, pointed tip

  c. Internal angle of blade is between 70 and 80 degrees

  d. Face is flat or curved

   (1) Straight sickle (also called a jacquette scaler) has a flat face

   (2) Curved sickle has a curved face

  e. Blade is effective in removing supragingival stain and calculus and up to 1mm subgingivally on remaining surfaces (Figure 8–51)

 4. Types

  a. Anterior—use on anterior dentition

   (1) Blade can be curved or straight and in the same plane as the handle (Figure 8–52)

   (2) Shank can be straight or slightly offset (e.g., H6/H7 or Nevi 1 scaler) (Figure 8–53)

  b. Universal—can be used throughout the entire dentition

   (1) Blade is curved or straight and not in same plane as the shank (Figure 8–54)

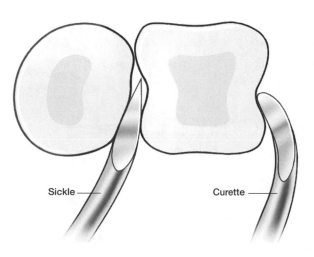

Sickle   Curette

Figure 8–51 Triangular-shaped tip of a sickle scaler cannot adapt to subgingival root concavities.

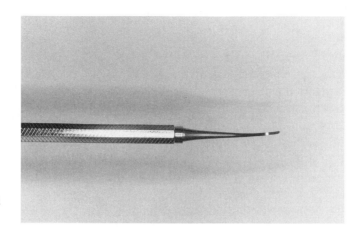

Figure 8–52   Sickle scaler blade in same plane as handle.

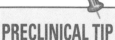

PRECLINICAL TIP

Adapting Your Knowledge: In determining the correct working end, make sure the terminal shank is not only parallel to the long axis of the tooth, but also that the instrument handle is directed toward the opening of the oral cavity.

    (2) Shank has contra-angled bend (e.g., 204SD and Nevi 2)

5. Determination of correct working end—accomplished when terminal shank is parallel to the long axis of the tooth; position handle toward opening of oral cavity (Figure 8–55)

6. Grasp
    a. Initially use a light grasp during exploratory stroke
    b. Apply a moderate grasp to remove light deposits
    c. Use a firmer grasp and fulcrum to remove more tenacious deposits

7. Instrumentation fulcrum
    a. Place palm toward arch to be instrumented
    b. Fulcrum with ring finger as close as possible to working area

8. Insertion—insert at or as near zero degrees as possible; blade is closed or tilted toward the tooth, so the tip is slipped under the free margin of the gingiva (Figure 8–56)

9. Adaptation
    a. Place 1mm to 2mm of tip flush against tooth (Figure 8–57)
    b. Use one of the following options to keep tip adapted to tooth and to prevent tissue trauma
        (1) Option 1—roll the scaler with thumb and support with index finger around line angles (Figures 8–58a and 8–58b)
        (2) Option 2—stop and reposition at line angles

10. Angulation—to remove or scale deposits, open blade by tilting it away from tooth, between 45 and 90 degrees (Figure 8–59)

Figure 8–53   Sickle scaler shank slightly offset.

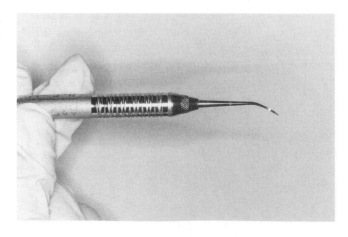

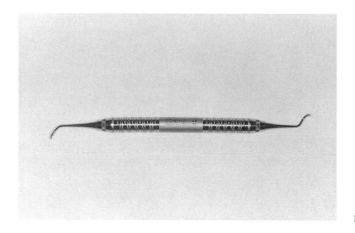

Figure 8–54   Sickle scaler blade not in same plane as shank.

11. Activation
    a. Begin at the distal line angle to instrument the distal interproximal contact
    b. Pivot on fulcrum to angle the cutting edge toward the tooth surface
    c. Rock the wrist and pivot hand on fulcrum following the rounded contour of the tooth surface
    d. Use short, overlapping vertical/oblique strokes, extending from base of the deposit coronally
    e. Finish with the tip of instrument under the contact
    f. Turn tip toward mesial
    g. Reposition instrument at the distal line angle and use oblique strokes to move instrument toward the mesial line angle
    h. Rock the wrist and pivot following the contour of the tooth
    i. Reposition at mesial line angle and finish stroke under the mesial contact
        Tip: Use same working end for facial surfaces in same sextant; use opposite end for lingual surfaces in same sextant, except for sextant 5.
12. Instrumentation pattern
    a. Sextant 1 (maxillary right)

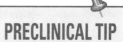

PRECLINICAL TIP

Adapting Your Knowledge: Calculus can be removed when pressure is applied against tooth. This can happen only when the blade is 45 to 90 degrees to the tooth. Most deposits are removed when the blade is open between 60 and 70 degrees.

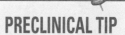

PRECLINICAL TIP

Adapting Your Knowledge: The purpose of repositioning is to keep the wrist in neutral position by keeping the hand straight with the arm.

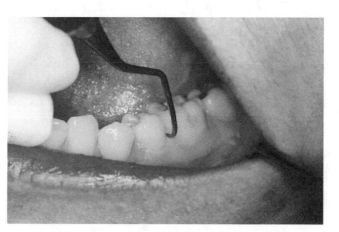

Figure 8–55   Determining correct working end of a sickle scaler. Place terminal shank parallel to long axis of the tooth. Handle of instrument is directed toward opening of oral cavity.

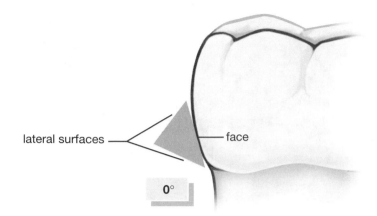

lateral surfaces —   — face

0°

Figure 8–56   Insertion of sickle scaler. Insert at zero degrees.

(1) Facial
  (a) Operator position—10:00 with arm at 9:00 (left-handed, 2:00 with arm at 3:00)
  (b) Patient's head—position slightly away from operator
  (c) Patient's chin—position up
  (d) Light—position over chest, angle up
  (e) Mirror—use for retraction when face of mirror is toward check; use illumination when face of mirror is toward teeth—usually to view distal surfaces
  (f) Instrument fulcrum—position as close as possible to working area
(2) Lingual
  (a) Operator position—10:00 to 11:30 (left-handed, 2:00 to 12:30); avoid excessive bending and/or leaning to avoid blocking light
  (b) Patient's head—position toward operator
  (c) Patient's chin—position up
  (d) Light—position over chest, angle up
  (e) Mirror—fulcrum on opposite maxillary premolar; use indirect vision and illumination
  (f) Instrument fulcrum—position as close as possible to working area
(3) Application

Figure 8–57   Adaptation of sickle scaler. Place 1–2 mm of tip flush against tooth.

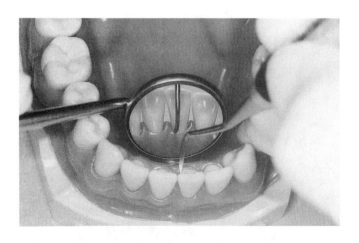

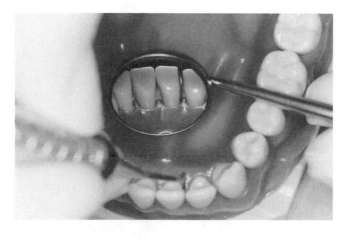

Figure 8–58A   Adaptation of sickle scaler, keeping tip against tooth at all times.

(a) Insert tip at distal line angle
(b) Activate vertical/oblique strokes toward distal, making sure to always keep tip against tooth
(c) Roll tip around line angle proximal surface, finishing under contact
(d) Turn tip toward mesial and reposition at distal line angle
(e) Reinsert at distal line angle and use vertical/oblique strokes to move instrument toward mesial line angle
(f) Stop at mesial line angle; use one of the following options to keep tip adapted to tooth and to prevent tissue trauma
  • Option 1—roll the scaler with thumb and support with index finger around line angle
  • Option 2—stop and reposition at line angle
(g) Proceed around line angle into proximal surface, finishing under contact

b. Sextant 2 (maxillary anteriors)—mentally divide each tooth down the center, surfaces from midline to interproximal toward operator are called *toward;* surfaces from midline to interproximal away from operator are called *away*
(1) Facial

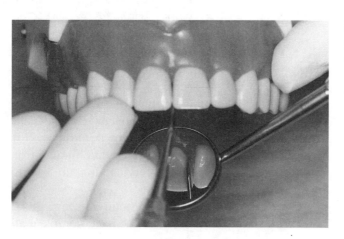

Figure 8–58B   Keep instrument tip adapted to tooth at all times to prevent tissue trauma.

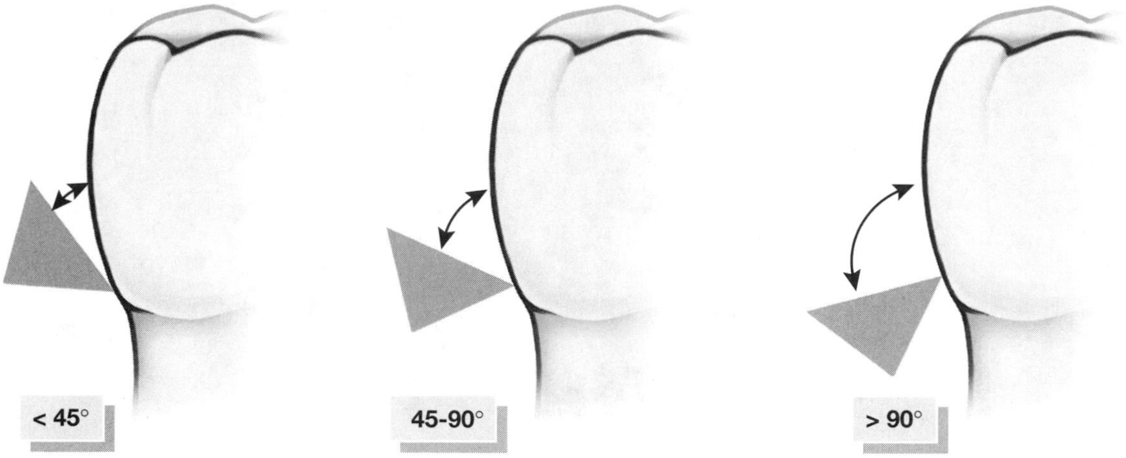

Figure 8–59 Working angulations. To scale deposits, open blade by tilting it away from the tooth between 45 and 90 degrees.

  (a) Operator position—11:00 to 11:30 (left-handed, 1:00 to 12:30)
  (b) Patient's head—position straight or slightly toward the operator
  (c) Patient's chin—position up
  (d) Light—position over chest, angle up
  (e) Mirror—in nondominant hand, palm mirror and retract lip with index finger; use direct vision
  (f) Instrument fulcrum—position as close as possible to working area
 (2) Lingual
  (a) Operator position—11:00 to 11:30 (left-handed, 1:00 to 12:30); avoid leaning and/or bending excessively over patient
  (b) Patient's head—position straight or slightly toward the operator
  (c) Patient's chin—position up
  (d) Light—position over chest, angle up
  (e) Mirror—fulcrum on maxillary left premolars; use indirect vision, illumination, and transillumination
  (f) Instrument fulcrum—position as close as possible to working area
 (3) Application—facial and lingual
  (a) Insert tip slightly past midline of tooth
  (b) Activate vertical/oblique strokes toward operator, across cervical, making sure to always keep tip against tooth
  (c) Roll tip around line angle into proximal surface, finishing under contact; complete all surfaces toward operator
  (d) Reposition tip at midline of tooth
  (e) Activate vertical/oblique strokes away from operator, across cervical, making sure to always keep tip against tooth
  (f) Roll tip around line angle into proximal surface, finishing under contact; complete all surfaces away from operator

c. Sextant 3 (maxillary left)
   (1) Facial
      (a) Operator position—9:00 to 11:30 (left-handed, 3:00 to 12:30)
      (b) Patient's head—position toward operator
      (c) Patient's chin—position up
      (d) Light—position over chest, angle up
      (e) Mirror—retract cheek with mirror face toward teeth for indirect vision; use direct vision for premolars; avoid resting rim of mirror on gingiva or alveolar bone
      (f) Instrument fulcrum—position as close as possible to working area without blocking light
   (2) Lingual
      (a) Alternate position A
         • Operator position—9:00 (left-handed, 3:00)
         • Patient's head—position up and away from operator
         • Patient's chin—position up
         • Light—position over chest, angle up
         • Mirror—fulcrum on opposite maxillary premolars; use indirect vision and illumination
         • Instrument fulcrum—position as close as possible to working area
      (b) Alternate position B
         • Operator position—10:00 to 11:30 (left-handed, 2:00 to 12:30)
         • Patient's head—position toward operator
         • Patient's chin—position up
         • Light—position over chest, angle up
         • Mirror—position on the opposite maxillary premolar area
               Tip: If the operator fulcrums on the facial surfaces of the opposite maxillary premolar teeth, it helps retract the lip, allowing for greater illumination.
         • Instrument fulcrum—using the pen grasp, position on the maxillary anteriors, making sure to place grasp toward middle of handle
   (3) Application (facial and lingual)
      (a) Insert tip at distal line angle
      (b) Activate vertical/oblique strokes toward distal, making sure to keep tip against tooth at all times
      (c) Roll tip around line angle into proximal surface, finishing under contact
      (d) Turn tip toward mesial and reposition at distal line angle
      (e) Reinsert at distal line angle and use vertical/oblique strokes to move instrument toward mesial line angle
      (f) Stop at mesial line angle; use one of the following options to keep tip adapted to tooth and to prevent tissue trauma
         • Option 1—roll the scaler with thumb and support with index finger around line angle

---

PRECLINICAL TIP

Adapting Your Knowledge: When working in areas with limited direct vision, keep face of mirror toward the teeth so distal surfaces can be viewed. Neutral body positions should always be maintained.

- Option 2—stop and reposition at line angle

    (g) Proceed around line angle into proximal surface, finishing under contact

d. Sextant 4 (mandibular left)

    (1) Facial

        (a) Operator position
- Distals—9:00 (left-handed, 3:00)
- Mesials—11:30 (left-handed, 12:30)

        (b) Patient's head—position toward operator

        (c) Patient's chin—position down

        (d) Light—position over mouth

        (e) Mirror—retract cheek with mirror face toward teeth for molars; retract for premolars using direct vision

        (f) Instrument fulcrum—position as close as possible to working area

    (2) Lingual

        (a) Operator position—7:30 to 9:00 (left-handed, 4:30 to 3:00)
- Position 1—7:30 (left-handed, 4:30)—place knees together at side of chair facing 12:00 position
- Position 2—9:00 (left-handed, 3:00)—straddle chair with weight evenly distributed

        (b) Patient's head—position away from operator

        (c) Patient's chin—position down

        (d) Light—position over mouth

        (e) Mirror—fulcrum on opposite mandibular premolar area; retract tongue with mirror face toward teeth; use indirect vision and illumination

        (f) Instrument fulcrum—position as close as possible to working area

    (3) Application (facial and lingual)

        (a) Insert tip at distal line angle

        (b) Activate vertical/oblique strokes toward distal, making sure to always keep tip against tooth

        (c) Roll tip into proximal surface, finishing under contact

        (d) Turn tip toward mesial and reposition at distal line angle

        (e) Reinsert at distal line angle and use vertical/oblique strokes to move instrument toward mesial line angle

        (f) Stop at mesial line angle; use one of the following options to adapt tip to tooth and to prevent tissue trauma
- Option 1—roll the scaler with thumb and support with index finger around line angle
- Option 2—stop and reposition at line angle

        (g) Proceed around line angle into proximal surface, finishing under contact

e. Sextant 5 (mandibular anterior)

    (1) Facial and lingual (surfaces toward)

        (a) Operator position—7:30 to 9:00 (left-handed, 4:30 to 3:00)

        (b) Patient's head—position straight or slightly away

        (c) Patient's chin—position down

(d) Light—position over mouth

(e) Mirror—use palm grasp and retract lip with index finger of nondominant hand for facial surfaces; use indirect vision for lingual surfaces

(f) Instrument fulcrum—position as close as possible to working area

(2) Facial and lingual (surfaces away)

   (a) Operator position—11:30 (left-handed, 12:30)

   (b) Patient's head—position straight or slightly toward

   (c) Patient's chin—position down

   (d) Light—position over mouth

   (e) Mirror—use palm grasp and retract lip with index finger of nondominant hand for facial surfaces; use indirect vision for lingual surfaces

   (f) Instrument fulcrum—position as close as possible to working area

(3) Application

   (a) Surfaces toward operator (facial and lingual)

     • Insert tip past midline

     • Activate vertical/oblique strokes toward operator, across cervical, making sure to always keep tip against tooth

     • Roll tip around line angle into proximal surface, finishing under contact (Figure 8–60)

   (b) Surfaces away from operator (facial and lingual)

     • Reposition tip at midline of tooth

     • Activate vertical/oblique strokes away from operator, across cervical, making sure to always keep tip against tooth

     • Roll tip around line angle into proximal surface, finishing under contact

f. Sextant 6 (mandibular right)

(1) Facial

   (a) Operator position—7:30 to 9:00 (left-handed, 4:30 to 3:00)

     • Position 1—7:30 (left-handed, 4:30)—place knees together at side of chair facing 12:00 position

---

PRECLINICAL TIP

Adapting your Knowledge: To increase time efficiency, complete all facial surfaces towards you, then complete all lingual surfaces toward you before instrumenting the surfaces away.

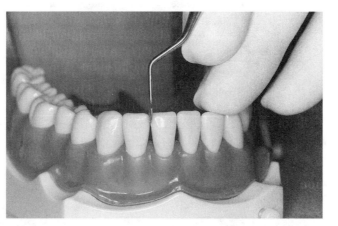

Figure 8–60   Roll instrument tip to finish under contact.

- Position 2—9:00 (left-handed, 3:00)—straddle chair with weight evenly distributed

(b) Patient's head—position slightly away

(c) Patient's chin—position down

(d) Light—position over mouth

(e) Mirror—retract cheek; use indirect vision for molars, direct vision for premolars

(f) Instrument fulcrum—position on incisal/occlusal of mandibular canine/premolar area

(2) Lingual

(a) Operator position

- Distals—9:00 (left-handed, 3:00)
- Mesials—11:30; (left-handed, 2:30)

(b) Patient's head—position toward operator

(c) Patient's chin—position down

(d) Light—position over mouth

(e) Mirror—retract cheek with mirror face toward teeth for molars; retract for premolars using direct vision

(f) Instrument fulcrum—position as close as possible to working area

(3) Application

(a) Insert tip at distal line angle

(b) Activate vertical/oblique strokes toward distal, making sure to always keep tip against tooth

(c) Roll tip around line angle into proximal surface, finishing under contact

(d) Turn tip toward mesial and reposition at distal line angle

(e) Reinsert at distal line angle and use vertical/oblique strokes to move instrument toward mesial line angle

(f) Stop at mesial line angle; use one of the following options to adapt tip to tooth and to prevent tissue trauma

- Option 1—roll the scaler with thumb and support with index finger around line angle
- Option 2—stop and reposition at line angle

(g) Proceed around line angle into proximal surface, finishing under contact

See Scaling Instrument Task Skill Sheet at end of chapter.

E. Universal curette

1. A rounded, curved, scaling instrument used on any tooth for scaling

2. Used to remove supra- and subgingival calculus from anterior and posterior teeth in the proximal surfaces as well as facial and lingual surfaces—all with the convenience of using one instrument

3. Characteristics

a. Internal angle between 70 and 80 degrees (refer to 8–5b)

b. Blade at 90-degree angle to the shank of the instrument (perpendicular)

c. Two parallel cutting edges that curve around and meet at the round toe; both cutting edges are utilized

    d. Cutting edges form at the junction of the lateral surfaces and facial surface on either side

    e. Cross-section is half-moon shape

    f. Rounded back where the lower portions of the lateral surfaces meet; remains next to the soft tissue

    g. Curved face

    h. Paired mirror image working ends

4. Types: All universal instruments are designed to use throughout the entire dentition, which is convenient. The anterior and posterior designation actually refers to variations in shank length. Some universal curettes are designed with more angle than others. Examples include the Barnhart 1-2 and Barnhart 5-6 (Figure 8–61). Both are universal curettes and used throughout the mouth, but the Barnhart 1-2 has a straighter, longer shank than the Barnhart 5-6, which looks shorter and more curved. Other examples of universal curettes include

    a. Columbia 13/14

    b. Columbia 2R/2L

    c. Columbia 4R/4L

    d. Younger Good 7/8

    e. McCall's 13/14

    f. Langer 1/2, 3/4, 5/6

5. Determination of correct working end

    a. Place toe of instrument into interproximal—align terminal shank parallel to interproximal surface; position handle toward opening of oral cavity

    b. When the correct end is adapted, most of the face of the instrument *cannot* be seen

      (1) If the face can be seen, the wrong end is being adapted—to correct, switch ends

      (2) Blade should curve toward the tooth

6. Grasp—use modified pen grasp

7. Instrument fulcrum—place an intraoral fulcrum as close as possible to the working area

8. Insertion—insert at or as near zero degrees as possible; blade is closed, or tilted toward the tooth, as the rounded back is slipped under the free margin of the gingiva (refer to 8–56)

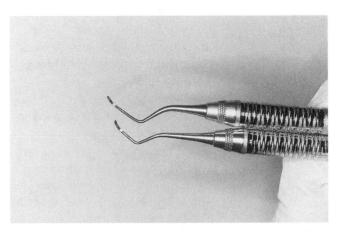

Figure 8–61   Barnhart 1-2 and Barnhart 5-6.

9. Adaptation: Place 1 mm to 2mm of toe flush against tooth; use one of the following options to adapt toe to tooth and to prevent tissue trauma
   a. Option 1—roll instrument with thumb and index finger around line angles
   b. Option 2—stop and reposition at line angles
      Tip: This instrument has two cutting edges. When not properly adapted, trauma to the soft tissue can occur.
10. Angulation—to remove or scale deposits, open blade by tilting away from tooth, between 45 and 90 degrees
11. Activation
    a. Begin at the distal line angle to instrument the distal interproximal contact
    b. Pivot on fulcrum to angle the cutting edge toward the tooth surface
    c. Rock the wrist and pivot hand on fulcrum following the rounded contour of the tooth surface
    d. Use short, overlapping vertical/oblique strokes, extending from base of the deposit coronally
    e. Finish with the toe of instrument under the contact
    f. Turn toe toward mesial
    g. Reposition instrument at the distal line angle and use oblique strokes to move instrument toward the mesial line angle
    h. Rock the wrist and pivot following the contour of the tooth
    i. Reposition at mesial line angle and finish stroke under the mesial contact
       Tip: Use same working end for facial surfaces in same sextant; use opposite end for lingual surfaces in same sextant, except for sextant 5
12. Instrument pattern
    a. Sextant 1 (maxillary right)
       (1) Facial
           (a) Operator position—10:00 with arm at 9:00 (left-handed, 2:00 with arm at 3:00)
           (b) Patient's head—position slightly away from operator
           (c) Patient's chin—position up
           (d) Light—position over chest, angle up
           (e) Mirror—use for retraction when face of mirror is toward cheek; use illumination when face of mirror is toward teeth—usually to view distal surfaces
           (f) Instrument fulcrum—position as close as possible to working area without blocking light
       (2) Lingual
           (a) Operator position—10:00 to 11:30 (left-handed, 2:00 to 12:30); avoid excessive bending and/or leaning for vision
           (b) Patient's head—position toward operator
           (c) Patient's chin—position up
           (d) Light—position over chest, angle up
           (e) Mirror—fulcrum on opposite maxillary premolar; use indirect vision and illumination

(f) Instrument fulcrum—position as close as possible to working area

(3) Application (facial and lingual)

   (a) Insert toe at distal line angle

   (b) Activate vertical/oblique strokes toward distal, making sure to keep toe against tooth at all times

   (c) Roll toe around proximal surface, finishing under contact

   (d) Turn toe toward mesial and reposition at distal line angle

   (e) Reinsert at distal line angle

   (f) Reactivate vertical/oblique strokes to move instrument across cervical toward mesial line angle

   (g) Stop at mesial line angle; use one of the following options to adapt toe to tooth and to prevent tissue trauma

   • Option 1—roll the curette with thumb and support with index finger around line angle

   • Option 2—stop and reposition at line angle

   (h) Proceed around line angle into proximal surface, finishing under contact

b. Sextant 2 (maxillary anteriors)—mentally divide each maxillary anterior tooth down the center; surfaces from midline to interproximal toward operator are called *toward*, surfaces from midline to interproximal away from operator are called *away*

(1) Facial

   (a) Operator position—11:00 to 11:30 (left-handed, 1:00 to 12:30)

   (b) Patient's head—position straight or slightly toward the operator

   (c) Patient's chin—position up

   (d) Light—position over chest, angle up

   (e) Mirror—in nondominant hand, palm mirror and retract lip with index finger; use direct vision

   (f) Instrument fulcrum—position as close as possible to working area

(2) Lingual

   (a) Operator position—11:00 to 11:30 (left-handed, 1:00 to 12:30); avoid leaning and/or bending excessively over patient

   (b) Patient's head—position straight or slightly toward the operator

   (c) Patient's chin—position up

   (d) Light—position over chest, angle up

   (e) Mirror—fulcrum on maxillary left premolars; use indirect vision, illumination, and transillumination

   (f) Instrument fulcrum—position as close as possible to working area

(3) Application (facial and lingual)

   (a) Insert toe slightly past midline of tooth

   (b) Activate vertical/oblique strokes toward operator, across cervical, making sure to always keep toe against tooth

PRECLINICAL TIP

Adapting Your Knowledge: To increase time efficiency, complete all facial surfaces towards you, then complete all lingual surfaces toward you before instrumenting the surfaces away.

(c) Roll toe around line angle into proximal surface, finishing under contact; complete all surfaces toward operator

(d) Reposition toe at midline

(e) Activate vertical/oblique strokes away from operator, across cervical

(f) Roll toe around line angle into proximal surface, finishing under contact; complete all surfaces away from operator

c. Sextant 3 (maxillary left)

   (1) Facial

     (a) Operator position—9:00 to 11:30 (left-handed, 3:00 to 12:30)

     (b) Patient's head—position toward operator

     (c) Patient's chin—position up

     (d) Light—position over chest, angle up

     (e) Mirror—retract cheek with mirror face toward teeth for indirect vision; use direct vision for premolars; avoid resting rim of mirror on gingiva or alveolar bone

     (f) Instrument fulcrum—position as close as possible to working area without blocking light

   (2) Lingual

     (a) Alternate position A
- Operator position—9:00 (left-handed, 3:00)
- Patient's head—position up and away from operator
- Patient's chin—position up
- Light—position over chest, angle up
- Mirror—fulcrum on opposite maxillary premolars; use indirect vision and illumination
- Instrument fulcrum—position as close as possible to working area

     (b) Alternate position B
- Operator position—10:00 to 11:30 (left-handed, 2:00 to 12:30)
- Patient's head—position toward operator
- Patient's chin—position up
- Light—position over chest, angle up
- Mirror—fulcrum on opposite maxillary premolar area

       Tip: If the operator fulcrums on the facial surfaces of the opposite maxillary premolar teeth, it helps retract the lip, allowing for greater illumination.
- Instrument fulcrum—using the pen grasp, position on the maxillary anteriors, making sure to place grasp toward middle of handle

   (3) Application (facial and lingual) (Figure 8–62)

     (a) Insert toe at distal line angle

     (b) Activate vertical/oblique strokes toward distal, making sure to keep toe against tooth at all times

     (c) Roll toe around proximal surface, finishing under contact

---

PRECLINICAL TIP

Adapting Your Knowledge: When working in areas with limited direct vision, keep face of mirror toward the teeth so distal surfaces can be viewed. Neutral body positions should always be maintained.

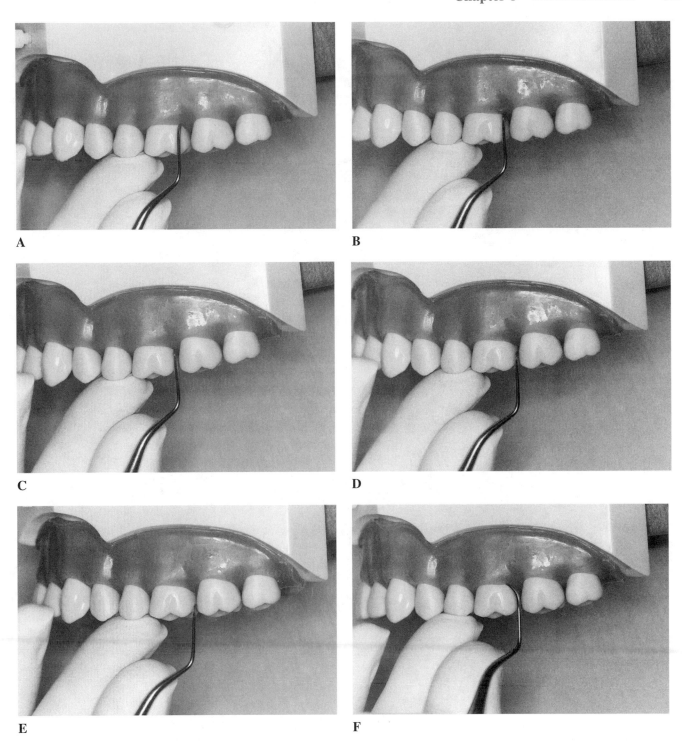

Figure 8–62   Application of Barnhart 1-2.

(d) Turn toe toward mesial and reposition at distal line angle
(e) Reinsert at distal line angle
(f) Reactivate vertical/oblique strokes to move instrument across cervical toward mesial line angle

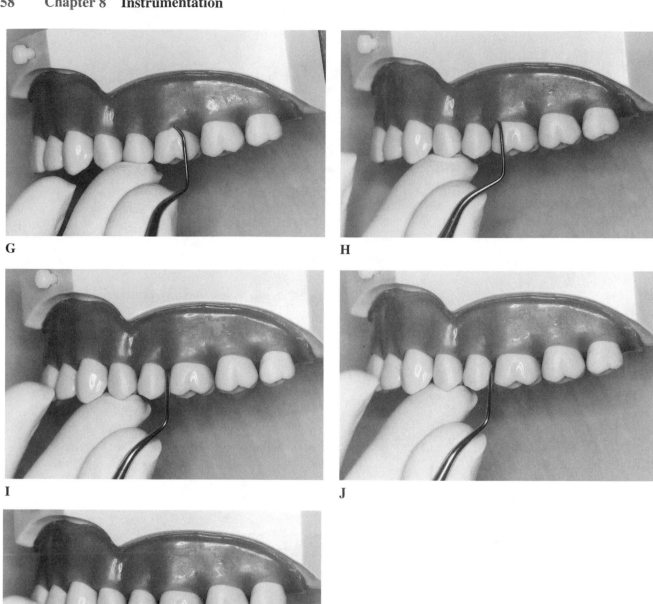

G

H

I

J

K

Figure 8–62   Continued.

(g) Stop at mesial line angle; use one of the following options to adapt toe to tooth and to prevent tissue trauma
  • Option 1—roll the curette with thumb and support with index finger around line angle
  • Option 2—stop and reposition at line angle
(h) Proceed around line angle into proximal surface, finishing under contact
d. Sextant 4 (mandibular left)
   (1) Facial
     (a) Operator position

- Distals—9:00 (left-handed, 3:00)
- Mesials—11:30 (left-handed, 12:30)
  (b) Patient's head—position toward operator
  (c) Patient's chin—position down
  (d) Light—position over mouth
  (e) Mirror—retract cheek with mirror face toward teeth for molars; retract for premolars using direct vision
  (f) Instrument fulcrum—position as close as possible to working area
(2) Lingual
  (a) Operator position—7:30 to 9:00 (left-handed, 4:30 to 3:00)
- Position 1—7:30 (left-handed, 4:30)—place knees together at side of chair facing 12:00 position
- Position 2—9:00 (left-handed, 3:00)—straddle chair with weight evenly distributed
  (b) Patient's head—position away from operator
  (c) Patient's chin—position down
  (d) Light—position over mouth
  (e) Mirror—fulcrum on opposite mandibular premolar area; retract tongue with mirror face toward teeth; use indirect vision and illumination
  (f) Instrument fulcrum—position as close as possible to working area
(3) Application (facial and lingual)
  (a) Insert toe at distal line angle
  (b) Activate vertical/oblique strokes toward distal, making sure to keep toe against tooth at all times
  (c) Roll toe around proximal surface, finishing under contact
  (d) Turn toe toward mesial and reposition at distal line angle
  (e) Reinsert at distal line angle
  (f) Reactivate vertical/oblique strokes to move instrument across cervical toward mesial line angle
  (g) Stop at mesial line angle; use one of the following options to adapt toe to tooth and to prevent tissue trauma
- Option 1—roll the curette with thumb and support with index finger around line angle
- Option 2—stop and reposition at line angle
  (h) Proceed around line angle into proximal surface, finishing under contact
e. Sextant 5 (mandibular anterior)
  (1) Facial and lingual (surfaces toward)
    (a) Operator position—7:30 to 9:00 (left-handed, 4:30 to 3:00)
    (b) Patient's head—position straight or slightly away
    (c) Patient's chin—position down
    (d) Light—position over mouth
    (e) Mirror—use palm grasp and retract lip with index finger of nondominant hand for facial surfaces; use indirect vision for lingual surfaces

PRECLINICAL TIP

Adapting your Knowledge: In an effort to increase time efficiency, complete all facial surfaces towards you, then complete all lingual surfaces toward you before instrumenting the surfaces away.

      (f) Instrument fulcrum—position as close as possible to working area

  (2) Facial and lingual (surfaces away)

    (a) Operator position—11:30 (left-handed, 12:30)

    (b) Patient's head—position straight or slightly toward

    (c) Patient's chin—position down

    (d) Light—position over mouth

    (e) Mirror—use palm grasp and retract lip with index finger of nondominant hand for facial surfaces; use indirect vision for lingual surfaces

    (f) Instrument fulcrum—position as close as possible to working area

  (3) Application

    (a) Surfaces toward operator (facial and lingual)

- Insert toe past midline
- Activate vertical/oblique strokes toward operator, across cervical, making sure to always keep toe against tooth
- Roll toe around line angle into proximal surface, finishing under contact

    (b) Surfaces away from operator (facial and lingual)

- Reposition toe at midline of tooth
- Activate vertical/oblique strokes away from operator, across cervical, making sure to always keep toe against tooth
- Roll toe into proximal surface, finishing under contact

f. Sextant 6 (mandibular right)

  (1) Facial

    (a) Operator position—7:30 to 9:00 (left-handed, 4:30 to 3:00)

- Position 1—7:30 (left-handed, 4:30)—place knees together at side of chair facing 12:00 position
- Position 2—9:00 (left-handed, 3:00)—straddle chair with weight evenly distributed

    (b) Patient's head—position slightly away

    (c) Patient's chin—position down

    (d) Light—position over mouth

    (e) Mirror—retract cheek; use indirect vision for molars, direct vision for premolars

    (f) Instrument fulcrum—position on incisal/occlusal of mandibular canine/premolar area

  (2) Lingual

    (a) Operator position

- Distals—9:00 (left-handed, 3:00)
- Mesials—11:30 (left-handed, 12:30)

    (b) Patient's head—position toward operator

    (c) Patient's chin—position down

    (d) Light—position over mouth

    (e) Mirror—retract cheek with mirror face toward teeth for molars; retract for premolars using direct vision

(f) Instrument fulcrum—position as close as possible to working area

(3) Application (facial and lingual)

(a) Insert toe at distal line angle

(b) Activate vertical/oblique strokes toward distal, making sure to keep toe against tooth at all times

(c) Roll toe around proximal surface, finishing under contact

(d) Turn toe toward mesial and reposition at distal line angle

(e) Reinsert at distal line angle

(f) Reactivate vertical/oblique strokes to move instrument across cervical toward mesial line angle

(g) Stop at mesial line angle; use one of the following options to adapt toe to tooth and to prevent tissue trauma

• Option 1—roll the curette with thumb and support with index finger around line angle

• Option 2—stop and reposition at line angle

(h) Proceed around line angle into proximal surface, finishing under contact

See Scaling Instrument Task Skill Sheet at end of chapter.

VII. Air/water syringe

A. Grasp (Figure 8–63): Palm grasp—hold air/water syringe in palm of dominant hand, wrap fingers around the handle, and activate the buttons on top with pad of thumb

B. Uses of air

1. Caries examination and detection—dry teeth thoroughly to increase visibility

2. Calculus examination and detection

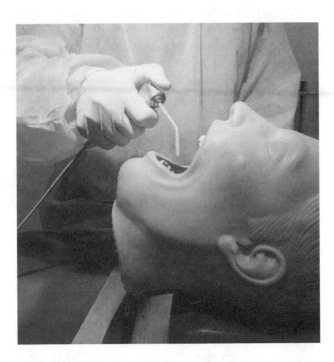

Figure 8–63   Using palm grasp to hold air/water syringe.

a. Use strong steady stream of air—dehydrates supragingival calculus, which appears chalky white

b. Deflect tissue to view subgingival calculus

3. Contraindications—use with caution on patients with hypersensitive teeth

C. Uses of water

1. Increases visibility

2. Clears field of operation of debris, saliva, and blood

3. Provides moisture for patient comfort

D. Air/water mixture—created by depressing both air/water simultaneously

1. Helps dislodge blood clots when field of vision needs to be cleared

2. Caution: Creates an aerosol, so use universal precautions

VIII. **Summary of Instrumentation**

Instrumentation is one of the most challenging tasks to be learned in dental hygiene. It is rewarding to see the before's and after's of scaling and have the patient notice the difference in the way the mouth feels and looks. It is one of the most important tasks to accomplish in dental hygiene, because removal of hard and soft deposits stimulates healing and improves oral health. Ultimately, the patient is in control of his or her oral hygiene through the preventive measures employed; however, thorough instrumentation can provide patient motivation needed to maintain health.

Excellent instrumentation skills are developed with time and experience. Following and building on solid foundational principles will lead to success and increased competence in using instruments. Becoming an excellent clinician is more than being good at instrumentation; it is also adopting an attitude of wanting to constantly learn new techniques and advanced concepts. Mastering the principles of instrumentation will bring much reward and satisfaction to the career of dental hygiene.

IX. **Instrument Sharpening**

Sharpening is an important maintenance step for scaling instruments and helps the dental hygienist achieve the best performance possible. Ideally, instruments should be sharpened after sterilization.

A. Objective of sharpening: Produce a sharp cutting edge without changing the original design of the instrument[13]

B. Rationale for sharpening

1. Keeps instruments sharp[2] and true to their original design by preserving the correct angulation between the instrument face and the lateral surface(s)

2. Enhances job efficiency and quality of care to patient, as sharp instruments reduce appointment time

3. Improves tactile sensitivity, because a sharp instrument allows the use of a relaxed grasp and a controlled stroke

4. Reduces operator fatigue, since fewer strokes are needed; dull instruments must be used with excessive pressure

5. Increases comfort to patient due to fewer strokes needed

C. Sharpening stones

1. Description (Figure 8–64): Sharpening stones are abrasive devices used to restore the cutting edge on a dull instrument without changing its original design. They are made of gritty, abrasive particles compressed into a solid piece that is harder than the metal of the in-

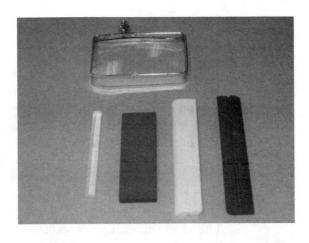

Figure 8–64 Sharpening stone, plastic testing stick, and magnifying glass.

strument. Coarse stones have large particles that cut rapidly. Fine stones have smaller particles that cut more slowly. (See Table 8–4)

a. Fine-to-medium stones
   (1) Arkansas stone—fine-grained, natural stone quarried from natural mineral deposits
       (a) Available in flat, rectangular, wedge, cylindrical, or round shapes; flat, rectangular, or wedge-shaped stones may have grooves for the special adaptation of curved blades, used for routine sharpening
       (b) Edges may be rounded or square
   (2) I (India) stone—synthetic (man-made), medium-textured stone used to sharpen dull cutting edges
   (3) Ceramic stone—fine-grained synthetic stone used for routine sharpening

b. Coarse (Composition) stone—synthetic, coarse-grained stone used for extensive sharpening and reshaping of working ends that have dull or worn cutting edges; especially good for blades that have been improperly sharpened

2. Stone design: Sharpening stones are available in varying sizes, shapes, and textures. Many come with a guide and manufacturer's instructions that must be followed for best results. Samples can be seen at professional meetings where vendors display their products. Manufacturers frequently advertise new designs and products in professional journals. Types of unmounted sharpening stones include:

a. Rectangular or flat—used to sharpen the blade of the instrument in three sections—heel third, middle third and lower third of blade

Table 8–4 Sharpening Stone Comparison Chart

Name	Origin	Method	Lubricant	Texture	Application
Arkansas Stone	Natural	Unmounted, mounted, or rotary	Oil	Fine	Routine sharpening and finishing
I Stone	Synthetic	Unmounted	Water or oil	Medium	Sharpening of excessively dull instruments or those requiring recontouring
Ceramic Stone	Synthetic	Unmounted	Water or dry	Fine	Routine sharpening and finishing
Composition Stone	Synthetic	Mounted	Water	Coarse	Reshaping of excessively worn instruments

*Mounting refers to stones that can be mounted on a slow-speed handpiece; beginning students should use with caution. This chart is used with courtesy from Hu-Friedy Manufacturing Company, 3232 N. Rockwell Street, Chicago, IL.[4]

b. Cylindrical or cone-shaped—useful when sharpening the face of curettes or curved sickle scalers; most often used to remove wire edges (minute metal projections) that can form when the lateral sides are sharpened

c. Grooved—designed to help cutting edge stay in proper angulation

d. Wedge—contains a rounded side that can be used like the cylindrical stone to remove wire edge or to sharpen the face of the blade; flat side is used to sharpen the lateral borders of the blade or cutting edges

D. Armamentarium

1. Stone

2. Lubricant (mineral oil or water)

   a. Application—apply with cotton tip applicator or gauze square

   b. Purpose

      (1) Facilitates movement of the instrument over the stone

      (2) Reduces frictional heat

      (3) Prevents clogging of metal shavings on the surface of the stone; use gauze square to remove the residue, called sludge, created by metal shavings and oil/water

   c. Refer to Table 8–4 to determine which agent should be used for each stone

3. Light source—use a good light source, such as the dental unit or a lab bench, since a sharp cutting edge does not reflect light; a dull cutting edge appears as a white area at the junction of the face and lateral surfaces

4. Magnification—magnifying glass or magnification loupes can help identify cutting edge and dull edges

5. Plastic testing stick—use to determine instrument sharpness

   a. Grasp stick with nondominant hand at waist level

   b. Fulcrum on the top of the stick with dominant hand

   c. Adapt the cutting edge against the stick at the same angle used to scale a tooth

   d. Position the lower shank of the instrument parallel to the long axis of the stick

   e. Cut into stick with blade

      (1) Sharp instrument will bite into the stick, and a pinging metallic noise can be heard

      (2) Dull instrument will glide over the stick and not catch plastic[13]

   f. Apply all three areas (heel third, middle third, and lower third of blade) of the cutting edge to test for sharpness; resharpen any portion of the blade that does not bite or grab into the stick

   g. Autoclave plastic testing sticks with sharpening stones

6. Personal protective equipment (PPE);

   a. Protective eyewear to prevent metal shavings from becoming lodged in eye

   b. Gloves for protection

   c. Mask if instruments are contaminated

7. Use clock positions as a reference to determine the proper positioning of the instrument and stone[11]

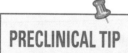

PRECLINICAL TIP

Adapting Your Knowledge: Light reflects from a dull surface. The cutting edge of a sharp instrument has length but no width, since it is a narrow line.[13]

E. Signs of instrument dullness: Repeated use of a dental instrument wears away minute particles of metal from the blade, causing the cutting edge to take on a rounded shape and resulting in a dull, ineffective blade.[12] Instruments should be sharpened at the first sign of dullness, which may include one of the following

1. Instrument not biting into plastic test stick, but instead gliding over it—not catching
2. White line along cutting edge due to the reflection of the light; best viewed under lighted magnification (Figure 8–65b)
3. Cutting edge showing thickness and more depth; when an instrument is sharp, the cutting edge is only a line
4. Scaling procedures taking longer due to inefficiency of cutting edge

F. Technique for sharpening sickle scalers (moving stone)

1. Grasp instrument in nondominant hand
2. Stabilize back of fingers and instrument against a hard surface, such as a tabletop or a lab bench, to prevent slipping (Figure 8–66)
3. Use clock positions (1:00 and 11:00)—provides an easy way to visualize the 110-degree angulation necessary between the blade and stone for sharpening to occur (Figures 8–67a and 8–67b)
4. Identify cutting edges—cutting edges are formed at the junction of the lateral sides and face of blade; lateral surfaces and face of sickle scalers meet at an internal angle between 70 and 80 degrees
5. Position face of instrument parallel to floor
6. Face tip toward operator
7. Divide the blade into thirds—heel, middle, and tip; at 12:00 position, apply stone to heel of blade; open stone to 1:00; then, using light pressure, move the stone up and down with strokes that are one-quarter to one-half inch in length (Figures 8–68a and 8–68b)
8. Continue moving stone to middle third of blade

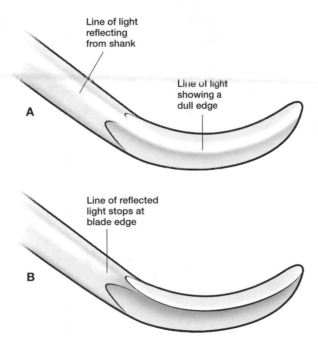

Figure 8–65A Line of light showing a dull edge. 8-65B Line of light showing a sharp edge.

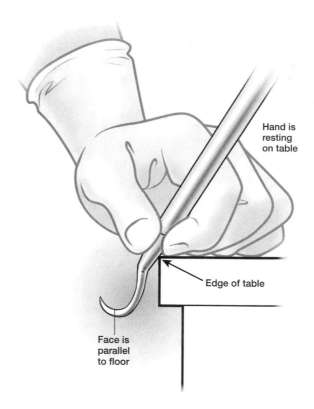

Figure 8–66   Stabilize hand against hard surface when sharpening.

9. Follow to tip third of blade, finishing with down stroke to avoid creating a wire edge[13] (Figure 8–69)

10. Apply stone to *opposite* side of blade at 11:00 position and sharpen entire blade in thirds once again

11. Sharpening the face—use round or conical stone for curved face, such as the modified sickle scaler; use flat stone for instrument with straight face, such as the jacquette sickle scaler

NOTE: Sides are most often sharpened, although face can occasionally be sharpened. Sharpening only the face and not the lateral surfaces can weaken the blade; therefore, it is best to sharpen the cutting surfaces equally in order to preserve the contour of the instrument

a. Stabilize instrument with the tip toward the operator

b. Sharpen curved face of blade—moving toward the tip, roll the conical or round stone, using light, even pressure, toward the operator, beginning at the intersection of the shank and working end (Figure 8–70)

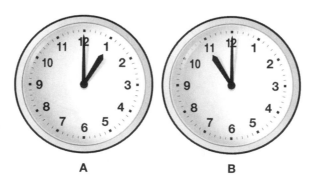

Figure 8–67   Clock positions used during instrument sharpening. A. One o'clock B. Eleven o'clock.

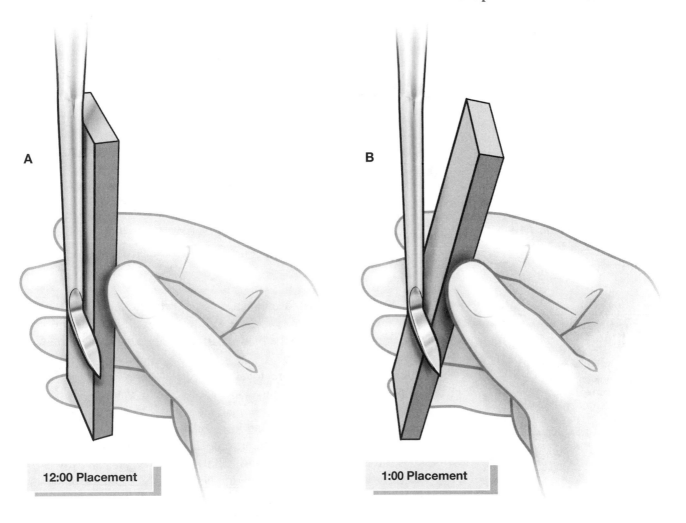

A   12:00 Placement

B   1:00 Placement

Figure 8–68A   Applying sharpening stone to sickle scaler at twelve o'clock position. 8-68B Applying sharpening stone to sickle scaler at one o'clock position.

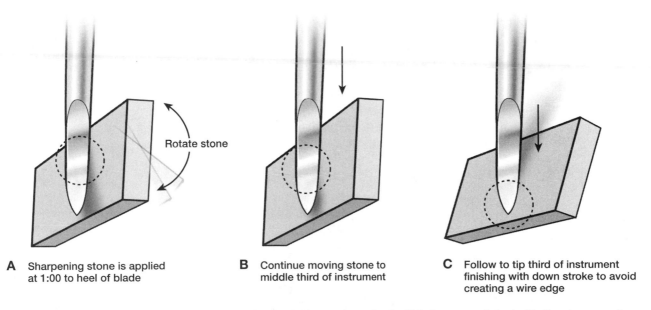

Rotate stone

A   Sharpening stone is applied at 1:00 to heel of blade

B   Continue moving stone to middle third of instrument

C   Follow to tip third of instrument finishing with down stroke to avoid creating a wire edge

Figure 8–69   Sharpening sickle scaler. A. Apply sharpening stone to heel of blade at one o'clock. B. Continue moving stone to middle third of blade C. Follow to tip of blade finishing with a down stroke to avoid creating a wire edge.

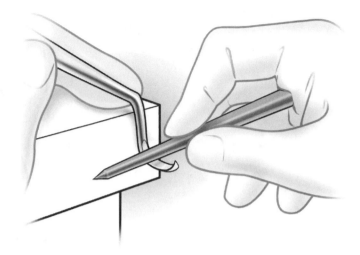

Figure 8–70 Sharpening the face
of a curved sickle scaler.

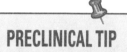

c. Sharpen straight face of blade—adapt flat stone to the flat face; move the stone in horizontal strokes, using light, even pressure across the face of the blade; perform only periodically to avoid weakening the blade

12. Test for sharpness as previously described
G. Technique for sharpening universal curette (moving stone)
1. Grasp instrument in nondominant hand
2. Stabilize back of fingers and instrument against a hard surface like a tabletop or a lab bench to prevent slipping
3. Use clock positions (1:00 and 11:00)—provides an easy way to visualize the 110-degree angulation necessary between the blade and stone for sharpening to occur (see Figures 8–68a and 8–68b)
4. Identify cutting edges—formed at the junction of the lateral sides and face of blade; lateral surfaces and face of universal curettes meet at an internal angle between 70 and 80 degrees

Figure 8–71 Sharpening curette blade at one o'clock position.

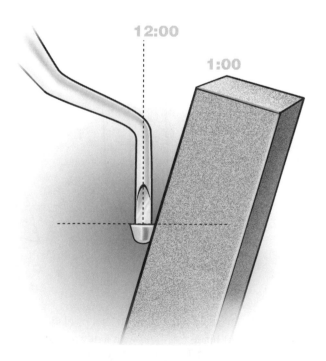

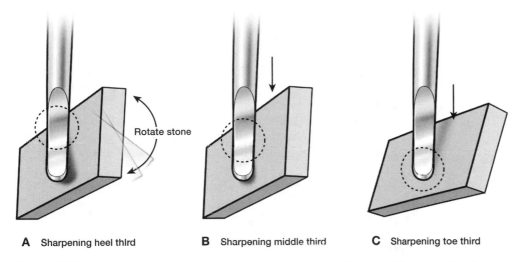

A Sharpening heel third   **B** Sharpening middle third   **C** Sharpening toe third

Figure 8–72   Sharpening curette scaler. A. Apply stone to heel third of blade. B. Continue moving stone to middle third of blade. C. Follow to toe third of blade and finish with a down stroke.

5. Position face of instrument parallel to floor
6. Face toe toward operator
7. Divide the blade into thirds—heel, middle, and toe
8. At 12:00 position, apply stone to heel of blade, then open stone to 1:00 position; using light pressure, move stone up and down with strokes that are one-quarter to one-half inch in length, using light pressure (Figure 8–71)
9. Continue moving stone to middle third of blade (Figure 8–72).

PRECLINICAL TIP

Adapting Your Knowledge: An excellent way to sharpen the toe is to use a grooved stone at a 45-degree angle.

Figure 8–73   Sharpening opposite side of curette blade at eleven o'clock position.

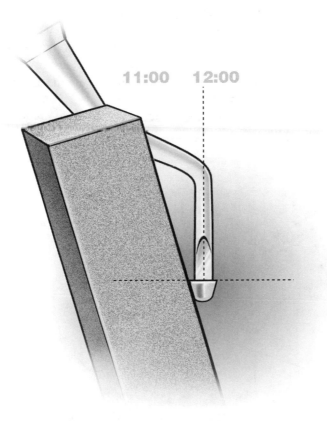

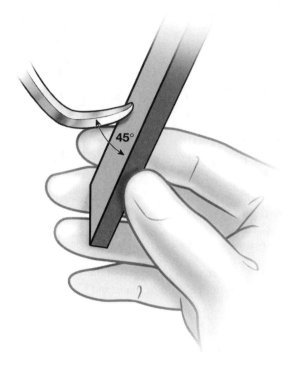

Figure 8–74   Rounding toe at forty-five degrees with sharpening stone.

10. Follow to toe third of blade, finishing with down stroke to avoid creating a wire edge
11. Apply stone to *opposite* side of blade at 11:00 position and sharpen entire blade in thirds once again (Figure 8–73)
    a. Sharpening and rounding toe
    b. Continue the stroke around the toe to preserve its rounded contour by decreasing the stone angle to 45 degrees (Figure 8–74); sharpening only the lateral borders will result in the toe losing its roundness and taking on a pointed shape
12. Sharpening the face—use round or conical stone (Figure 8–75)
    a. Roll the conical or round stone, using light, even pressure, toward the operator, beginning at the intersection of the shank and working end
    b. Move toward the toe so both cutting edges are contacted at the same time

Figure 8–75   Sharpening the face of the curette with a conical stone.

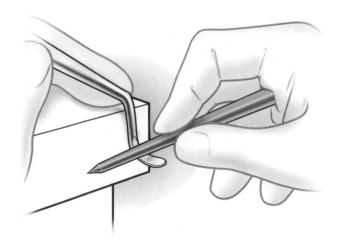

     c. Perform periodically to avoid weakening the blade and shortening the life of the instrument

    13. Test for sharpness as previously described

H. Care of sharpening stones

    1. Handle stones with care, since they break easily when dropped

    2. After use, clean stones in the ultrasonic cleaner to remove metal particles that become embedded into the surface of the stone during use; this also removes the oily layer that might have been applied prior to sharpening

    3. Wrap sharpening stone in gauze for protection, and autoclave

    4. Follow lubrication recommendation for the particular stone used, according to manufacturer's instructions

    5. Rotate area of use on stone to prevent grooving

Sharpening stones will last for many years with proper care. Regular cleaning to remove metal particles will prevent stones from developing a smooth glaze. Also, the entire stone should be utilized to prevent grooving. In addition, proper packaging and handling will prevent stone breakage.

QUESTIONS

1. The part of the instrument that joins the handle and the working end is the
   a. tip.
   b. blade.
   c. face.
   d. shank.

2. The cross-section of a sickle scaler is a
   a. circle.
   b. half circle.
   c. triangle.
   d. hexagon.

3. The MOST sensitive instrument to use for tactile sensitivity is the
   a. probe.
   b. explorer.
   c. curette.
   d. sickle scaler.

4. For proper adaptation of a universal curette, the lower shank should be placed in what position to the long axis of the tooth?
   a. Parallel
   b. Perpendicular
   c. Oblique
   d. Horizontal

5. Which type of grasp and fulcrum is BEST when using the periodontal probe?
   a. Light grasp and fulcrum
   b. Light grasp, moderate fulcrum
   c. Moderate grasp, light fulcrum
   d. Moderate grasp and fulcrum

6. All of the following are functions of a dental mirror EXCEPT one. Which one is the EXCEPTION?
   a. Retraction
   b. Fulcrum
   c. Transillumination
   d. Indirect vision

7. Which of the following instruments is used with a walking stroke or a bobbing motion?
   a. Explorer
   b. Probe
   c. Sickle scaler
   d. Curette

8. The lateral sides of the sickle scaler meet to form a
   a. rounded tip.
   b. sharp pointed tip.
   c. wire point.
   d. calibrated measuring stick.

9. Which part of the curette blade is adapted during scaling?
   a. Toe-third
   b. Lateral sides
   c. Face
   d. Tip

10. The BEST position for the dental light when working on the mandibular arch is
    a. angled upward.
    b. directly overhead.
    c. 12 inches from the patient's face.
    d. directed on the patient's chin.

11. The BEST position for the dental light when working on the maxillary arch is
    a. angled upward.
    b. directly overhead.
    c. 12 inches from the patient's face.
    d. directed on the patient's chin.

12. The cutting edge of the sickle or curette scalers must be sharpened in three sections. This helps maintain the original contour of the blade.
    a. Both statements are TRUE.
    b. Both statements are FALSE.
    c. The first statement is TRUE. The second statement is FALSE.
    d. The first statement is FALSE. The second statement is TRUE.

13. The universal curette has
    a. one cutting edge.
    b. two cutting edges that are parallel.
    c. offset cutting edges.
    d. a cutting edge that converges in a point.

14. A final downstroke is made when sharpening instruments to
    a. preserve the original instrument design.
    b. round the toe.
    c. prevent the formation of a wire edge.
    d. remove sludge.

15. Which instrument should be used to help determine the amount of subgingival calculus on the teeth?
    a. Probe
    b. ODU 11/12 explorer
    c. #23 explorer
    d. Sickle scaler
    e. Universal curette

16. The working end of a sickle scaler is formed by the
    a. rounded back and sides.
    b. lateral sides and face.
    c. back and face.
    d. lateral sides and back.

17. How many measurements are made for each tooth during the periodontal charting?
    a. Two
    b. Four
    c. Six
    d. Eight

18. With which of the following instruments is dental caries BEST detected?
    a. ODU 11/12 explorer
    b. Periodontal probe
    c. Dental mirror
    d. #23 explorer

19. How much force, in grams, should be applied when using the periodontal probe?
    a. 25
    b. 50
    c. 75
    d. 100

20. The line where two surfaces meet on an instrument is called the
    a. face.
    b. shank.
    c. cutting edge.
    d. handle.

21. How much pressure should be used during the exploratory stroke?
    a. Light
    b. Moderate
    c. Heavy
    d. Alternating moderate and heavy

22. During instrument sharpening with a flat stone, what should be the proper angulation, in degrees, between the instrument and stone?
    a. 80 to 90
    b. 90 to 100
    c. 100 to 110
    d. 110 to 120

23. To open the angulation of the curette blade when scaling, the shank should be placed
    a. parallel to the tooth.
    b. perpendicular to the tooth.
    c. away from the tooth.
    d. toward the tooth.
    e. near the tooth.

24. Where is the BEST place for the dominant hand to fulcrum when instrumenting the facial surfaces of Sextant 1?
    a. Sextant 2
    b. Sextant 3
    c. Sextant 6
    d. As close as possible to the working area without blocking the light

25. A sharp instrument increases efficiency of the operator. It also aids in reducing appointment time and operator fatigue, and increases the quality of care to the patient.
    a. Both statements are TRUE.
    b. Both statements are FALSE.
    c. The first statement is TRUE. The second statement is FALSE.

d. The first statement is FALSE. The second statement is TRUE.

26. When rounding the toe of the universal curette during instrument sharpening, what angulation, in degrees, should be utilized?
    a. 45
    b. 90
    c. 110
    d. 180

27. To engage lateral pressure when scaling, it is necessary to increase pressure on the fulcrum and keep the grasp light to moderate.
    a. Both statement and reason are CORRECT.
    b. Both the statement and reason are INCORRECT.
    c. The statement is CORRECT, but the reason is INCORRECT.
    d. The statement is INCORRECT, but the reason is CORRECT.

28. The glare test, or visual inspection, is one way to test for instrument sharpness. A sharp instrument will reflect light on the cutting edge and appear shiny.
    a. Both statements are TRUE.
    b. Both statements are FALSE.
    c. The first statement is TRUE. The second statement is FALSE.
    d. The first statement is FALSE. The second statement is TRUE.

29. The relationship between the instrument and surface of the tooth is known as
    a. insertion.
    b. angulation.
    c. adaptation.
    d. stroke.

30. Which part of the instrument is MOST useful in determining the correct end of the instrument?
    a. Handle
    b. Functional shank
    c. Terminal shank
    d. Working end

REFERENCES

1. Wilkins, E. *Clinical Practice of the Dental Hygienist,* 8th ed. Baltimore: Lippincott, Williams, & Wilkins, 1999.

2. Cooper, M. D. Keeping the Sharper Edge. *RDH,* 19(4), 46, 49–50, 1999.

3. Guignon, A. N. Let Fingers Do the Talking. *RDH,* 21(10), 72, 107, 2001.

4. Hu-Friedy Catalog, 3rd ed. Hu-Friedy Manufacturing Company, Chicago, IL, 2000.

5. Schmidt, C. R. Task Analysis of the Nevi 1 and Nevi 2 Periodontal Instruments. *Journal of Practical Hygiene,* 11(2), 15–19, 2002.

6. Boyden, S. Hu-Friedy Manufacturing Company. Chicago, IL, 2002. Interview July 2003.

7. Finkbeiner, B. L. Four-Handed Dentistry: Instrument Transfer. *Journal of Contemporary Dental Practice,* (2)1, 57–76, 2001.

8. Schoen, D. H. Instrument Effects on Smoothness Discrimination. *Journal of Dental Education,* 56(11), 741–745, 1992.

9. Huennekens, S. C., & S. J. Daniel. Task Analysis of the ODU 11/12 Explorer. *Journal of Dental Hygiene,* 66(1), 24–26, 1992.

10. Garnick, J. J., & L. Silverstein. Periodontal Probing: Probe Tip Diameter. *Journal of Periodontology,* 71(1), 96–103, 2000.

11. Burns, S. *It's About Time.* Published by Hu-Friedy, Chicago, 1995.

12. Sharpening Page. Hu-Friedy Manufacturing Company. 7 October 2002. Online: http://www.hufriedy.com/PGprosha.htm

13. Ellingson, P. Instrument Sharpening: How to Solve Your Sharpening Problems. *Journal of Practical Hygiene,* 2(6), 23–25, 1993.

MIRROR SKILL SHEET

Student _____

Date _____

Instructor _____

Re-evaluation

Instr: _____

Date _____

Instr: _____

Date _____

	S	U	Comments	S	U	Comments	S	U	Comments
GRASP									
1. Utilizes modified pen grasp in nondominant hand.									
2. Palms mirror when using finger retraction.									
FULCRUM									
3. Fulcrums, when appropriate, avoiding discomfort or trauma.									
4. Keeps ring finger straight.									
RETRACTION									
5. Avoids pinching lip/cheek while retracting buccal mucosa.									
6. Avoids striking teeth during insertion and placement.									
7. Avoids resting mirror on gingiva or alveolar bone.									
ILLUMINATION/INDIRECT VISION; uses									
8. Indirect vision when areas are not easily visible.									
9. Illumination.									
10. Direct vision, when appropriate.									
11. Transillumination for anterior teeth to view caries, deposits, and restorations.									
ERGONOMICS; utilizes proper									
12. Patient/operator positioning.									
13. Lighting.									

Courtesy of Indiana University Purdue University Fort Wayne Dental Hygiene Program.

CARIES-DETECTION EXPLORER SKILL SHEET

Student _____

Date _____

Instructor _____

	S	U	Comments
GRASP			
1. Stacks fingers together.			
2. Bends fingers slightly.			
3. Bends thumb knuckle out.			
4. Holds instrument on side of fat pad.			
5. Holds instrument between 2nd & 3rd knuckles.			
FULCRUM			
6. Keeps fulcrum extended straight.			
7. Stabilizes ring finger on occlusal/incisal surfaces.			
ADAPTATION-ANGULATION			
8. Keeps terminal shank 90° to surface being checked.			
9. Uses firm pressure.			
10. Properly checks the following surfaces:			
a. Occlusal (posterior)			
b. Mesial/distal (anterior)			
c. Facial/lingual			
d. Around restoration, if present			
DENTAL MIRROR; uses proper			
11. Grasp/fulcrum.			
12. Retraction.			
13. Reflection/illumination/transillumination.			
ERGONOMICS; utilizes proper			
14. Patient/operator positioning.			
15. Lighting.			

Courtesy of Indiana University Purdue University Fort Wayne Dental Hygiene Program.

11/12 CALCULUS-DETECTING EXPLORER SKILL SHEET

Student _____
Date _____
Instructor _____

Re-evaluation
Instr: ___
Date ___

Instr: ___
Date ___

	S	U	Comments	S	U	Comments	S	U	Comments
GRASP									
1. Stacks fingers together.									
2. Bends fingers slightly.									
3. Bends thumb knuckle out.									
4. Places instrument on side of fat pad.									
5. Holds instrument between 2nd & 3rd knuckles.									
FULCRUM									
6. Keeps finger straight.									
7. Stabilizes ring finger.									
8. Repositions to change areas/pivots toward tooth.									
HAND									
9. Keeps straight with forearm.									
10. Positions palm toward occlusal/incisal plane.									
ADAPTATION-ANGULATION									
11. Keeps 1-2 mm of tip on tooth.									
12. Keeps tip parallel to occlusal/incisal to occlusal/incisal (facial/lingually).									
13. Keeps tip at 80° to long axis of tooth (mesial/distally).									
14. Repositions at line angles.									
EXPLORING STROKE									
15. Uses wrist/forearm action to move instrument.									
16. Uses light grasp to check for calculus.									
17. Uses short-overlapping-channel strokes.									
18. Rolls/pivots instrument - keeps tip on tooth interproximally.									
19. Explores subgingivally.									
20. Finishes under contacts.									
DENTAL MIRROR; utilizes proper									
21. Grasp/fulcrum.									
22. Retraction.									
23. Reflection/illumination/transillumination.									
ERGONOMICS; utilizes proper									
24. Patient/operator positioning.									
25. Lighting.									

Courtesy of Indiana University Purdue University Fort Wayne Dental Hygiene Program.

PROBE SKILL SHEET

Student _____

Date _____

Instructor _____

Re-evaluation

Instr: _____

Date _____

Instr: _____

Date _____

	S	U	Comments		S	U	Comments		S	U	Comments
GRASP											
1. Stacks fingers together.											
2. Bends fingers slightly.											
3. Bends thumb knuckle out.											
4. Places instrument on side of fat pad.											
5. Holds instrument between 2nd & 3rd knuckles.											
FULCRUM											
6. Keeps finger straight.											
7. Stabilizes "ring" finger.											
8. Repositions to change areas/pivots towards tooth.											
HAND											
9. Keeps straight with forearm.											
ADAPTATION-ANGULATION											
10. Inserts probe at line angle.											
11. Places probe in contact against root/tooth surface.											
12. Moves tip up and down (walking strokes) of 1 to 2 mm.											
13. Touches attachment area gently with each down stroke.											
EXPLORED-WORKING STROKE											
14. Walks probe interproximally until it touches the contact area.											
15. Lifts probe SLIGHTLY off base while remaining in sulcus.											
16. Angles probe under contact area.											
17. Reinserts the probe at the line angle and walks across the middle third.											
18. Repositions probe to evaluate interproximal aspect; then angles under contact.											
19. Covers entire circumference of tooth.											
20. Uses wrist/forearm action to move instrument.											
DENTAL MIRROR; utilizes proper											
21. Retraction.											
22. Reflection/illumination/transillumination.											
ERGONOMICS; utilizes proper											
23. Patient/operator positioning.											
24. Lighting.											

Courtesy of Indiana University Purdue University Fort Wayne Dental Hygiene Program.

SCALING INSTRUMENT SKILL SHEET

Student _____

Date _____

Instructor _____

Re-evaluation
Instr: _____
Date _____

Instr: _____
Date _____

	S	U	Comments	S	U	Comments	S	U	Comments
GRASP									
1. Stacks fingers together.									
2. Bends fingers slightly.									
3. Bends thumb knuckle out.									
4. Places instrument on side of fat pad.									
5. Holds instrument between 2nd & 3rd knuckles.									
FULCRUM									
6. Keeps finger straight.									
7. Stabilizes "ring" finger.									
8. Repositions to change areas/pivots toward tooth.									
HAND									
9. Keeps straight with forearm.									
10. Positions palm toward occlusal/incisal plane.									
ADAPTATION-ANGULATION									
11. Keeps 1-2 mm of blade on tooth.									
12. Positions face of blade parallel to occlusal/incisal (facial/lingually).									
13. Keeps face of blade - 80° to long axis (mesial/distally).									
14. Repositions at line angles.									
EXPLORING - WORKING STROKE									
15. Uses wrist/forearm action to move instrument.									
16. Uses light grasp to check for calculus.									
17. Uses short-overlapping-channel strokes.									
18. Rolls/pivots instrument—keeps tip on tooth.									
19. Scales subgingivally.									
20. Engages calculus; uses lateral pressure.									
21. Finishes under contacts.									
22. Re-explores for calculus removal.									
DENTAL MIRROR; utilizes proper									
23. Grasp/Fulcrum.									
24. Retraction.									
25. Reflection/illumination.									
ERGONOMICS; utilizes proper									
26. Patient/operator positioning.									
27. Lighting.									

Courtesy of Indiana University Purdue Fort Wayne University Dental Hygiene Program.

INSTRUMENT SHARPENING SKILL SHEET

Student _____
Date _____
Instructor _____

Instrument: _____

Re-evaluation
Instr: _____
Date _____

Instr: _____
Date _____

	S	U	Comments	S	U	Comments	S	U	Comments
1. Assembles armamentarium in area with good lighting.									
2. Applies lubrication (oil for natural stone, water for synthetic stone).									
3. Identifies dull edge with plastic test stick or with visual test.									
GRASP (Stable instrument, moving stone technique)									
4. Uses palm grasp for sterile instrument in non-dominant hand.									
FULCRUM									
5. Stabilizes instrument against hard surface so face is parallel to countertop.									
HAND									
6. Hold stone in dominant hand.									
ADAPTATION-ANGULATION									
7. Places stone perpendicular to face of instrument.									
8. Moves stone to establish 110° angulation between stone and face of blade.									
WORKING STROKE									
9. Applies short up and down strokes.									
• Begins at heel third of blade.									
• Moves stone to middle third.									
• Continues to the end third of blade.									
• Finishes on down stroke.									
UNIVERSAL CURETTE									
10. Sharpens both edges using steps in #9.									
11. Sharpens toe with stone at 45° angle.									
EVALUATION									
12. Visually determines sharpness of blade.									
13. Utilizes plastic testing stick.									

Courtesy of Indiana University Purdue University Fort Wayne Dental Hygiene Program

Chapter 9

Polishing

Lauri Wiechmann, RDH, MPA

MediaLink

A companion CD-ROM, included free with each new copy of this book, supplements the procedures presented in each chapter. Insert the CD-ROM to watch video clips and view a large collection of color images that is also included. This multimedia library is designed to help you add a new dimension to your learning.

KEY TERMS

abrasion. Wearing away or removal of material by mechanical means.

abrasive. Object that produces abrasion.

aluminum oxide. Hard abrasive agent that can be mixed into a paste and used to polish acrylic and composites.

high-velocity (volume) evacuation (HVE). Evacuation device that operates with high suction.

nylon brush. Attaches to the prophy angle and is used to clean surfaces such as the occlusals of posterior teeth.

polishing paste. Agent used to cleanse and polish the tooth surface.

prophy angle. Attaches to the handpiece and holds the polishing cup or nylon brush used to polish teeth.

pumice. A silica-like volcanic glass abrasive used as a polishing agent for enamel, gold foil, and amalgam.

rubber cup. Polishing cup that attaches to the prophy angle; used to apply abrasive agent to tooth.

saliva ejector. Evacuation device that operates with low suction.

selective polishing. Polishing teeth on an as-needed basis when stain is present that is not removed during instrumentation.

silex. A silica-like material used for polishing gold alloys.

slow-speed handpiece. An engine device used in dentistry for polishing teeth, finishing and polishing restorations, and some steps in the preparation of restorations.

tin oxide. Low-abrasive agent used to polish metallic and composite restorations.

zirconium silicate. A natural mineral abrasive with a high degree of abrasiveness found in commercial polishing pastes.

LEARNING OBJECTIVES

After reading this chapter, the student will be able to:

- discuss the clinical considerations of a bacteremia being produced;
- identify ways to reduce aerosol;
- discuss ways to reduce and purposes of reducing drag of the handpiece cord respectively;
- discuss the armamentarium needed for polishing;
- compare the different attachment mechanisms of a polishing cup;
- contrast the types of polishing cups;
- differentiate between the abrasive agents, examining the degree of hardness and the intended surface for which they are to be used;

- discuss how the shape and size of the abrasive material affect the tooth structure being polished;
- explain the effect of abrasives on different restorative materials;
- state the importance of using light pressure during the polishing procedure for the operator, patient, and tooth structure;
- contrast the effects low and high speed have on the tooth during polishing;
- explain the rationale of using a wetting agent instead of a dry agent during polishing;
- compare and contrast polishing versus selective polishing;
- list and discuss each procedural step for polishing.

I. Introduction

Polishing involves using a rubber cup or nylon brush with an abrasive agent to get the tooth clean. The American Dental Hygienists' Association cites that a change has occurred in the philosophy of polishing in recent years and provides excellent background and scientific inquiries into the sometimes controversial topic of polishing.[1] While dental hygienists provide a rubber cup polish for each patient, others incorporate selective polishing within their treatment regime. While the philosophy for polishing varies among clinicians, the rationale for polishing remains the same—removing stain in order to make the tooth surface smooth.

II. Armamentarium

A. Slow-speed handpiece: An engine device that most commonly operates by an electric motor or compressed air and is activated by a rheostat, or foot pedal. It is connected from a hose on the delivery mechanism system to the air-turbine handpiece. The slow-speed handpiece is used for finishing and polishing restorations, some steps in restorative preparation, and polishing teeth. (Figure 9–1)

1. Weight of handpiece
   a. Available in a variety of weights ranging from 3 ounces to more than 9 ounces
   b. Use a lightweight handpiece (under 6 oz) and eliminate drag of the cord to prevent operator fatigue; ways to eliminate drag of cord include
      (1) Secure between leg and patient chair
      (2) Drape over "pinky" finger
      (3) Wrap around forearm
2. Activate handpiece by using the rheostat
3. Maintenance
   a. Autoclave after each use
   b. Clean and lubricate according to manufacturer's recommendations to ensure quality maintenance and longevity of the handpiece

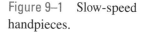

PRECLINICAL TIP

Polishing Your Knowledge: The slow-speed handpiece operates in the range of 6,000 to 10,000 revolutions per minute, whereas the high-speed handpiece operates in the range of 310,000 to 440,000 revolutions per minute.

Figure 9–1   Slow-speed handpieces.

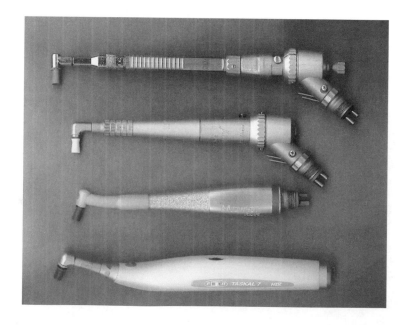

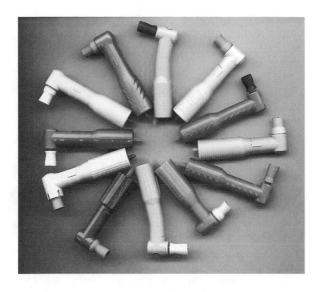

Figure 9–2 Disposable prophy angles.

B. Prophy angle: Angle attaches to the handpiece and holds the polishing cup or nylon brush used to polish the teeth. Its design is straight, contra-angled or right-angled, and disposable or autoclavable (Figure 9–2). Air pressure, generally greater than 20 pounds per square inch (p.s.i.), is required for a disposable prophy angle when using a firm cup. Air pressure, less than 20 p.s.i., is required when using a disposable angle with a soft cup.[2]

C. Polishing cups (latex or latex-free): Used to apply an abrasive material or polishing agent for the purpose of cleaning tooth surfaces. Polishing cups are components of disposable prophy angles or separate entities that attach onto nondisposable (autoclavable) prophy angles (screw-on type [threaded] or slip-on types)
 1. Types (Figure 9–3)

> **PRECLINICAL TIP**
>
> **Polishing Your Knowledge:** Watch the gauge, found on the delivery mechanism of the dental unit, to help monitor the amount of air pressure used.

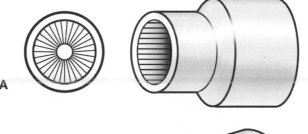
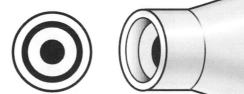
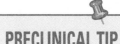
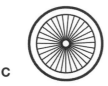
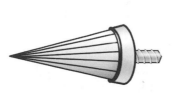

A

B

C

Figure 9–3 Types of polishing cups. A. Webbed B. Non-webbed C. Pointed

a. Webbed
(1) Refers to the design on the internal surface of the cup; contributes to the cup's degree of flexibility—less flexible than non-webbed cups
(2) Available in a variety of styles
b. Non-webbed
(1) Design lacks webbing on the internal surface of the cup
(2) Provides more flexibility and therefore produces greater flare of the cup periphery when pressure is applied
c. Pointed shape is conical and tapers to a narrow tip; designed for access around the brackets and under arch wires with orthodontia
d. Flat design resembles a cylinder and has a flat or blunt appearance at the terminal end; designed for polishing large areas of the tooth

2. Rigidity classifies the firmness of the polishing cup—hard (firm), medium, or soft
a. Hard (firm)—rigid, not as flexible as the other types; removes stain at a faster rate
b. Soft—provides more flexibility and flares more at the periphery when pressure is applied; as a result, it decreases operator fatigue, since less pressure is required to flare the cup into interproximal or subgingival areas

3. Parts of the polishing cup
a. Rim—used during polishing when cup is properly flared
b. Center—holds polishing paste

4. Attachment mechanism—method of attaching the polishing cup to the prophy angle depends on the type of prophy angle used
a. Types (Figure 9–4)
(1) Screw-in

PRECLINICAL TIP

Polishing Your Knowledge: Many manufacturers color code the polishing cup to make it easier to determine its firmness.

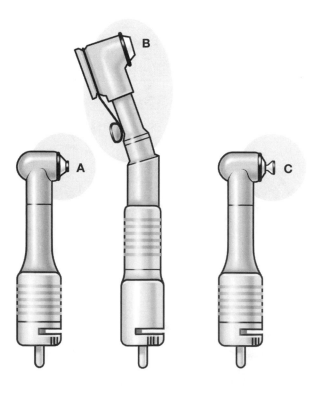

Figure 9–4   Types of prophy angles. A. Right angle for screw-in attachments. B. Latch-type contra-angle for use with mandrel mounted attachments. C. Right angle for snap-on attachments.

(a) Threaded into nondisposable (autoclavable) prophy angles

(b) When attaching, make sure the prophy angle is spinning in a forward direction; if the angle is spinning in reverse, the polishing cup can disengage into the patient's mouth when contact is made with the tooth

(2) Latch design consists of a post with a special end that is placed and latched in the prophy angle by a lever; post must be positioned and latched properly, or the polishing cup can disengage into the patient's mouth

(3) Snap on—the prophy angle has a larger ended post where the polishing cup attaches; polishing cup has an opening on one side that, once placed over the post, fits securely

D. Nylon brushes: Nylon brushes attach to the prophy angle and aid in the removal of debris from pits and fissures of teeth, especially when preparing for sealant placement. They are most commonly available in the screw-in or latch types and disposables.

1. Types (Figure 9–5)

a. Tapered shape is conical, which allows for the bristles to get into pits and fissures better than a flat brush

b. Flat design is cylindrical, which allows for the maximum number of bristles to be in contact with the tooth surface at one time

2. Risk—use may cause abrasion to the gingiva and loss of enamel structure

E. Polishing pastes: Polishing pastes include agents used to cleanse and polish the tooth surface. They vary in both cleansing and polishing ability.

1. Ideal paste

a. Contains abrasives that start with an irregular shape, for cleaning ability, and become rounded in shape as polishing continues[5]

b. Should be able to cleanse and polish the teeth with the least amount of abrasivity

2. Concern: Abrasives are known to cause abrasion of hard dental tissues;[6] to determine the correct abrasive to use, evaluate the type of debris to be removed and specific teeth that need to be polished

III. Abrasion and Abrasives

A. Abrasion: Wearing away or removal of material by mechanical means; factors affecting level of abrasion include the following

1. Shape of particle: An irregular shape in the polishing material increases the cutting efficiency; contains higher abrasion

PRECLINICAL TIP

Polishing Your Knowledge: An evaluation of the medical history is vital to determine if the patient is sensitive to or has a latex allergy, since many polishing cups contain latex. If the patient has an allergy to latex or is latex-sensitive, a latex-free polishing cup is indicated. It is also recommended to schedule those with latex allergies first thing in the morning, before latex has been used in the office.

PRECLINICAL TIP

Polishing Your Knowledge: The size of the nylon bristle is larger than the pits and fissures on the tooth surface. As with toothbrush bristles, the deepest parts of the fissure may *not* be accessible.

PRECLINICAL TIP

Polishing Your Knowledge: Bristle brushes remove more enamel than the polishing cup.[3]

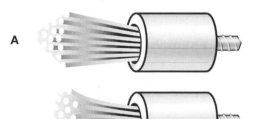

Figure 9–5   Types of nylon brushes. A. Tapered. B. Flat

a. As the material is used during the polishing procedure, the irregular shape is transposed into one with smoother edges, reducing its cutting efficiency, since it has low abrasion

    b. As the agent develops smoother edges, it polishes the tooth surface

2. Size of particle: Affects the rate at which the surface is abraded; commercial polishing pastes are classified by manufacturers as fine, medium, coarse, and plus grits

    a. Larger particle size wears away at the material and/or surface at a faster rate;[7] removes stain faster, but at the expense of creating deep scratches

    b. Smaller particle size removes the scratches previously placed by the larger particle size agent; smooths the tooth surface

3. Pressure of application: Amount of pressure applied to the surface/material affects the depth of the scratches and the rate at which the surface/material is removed; therefore, use light pressure

    a. Pressure that is too heavy limits uniform removal of the surface and/or material resulting in an uneven surface;[7] however, it does remove stain from the tooth surface at a faster rate

    b. Concern with using heavy pressure results in

       (1) Operator fatigue

       (2) Patient discomfort—excess pressure on the patient's mandible

       (3) Tissue trauma

       (4) Irreversible damage to the tooth structure due to heat build-up inside the tooth

4. Speed of application: Pertains to the rate at which the polishing device is rotating

    a. Maintain a slow speed to help control the rate of abrasion to the hard tissues of the tooth and produce less heat to tooth structure[8]

    b. As speed increases, the rate of abrasion increases and heat is generated, causing frictional heat, which can damage the pulp as well as cause patient discomfort

5. Wetting agents or lubricants: Examples include liquid, such as water, glycerin, or alcohol; mix with a dry abrasive agent

    a. Minimizes heat build-up and reduces frictional resistance

    b. Most pastes come prepackaged and don't require mixing

    c. When needed, to form a slurry mixture (thickened powder-water mixture), always add a lubricating agent, because using only a dry agent will increase the frictional resistance between the agent and the tooth structure[9]

B. Abrasive: Object that produces the abrasion; abrasive materials range from fine to coarse

    1. Types

      a. Aluminum oxide

        (1) Consists of an extremely hard abrasive

        (2) Can be mixed into a paste

        (3) Used to polish many types of restorations, such as acrylics and composites

      b. Pumice

        (1) Consists of a silica-like volcanic glass abrasive

        (2) Used as a polishing agent for enamel, gold foil, and amalgam

(3) Commonly found in polishing pastes

   c. Silex

     (1) Consists of a silica-like material, such as quartz or tripoli

     (2) Used for polishing gold alloys

   d. Tin oxide

     (1) Supplied in powder form

     (2) Mixed with water or glycerin to form slurry

     (3) Used to polish metallic restorations such as precious metal crowns and composite restorations

   e. Zirconium silicate

     (1) Comprised of a natural mineral

     (2) Possesses high abrasiveness

     (3) Found in commercial polishing pastes

     (4) Used for polishing tooth surfaces

2. Effect abrasives have on restorative materials

   a. All restorations exhibit some degree of roughness after polishing procedures;[5, 6] the least abrasive polishing agents must be selected to minimize roughness or to smooth the restoration; the finer the abrasive agent, the greater the polish

     (1) Give special attention to polishing composite surfaces;[10] use a product made especially for composite restorations; polish with aluminum silicate-coated disc after using polishing agent

     (2) Consider polishing gold restorations with toothpaste, since they lose their luster after polishing with latex or latex-free cup; toothpastes do not roughen the surface as do polishing agents[10]

     (3) Amalgam is moderately altered during polishing procedure; some polishing agents may remove the tarnish found on older amalgams[10]

   b. Consider polishing restorations with felt or foam polishing devices instead of polishing cups; firmness of the polishing cup does not allow for the polishing agent to work as designed[9]

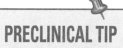

PRECLINICAL TIP

Polishing Your Knowledge: Placing a drop of hydrogen peroxide into a fine or medium grit polishing paste will help remove stain.

IV. Environmental Considerations

Creating an aerosol and "spatter": Since an aerosol is generated when using a dental handpiece with a polishing cup or nylon brush, utilize a means to keep the microbial count to a minimum.

A. Methods to minimize aerosol include

   1. High-velocity (volume) evacuation (HVE)

   2. Saliva ejector

   3. Rinsing with an antimicrobial agent prior to polishing to reduce the bacterial count present in the mouth

B. Avoid producing bacteremia

   1. Cause: Produced with any power-driven instrument during instrumentation or toothbrushing[11]

   2. Clinical considerations

     a. Review and/or update medical history—determine if patient has latex allergy; if yes, use latex-free materials; also make certain a condition is *not* present that could put the patient at risk for the development of a bacteremia, such as

       (1) Damaged or abnormal heart valves

       (2) Prosthetic valves

       (3) Joint replacements

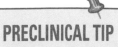

          (4) Rheumatic heart disease

          (5) Any other conditions that might warrant premedication, as recommended by the American Heart Association[12]

      b. Consult physician for antibiotic coverage—when receiving a prophylaxis, the patient may need antibiotic premedication[13]

V. Selective Polishing

    A. Indications

       1. Removes stain *not* accomplished during scaling/instrumentation

       2. Scale first, then polish using the finest abrasive agent to minimize damage to the tooth structure; use of a polishing cup first can cause unnecessary damage to the tooth surface

    B. Contraindications to polishing—excess polishing can result in more damage than was previously present; avoid polishing under certain conditions

       1. Xerostomia

         a. Signs and symptoms of concern include

           (1) Evidence of heavy bacterial plaque or other debris accumulation

           (2) Dental caries

           (3) Severely dry oral tissues

           (4) Soreness of the oral mucosa and tongue

         b. Recommended treatment includes using a toothbrush for plaque removal and instrumentation for stain removal

       2. Demineralized areas or dental caries—polishing an area with decay will cause more damage (refer to abrasion topic); recommended procedure includes toothbrush for plaque removal and instrumentation for stain removal

       3. Tooth sensitivity—avoid teeth that are sensitive due to exposed dentinal tubules; abrasive action of the prophylaxis procedure will create more wear on the tooth surface

       4. Newly erupted teeth—outer layer of a newly erupted tooth is not totally mineralized until approximately two years post eruption (known as period of maturation)

         a. Concerns

           (1) Polishing can interfere with the mineralization process

           (2) Excess heat can damage the pulp

           (3) Removes fluoride-rich outer layer; therefore, always use a polishing paste with fluoride to replenish fluoride lost during polishing

         b. Recommended polishing procedure includes toothbrushing for plaque removal and instrumentation for stain removal

       5. Severe gingivitis/gingiva that bleeds easily

         a. When the gingival tissues bleed, using a polishing cup can further damage the tissue

         b. Polishing immediately following nonsurgical periodontal therapy can delay wound healing and possibly cause an infection

       6. Lack of extrinsic stain and/or plaque—use selective polishing to remove stain *not* accomplished during instrumentation

       7. Contagious diseases—due to aerosols created

       8. Exposed root surfaces—due to decreased mineralization of cementum

       9. Respiratory disorders—includes asthma and emphysema

10. Patients susceptible to bacteremia[14]
C. Technique
1. Wear protective eyewear and a mask that covers the mouth and nose
2. Assemble handpiece and prophy angle according to the manufacturer's instructions
3. Check medical history for medical contraindications and possible latex allergy or sensitivity; choose latex-free polishing cup when indicated
4. Select appropriate abrasive material; use the least abrasive material indicated for the patient's dental condition
5. Hold the handpiece using the modified pen or pen grasp; try to eliminate drag of cord
6. Place abrasive material in polishing cup or on nylon brush
7. Establish firm fulcrum to enhance stability of the handpiece
8. Apply abrasive material to several teeth to help eliminate the first tooth from receiving most of the abrasive material
9. Activate handpiece by using the rheostat, maintaining a constant slow speed to control the rate of abrasion
10. Use HVE or saliva ejector throughout procedure to reduce aerosol
11. Apply polishing cup or nylon brush to tooth with light, intermittent pressure and slow, smooth, continuous motion, flaring the edges of the polishing cup (Figure 9–6)

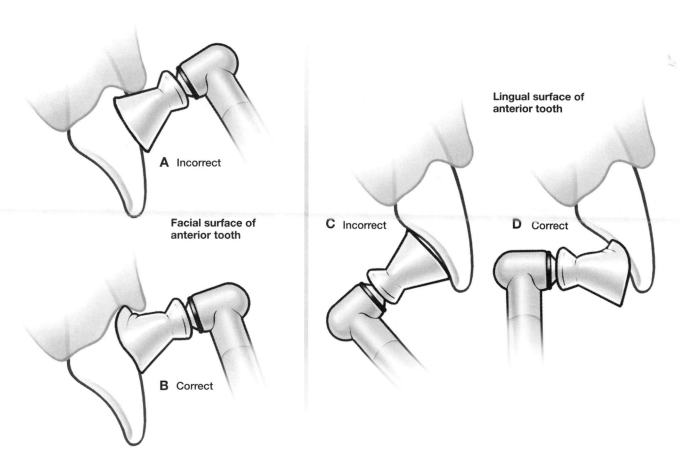

Figure 9–6   Proper polishing cup application. On facial surface of an anterior tooth. A. Incorrect. B. Correct. On lingual surface of an anterior tooth. C. Incorrect. D. Correct.

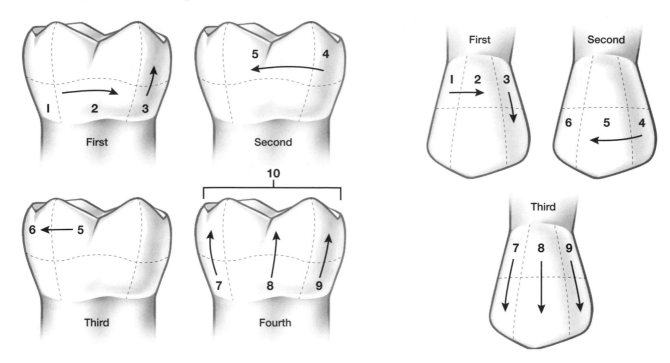

Figure 9–7   Polishing pattern on posterior and anterior teeth. 1, 2, 3 Polish cervical half; 4, 5, 6 Then polish occlusal/incisal half; 7, 8, 9 Finish with 3 to 4 oblique or vertical strokes; 10 Polish occlusal surfaces last.

12. Begin at distal line angle in the cervical half and push polishing cup into proximal area (Figure 9–7)
13. Reposition at distal line angle; use a pull stroke and polish along cervical half from distal line angle to mesial line angle
14. Push polishing cup into mesial proximal area (Figure 9–8)
15. Bring cup up mesial surface to complete occlusal/incisal half of tooth
16. Roll from mesial to distal contact
17. Finish with three to four oblique or vertical strokes (from gingiva to occlusal/incisal)
18. Polish occlusal surfaces (Figure 9–9)

Figure 9–8   Properly flaring prophy cup into proximals.

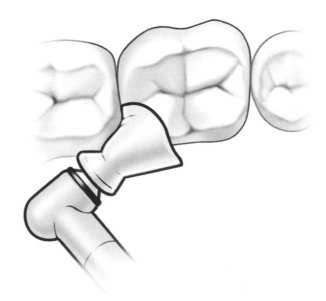

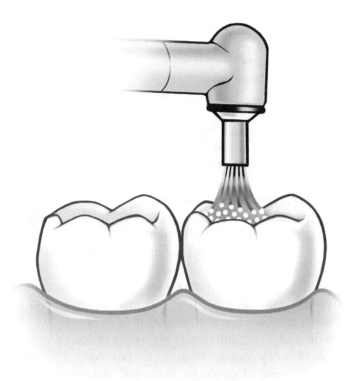

Figure 9–9   Polishing occlusal surface with nylon brush.

a. Use polishing cup or nylon brush
   (1) Polishing cup—use on occlusal surfaces that are restored
   (2) Brush—use on nonrestored occlusal surfaces
b. Polish one quadrant at a time
c. Follow cuspal inclines
   (1) Complete all facial inclines in one quadrant
   (2) Reposition and complete lingual inclines
19. Ensure removal of debris and then move to next tooth
20. Rinse teeth thoroughly
21. Continue with less abrasive agent if needed, using a new polishing cup
22. Floss patient to remove polishing particles that may remain interproximally
23. Provide patient with a final rinse

VI. **Air Polishing**

Consists of a slurry mixture of sodium bicarbonate and water that is applied to the tooth by a stream of air through a forced-air polishing device

A. Indications[15]
   1. Gently and precisely removes extrinsic stain faster than handscaling and using abrasives in rubber cups—3.15 times faster than hand curettes; use in place of rubber cup polishing[16]
   2. Prepares tooth for sealant
   3. During periodontal surgery as part of root preparation
   4. Removes soft debris around orthodontic appliances

B. Safety
   1. Removes less tooth structure than hand curette—10.68 microns in comparison to 27.09 microns with hand curette[16]

PRECLINICAL TIP

Polishing Your Knowledge: If using more than one degree of abrasive material during the polishing procedure, it is important to rinse the area thoroughly and use a new polishing cup before using the less abrasive agent. This rinsing procedure removes the previously used coarser abrasive and allows the finer agent to smooth the surface.[7] If the area is *not* rinsed thoroughly, the coarser agent will remain and continue to create deep scratches in the tooth surface.

2. Avoid loss of tooth structure by applying slurry for no more than 10 seconds on tooth surface[16]
3. Direct slurry away from soft tissues to avoid causing localized epithelial abrasion
4. Have patient remove contact lenses and wear safety glasses[15]

C. Contraindications[15]

1. If using sodium bicarbonate powder, *do not* use with patients on sodium-restricted diet for treatment of such conditions as hypertension or renal disease
2. Avoid use for patients with
   a. Communicable diseases
   b. Active periodontal conditions with soft, spongy gingiva
   c. Respiratory complications
   d. Metabolic disorders such as Cushing's disease or Addison's disease
   e. Long-term steroid therapy

Before polishing, thorough instrumentation should take place to remove calculus and as much extrinsic stain as possible. If polishing is indicated, the health history should be reviewed to determine if the patient has any contraindications for polishing. The operator must evaluate the type of debris on the teeth and select the most appropriate abrasive agent based on the existing conditions and presence of restorations.

QUESTIONS

1. What amount of pressure should be applied when removing stain with the polishing cup?
   a. Heavy consistent
   b. Heavy intermittent
   c. Light consistent
   d. Light intermittent

2. All of the following are styles of prophy angles EXCEPT one. Which one is the EXCEPTION?
   a. Straight
   b. Contra-angled
   c. Left-angled
   d. Disposable

3. Which of the following types of polishing cups decreases operator fatigue?
   a. Hard
   b. Firm
   c. Medium
   d. Soft

4. Which of the following describes what happens with the abrasive shape of an ideal polishing paste?
   a. Starts with a round shape and becomes irregular in shape
   b. Starts and remains with a round shape

   c. Starts and remains with an irregular shape
   d. Starts with an irregular shape and becomes rounded

5. All of the following are factors that affect the level of abrasion EXCEPT one. Which one is the EXCEPTION?
   a. Speed of application
   b. Drying agents
   c. Size of particle
   d. Pressure of application

6. As the speed of the handpiece increases, what is the effect on the tooth?
   a. Structure is removed.
   b. Surface becomes more polished.
   c. Surface cools.
   d. Surface becomes whiter.

7. Which of the following statements is TRUE regarding the use of abrasive agents on restorative materials?
   a. Use the coarsest material.
   b. Recommend a commercial prophylaxis paste for all restorative materials.
   c. Start with the finest abrasive agent and progress to the most abrasive agent.

d. Give individual attention to select the least abrasive agent for the specific type of restorative material.

8. The medical history needs to be consulted prior to polishing. Certain medical conditions put the patient at risk for the development of a bacteremia.
   a. Both statements are *TRUE*.
   b. Both statements are *FALSE*.
   c. The first statement is *TRUE*. The second statement is *FALSE*.
   d. The first statement is *FALSE*. The second statement is *TRUE*.

9. All of the following are methods of minimizing aerosol during polishing EXCEPT one. Which one is the EXCEPTION?
   a. Rinse with an antimicrobial agent prior to polishing.
   b. Run the polishing cup at a slow rate of speed.
   c. Use HVE during the procedure.
   d. Use the saliva ejector during the procedure.

10. The primary purpose of polishing teeth is to remove
   a. pellicle.
   b. calculus.
   c. plaque.
   d. stain.

11. Polishing demineralized areas is indicated. This strengthens the tooth structure by removing all plaque and its by-products from the area.
   a. Both statements are *TRUE*.
   b. Both statements are *FALSE*.
   c. The first statement is *TRUE*. The second statement is *FALSE*.

d. The first statement is *FALSE*. The second statement is *TRUE*.

12. Which of the following helps reduce operator fatigue during polishing?
   a. Use a medium-to-firm polishing cup.
   b. Secure the handpiece cord to eliminate drag.
   c. Use the saliva ejector during the procedure.
   d. Have the patient rinse with an antimicrobial agent prior to polishing.

13. All of the following are attachment mechanisms for the polishing cup to the prophy angle EXCEPT one. Which one is the EXCEPTION?
   a. Post
   b. Latch
   c. Screw-in
   d. Snap-on

14. All of the following can result from applying heavy pressure with the polishing cup EXCEPT one. Which one is the EXCEPTION?
   a. Patient discomfort
   b. Tissue trauma
   c. Operator fatigue
   d. Removal of calculus

15. During the polishing procedure, all of the following should be implemented to reduce operator aerosol contamination EXCEPT one. Which one is the EXCEPTION?
   a. Wear protective eye wear.
   b. Wear a mask.
   c. Retract with a mirror.
   d. Use a saliva ejector.

REFERENCES

1. American Dental Hygienists' Association Position on Polishing Procedures. American Dental Hygienists' Association, http//www.adha.org/profissues/polishingpaper.htm July 2003

2. Warren, D. P., H. C. Rice, D. K. McKitrick, J. A. McWherter, & J. M. Powers. Operating Air Pressure of Disposable Angles. *Journal of Dental Hygiene,* Summer 1999.

3. Thompson, R. E., & D. C. Way. Enamel Loss Due to Prophylaxis and Multiple Bonding/Debonding of Orthodontic Attachments. *American Journal of Orthodontics,* March 1981.

4. Lutz, F., B. Sener, T. Imfeld, F. Barbakow, & P. Schupbach. Self-Adjusting Abrasiveness: A New Technology for Prophylaxis Pastes. *Quintessence International,* 24(1), 1993.

5. Lutz, F., B. Sener, T. Imfeld, F. Barbakow, & P. Schupbach. Comparison of the Efficacy of Prophylaxis Pastes with Conventional Abrasives of a New Self-Adjusting Abrasive. *Quintessence International,* 24(3), 1993.

6. Neme, A., K. Frazer, L. Roeder, & T. Debner. Effect of Prophylactic Polishing Protocols on the Surface Roughness of Esthetic Restorative Material. *Operative Dentistry* 27(1) January–February 2002.

7. Craig, R., J. Powers, & J. Wataha. *Dental Materials, Properties and Manipulation,* 7th ed. Saint Louis: Mosby, 2000.

8. Gladwin, M., & M. Bagby. *Clinical Aspects of Dental Materials.* Philadelphia: Lippincott, Williams, and Wilkins, 2000.

9. Jefferies, S. R. The Art and Science of Abrasive Finishing and Polishing in Restorative Dentistry. *Dental Clinics of North America,* 42(4), October 1998.

10. Roulet, J. F., & T. K. Roulet-Mehrens. The Surface Roughness of Restorative Materials and Dental Tissues after Polishing with Prophylaxis and Polishing Pastes. *Journal of Periodontology,* April 1982.

11. Roberts, G. J., H. S. Holzel, M. R. Sury, N. A. Simmons, P. Gardner, & P. Longhurst. Dental Bacteremia in Children, *Pediatric Cardiology* January–February 1997.

12. Endocarditis Prophylaxis Information, American Heart Association, http://216.185.112.5/ presenter.jhtml?identifier= 11086

13. Roberts, G. J., P. Gardner, P. Longhurst, A. E. Black, & V. S. Lucas. Intensity of Bacteraemia Associated with Conservative Dental Procedures in Children. *British Dental Journal,* January 2000.

14. Lucas, V., & G. J. Roberts. Odontogenic Bacteremia Following Tooth Cleaning Procedures in Children. *Pediatric Dentistry,* March–April 2000.

15. Gutmann, M. Airpolishing: A Comprehensive Review of the Literature. *Journal of Dental Hygiene,* 72(3), 47–56, 1998.

16. Fong, C. Dispelling Air Polishing Myths. *Journal of Practical Hygiene,* 9(1), 25–27, 2000.

POLISHING PERFORMANCE SKILL SHEET

Student _____
Date _____
Instructor _____

Re-evaluation
Instr: _____
Date _____

	S	U	Comments	S	U	Comments	S	U	Comments
1. Uses sufficient polish.									
2. Applies polish to 2–3 teeth at a time.									
3. Uses secure/straight fulcrum.									
4. Keeps palm toward occlusal/incisal.									
5. Uses a slow rpm.									
6. Uses proper grasp—HP held on side of fat pad.									
7. Avoids splitting fingers.									
8. Pivots on fulcrum finger.									
9. Rolls handpiece slightly keeping thumb bent out.									
10. Flares rubber cup with light pressure on all surfaces									
Distal									
Cervical sweep									
Mesial									
11. Returns horizontal stroke from mesial to distal.									
12. Uses vertical finishing strokes.									
13. Rinses/evacuates mouth as needed.									
14. Uses rubber cup/brush on occlusals as instructed.									
15. Maintains aseptic technique throughout.									
16. Maintains correct posture/positions.									
17. Adjusts overhead light.									
Mirror: utilizes proper:									
18. Grasp.									
19. Fulcrum.									
20. Reflection.									
21. Retraction.									

Courtesy of Indiana University Purdue University Dental Hygiene Program.

Chapter 10

Fluorides

Mary D. Cooper, RDH, MSEd

MediaLink

A companion CD-ROM, included free with each new copy of this book, supplements the procedures presented in each chapter. Insert the CD-ROM to watch video clips and view a large collection of color images that is also included. This multimedia library is designed to help you add a new dimension to your learning.

KEY TERMS

acidogenic. Acid producing.

aciduric. Acid tolerant.

bactericidal. Capable of killing bacteria.

bacteriostatic. Inhibits growth or multiplication of bacteria.

carbonated hydroxyapatite. Inorganic mineral structure found in teeth.

cariogenic. Producing caries.

cariostatic. Interrupts the progress of dental caries.

cavitation. Formation of cavity.

fluorapatite. Results when all hydroxyl groups are replaced by fluoride.

fluorosis. Condition that results from excessive ingestion of fluoride during the developmental stage of the tooth.

paresthesia. Feeling of burning, tickling, or tingling.

tetany. Muscle twitches.

thixotropic. Property of certain gels of becoming less viscous.

LEARNING OBJECTIVES

After reading this chapter, the student will be able to:

- identify the bacteria involved in the caries process;
- explain the diet factors that play a role in the demineralization process;
- list the diseases, conditions, and drugs that cause xerostomia;
- compare and contrast professional topical fluorides;
- perform a professional topical fluoride application, to competency, using the tray technique;

- recall the amount of fluoride gel to dispense into a tray for children and adults;
- identify the different forms of fluorosis;
- identify the signs and symptoms of acute fluoride toxicity;
- list emergency treatment procedures for acute fluoride toxicity;
- differentiate the causes of acute and chronic toxicity.

I. Introduction

Dental caries is the most common dental disease seen in adult patients.[1] It is also the number one cause of tooth mortality in the United States.[2] Fluoride, a salt of hydrofluoric acid, has been known to battle this infectious disease for many years. It is primarily stored in the bones and teeth, and its roles include inhibiting demineralization and enhancing remineralization in the caries process by creating a crystalline structure on the surface of the tooth that is more acid resistant. Fluoride also plays a role in reducing the effect of acid-producing bacteria such as *mutans streptococci*.

The widespread use and availability of topical fluorides has made it possible for a decline in the prevalence of caries. A combined effort can be made with fluoride in drinking water, mouth rinses, dentifrices (toothpastes), and professional treatments.[3]

II. Composition of Teeth

A. Structures
  1. Enamel—least porous, followed by dentin, then cementum
     a. Hardest substance of the body—96 percent (by weight) mineralized (carbonated hydroxyapatite)
     b. Made up of mineral crystals housed in enamel rods
     c. Diffusion channels—small passageways between enamel rods filled with protein, lipid, and water
        (1) 85 percent (by volume) mineral
        (2) 15 percent is volume available for diffusion (breakdown)
  2. Dentin/cementum—made up of 47 percent by volume mineral and 53 percent lipid, protein, and water; 70 percent and 50 percent mineralized respectively

B. Carbonated hydroxyapatite—mineral of the tooth made up of defective calcium phosphate
  1. Rich in carbonate
  2. Contains calcium, phosphate, and hydroxyl ions
  3. More soluble in acid

C. Fluorapatite—results when all hydroxyl groups are replaced by fluoride, making the tooth less soluble in acid and therefore stronger

III. Caries Process

During the caries process, the tooth undergoes periods of demineralization and remineralization. Once the negative mineral balance produced by demineralization exceeds the remineralization balance, a carious lesion has formed.

A. Demineralization—dissolution of calcium and phosphate ions from the hydroxyapatite crystals of the tooth
  1. Development of carious lesions occurs in two stages
     a. Incipient lesion (also known as enamel, early and white spot lesions)—earliest stage of caries development; this stage can be arrested and reversed
        (1) Appears as a white or yellow-to-tan spot
        (2) Body of lesion—surface of enamel is relatively intact
     b. Overt (frank) lesion (also known as dentinal caries)—cavitation has occurred when demineralization is not stopped or reversed
  2. Cariogenic bacteria
     a. Two involved in the demineralization process are of special interest
        (1) *Mutans streptococci (MS)*—most common and abundant; include *Streptococcus mutans*
           (a) Bacteria associated with the initiation of caries; produce high amounts of acid
           (b) Gram-positive microorganisms
           (c) Adhere well to tooth surfaces
        (2) *Lactobacilli (LB)* species
           (a) Gram-positive microorganisms
           (b) Does not have the capability of dropping the pH in the oral cavity to initiate caries formation

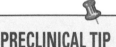

PRECLINICAL TIP

Strengthening Your Knowledge: Eighty percent of all children have dental decay by the time they are 18 years old.[3]

(c) Associated with the progression of caries; found in greater numbers in more advanced, smooth surface lesions

   b. Characteristics—both are acidogenic (acid producing) and aciduric (acid tolerant)

3. Process of demineralization includes

   a. Formation of pellicle—acellular glycoprotein, biofilm formed from saliva; will be covered by bacteria that forms plaque

   b. Acid-producing bacteria such as *MS* and *LB*

   c. Fermentable carbohydrates (e.g., glucose, sucrose, fructose, and starch)—used by bacteria for survival; by-products of their metabolism will be organic acids,[1] which include lactic, acetic, formic, and propionic

   d. Acids dissolve, through the pellicle, the calcium phosphate mineral in the enamel or exposed root surfaces

4. Factors that play a role in the demineralization process

   a. Diet

      (1) Frequency of intake of fermentable carbohydrates—*most* important factor, since exposure to carbohydrates results in teeth being constantly exposed to bacterial acids

      (2) Consistency of fermentable carbohydrates—"sticky" foods, such as dried fruits, tend to remain on the occlusal surfaces and are difficult to remove with brushing

      (3) Total amount of fermentable carbohydrates consumed

   b. Vomiting associated with eating disorders—induced vomiting increases the risk of acid exposure on the teeth

   c. Eating sugar-containing antacids, used for upset stomachs, increases caries risk

   d. Exposed root surfaces (recession) and root caries susceptibility—progression of root caries is 2.5 times faster than coronal caries

      (1) By age 70, adults have an average of three root lesions[5]

      (2) Root caries is more severe in males than females

      (3) Affects molar teeth more frequently than any other teeth

      (4) Critical pH level for dissolution is between 6.0 to 6.7 for cementum—higher than enamel, which is 4.5 to 5.5 pH

   e. Inadequate or poor oral hygiene—lack of plaque removal results in an increase in dental caries

   f. Lack of water fluoridation—low concentrations of fluoride in water helps reduce the incidence of dental caries; approximately 65 percent of U.S. communities have optimally fluoridated water[6]

   g. Orthodontic appliances—challenges proper plaque control

   h. Salivary dysfunction—decreases salivary flow, which can increase the progress of rampant caries; saliva is a natural defense mechanism against dental caries

      (1) Causes for decreased salivary flow, which result in xerostomia (dry mouth), include

         (a) Age-induced—salivary flow decreases with age

         (b) Chemo and/or radiation therapy for head and neck cancer—destroys the salivary glands, therefore decreasing salivary flow

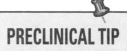

PRECLINICAL TIP

Strengthening Your Knowledge: Individuals with high levels of *MS*, greater than 1,000,000 per ml of saliva, should be considered at high risk for dental caries.[4]

PRECLINICAL TIP

Strengthening Your Knowledge: Four interrelated factors need to be present to initiate caries—*diet* (fermentable carbohydrates), *bacteria, decreased host resistance,* and *time* for the carious lesion to develop.

(c) Diabetes, leukemia, and pernicious anemia—patient experiences dehydration as a result of these conditions

(d) Sjögren's syndrome—congenital condition that is an autoimmune disorder of the salivary and lacrimal glands

(e) Use of over-the-counter (OTC) and prescription drugs can lead to increased plaque accumulation, soft tissue changes, and root caries; include
- Anticholinergics
- Antidepressants
- Antihistamines
- Antihypertensives
- Sedatives
- Tranquilizers

(2) Recommendations to patients with xerostomia

(a) Chew gum that contains xylitol and/or Recaldent™; does not promote tooth decay; stimulates salivary flow, enhances mineralization, and also has antibacterial effects

(b) Sip water to keep oral mucosa from drying

i. Use of bottled or filtered water—amount of fluoride in these products is often unknown or inconsistent

j. Tobacco—challenges the immune system; decreases salivary function

B. Remineralization: Occurs if, and when, acid is neutralized. There is an increase in calcium and phosphate ions in the saliva and plaque, which deposit into the demineralized areas, replacing lost minerals. This process occurs with combined efforts of fluoride and saliva. As a result, remineralized areas become stronger and more acid resistant.

IV. **Caries Prevention Strategies**

A. Preventive measures for plaque control include
1. Brushing
2. Flossing and use of other interdental aids as indicated
3. Using fluoride-containing dentifrices and mouth rinses
4. Using antimicrobial products through brushing, rinsing, or irrigating

B. Diet modification—note frequency and amount of cariogenic (fermentable carbohydrates) foods and drinks consumed by patient

C. Sealants—provide protection to the pits and fissures of teeth, especially occlusal surfaces of posterior teeth, where 88 percent of carious lesions occur

V. **Fluorides**

The incorporation of fluorides in community water systems as well as using topical fluoride applications have been proven to reduce dental caries. Water fluoridation was initially thought to have its greatest effect on the tooth surfaces prior to their eruption; however, it also demonstrates a positive effect topically—through ingestion and returning to the oral cavity via saliva.

Teeth are most susceptible to decay when they first erupt in the mouth. Therefore, it is important to incorporate preventive measures immediately.

Ingesting fluoridated water and using fluoridated toothpaste twice a day will help in the caries prevention process. Although fluoride is effective in the prevention and control of dental caries, it is important to protect against excess fluoride ingestion. Children should be supervised when using dental products so the proper amount of toothpaste is used and expectorated to avoid swallowing. In addition, as recommended by the American Dental Association, only individuals at moderate or high risk for caries should be given routine professional topical fluoride treatments.

A. Mechanism of action—topical fluorides prevent and inhibit caries progression in three ways: inhibit demineralization, enhance remineralization, and inhibit bacterial activity; fluorides are also used to control plaque accumulation, gingivitis, and dentinal hypersensitivity

   1. Inhibits demineralization, which involves the loss of calcium, phosphate, and carbonate, when it is present at the time of acid challenge

      a. Acts as a barrier against acid dissolution of the tooth surface; critical pH level for coronal and root caries is 4.5 to 5.5 and 6.0 to 6.7 respectively

      b. Fluoride, which absorbs to the crystal surface (hydroxyapatite), travels with the acid into the tooth forming fluorapatite, which protects the tooth surface from dissolution

   2. Enhances remineralization—recovers demineralized enamel

      a. Neutralizes acids

      b. Fluorides and fluorides in saliva are taken up, along with calcium and phosphate ions, back into the partially demineralized tooth; new crystals are formed, making the tooth stronger and more acid resistant; most fluoride is incorporated in the outer surface of the tooth

        (1) Role of saliva

          (a) Protects against caries by neutralizing (buffering) acids

          (b) Promotes remineralization and inhibits demineralization

          (c) Provides calcium and phosphate ions—the principle minerals that make up enamel

        (2) Outcome

          (a) New crystals take up fluoride and phosphate, forming fluorapatite

          (b) Makes enamel structure more acid resistant in areas of decalcification

   3. Inhibits activity of cariogenic bacteria; fluoride becomes toxic to bacteria after it enters cell wall

      a. Travels through cell wall into cariogenic bacteria in the form of hydrofluoric acid when pH values are lower; forms a calcium fluoride-like material in the enamel's surface

      b. In high concentrations (i.e., professional topical fluoride application), fluoride is bactericidal

      c. In low concentrations (i.e., daily at home topical application), fluoride is bacteriostatic

      d. Provides substantivity—ability to bind to pellicle and tooth structure and released over a period of time with retention of potency

PRECLINICAL TIP

Strengthening Your Knowledge: Critical pH is that level at which dissolution of the enamel and cementum may occur.

B. Systemic fluorides
1. Community water fluoridation—amount of fluoride is adjusted to an optimal level in domestic water supply
   a. Provides both systemic and topical effects—reducing caries rate significantly
   b. Optimal recommended concentration in community drinking water is 1 ppm, but can range from 0.7 ppm to 1.2 ppm—depending on the air temperature of the area—warmer climate, lower concentration level (.7 ppm); colder climate, higher concentration level (1.2 ppm)
      (1) Prevents fluorosis—a developmental defect of the enamel that occurs as a result of too much fluoride being ingested during enamel formation
      (2) Helps prevent decay by ensuring adequate fluoride bringing protection against bacteria
   c. Environmental Protection Agency (EPA)—monitors the fluoride concentration and quality and safety of drinking water
   d. Cost-effective—approximately $0.50/person/year
   e. Characteristics
      (1) Rapidly absorbed in the stomach and small intestine
      (2) Stored in the bones and teeth
      (3) Excreted through kidneys
   f. Effectiveness
      (1) Most effective against caries produced on smooth surfaces, least effective in pits and fissures
      (2) Most efficient method of bringing benefits of fluoride to community
      (3) Most effective in persons 6 months to 14 years of age
   g. Compounds used to fluoridate domestic water supplies include
      (1) Sodium silicofluoride
      (2) Sodium fluoride
      (3) Hydrofluorosilicic acid
2. Dietary fluoride supplements (tablets, lozenges or liquid)—designed to supplement dietary fluoride intake by children from 6 months to 14 years of age who live in areas with inadequate water fluoridation or do not consume the community's fluoridated water
   a. Prescribed for systemic and topical effects
   b. Intake based on age of child and concentration of fluoride in drinking water—water must be tested for fluoride content prior to prescribing supplement
   c. Recommended to supplement topical mechanism of fluoride (Table 10–1)

> **PRECLINICAL TIP**
>
> **Strengthening Your Knowledge:** In the United States, water and processed beverages can provide 75 percent of an individual's fluoride intake.[3]

Table 10–1   Supplemental Fluoride Dosage Schedule[4]

| Age | Based on Age and Concentration of Fluoride in Drinking Water Water Fluoride Concentration (ppm) | | |
	≤0.3 ppm	0.3–0.6 ppm	≥0.6 ppm
0–6 mo.	0	0	0
6 mo.–3 yrs.	0.25 mg/day	0	0
3–6 yrs.	0.50 mg/day	0.25 mg/day	0
6–16 yrs.	1.0 mg/day	0.50 mg/day	0

(1) Tablets and lozenges—manufactured with 1.0, 0.5, or 0.25 mg fluoride

(2) Recommended use—suck or chew supplement for 1 to 2 minutes before swallowing

3. Fluoride in foods—include tea and fish

4. Other effective products for antibacterial therapy—chlorhexidine gluconate—0.12%

   a. Initially use twice a day for two weeks

   b. Reduces levels of *mutans streptococci*

5. Fluoride recommendations: The recommendations in Table 10–2 were published in the 1995 *Journal of the American Dental Association (JADA)* special supplement on caries diagnoses and risk assessment regarding proper protocol when administering professional topical fluoride gels and foams[4]

C. Professional topical fluoride: Professional topical fluorides are high concentration fluoride systems that have been denoted as safe and effective in cariostatic and bactericidal benefits by the American Dental Association (ADA) as well as the Food and Drug Administration (FDA)—reducing caries by 30 percent. They are available as gels, rinses, foams, and varnishes, and include sodium, acidulated phosphate, and stannous fluorides. However, acidulated phosphate[7, 8] and neutral sodium fluorides are the most commonly applied professional fluorides in dental practices. Professional topical fluorides are applied on the tooth surfaces by brushing, using trays or the painting technique, and/or rinsing. Once applied, a temporary layer of calcium-like material is left on the tooth surface. High-concentration, in-office fluorides are recommended for those who are moderate to high risk for caries. For those at moderate risk, it is recommended to have applications twice a year. For those with high risk for caries, a quarterly application is recommended.

1. Types (Table 10–3)[9]

   a. Acidulated phosphate fluoride (APF)

      (1) Forms—include solution, gel, or foam

         (a) Thixotropic gels—set in a gel-like state, but not considered a true gel; act as a solution because they are easily forced into proximal areas

         (b) Foams—lighter in consistency and often are more acceptable to patients with a high gag reflex

      (2) Characteristics—acceptable taste, tissue compatible, nonstaining, stable, rapid uptake into the enamel, and ready to use

Table 10–2 Fluoride Recommendations

Water Fluoride Level	*Caries Status*		
	Caries-free	Active caries*	Rampant caries**
Deficient < 0.7 ppm	Apply topical 2x per year	Apply topical 2x per year	Apply topical 4x per year
Optimal	0	Apply topical 2x per year	Apply topical 2x per year

*Active means the patient has one or more carious lesions.
**Rampant means the patient has caries involving tooth surfaces not usually involved with caries, or the patient has lesions that are rapidly progressing.

Table 10–3   Comparison of Professionally Applied Fluorides

	Acidulated Phosphate Fluoride (APF) 1.23%	Neutral Sodium Fluoride (NaF) 2.0%	Varnish—Neutral Sodium Fluoride (NaF) 5.0%
Application Method	Tray, swab, or toothbrush	Tray, swab, or toothbrush	Swab or disposable brush
Contraindications	Hypersensitivity to fluoride or other ingredients; not indicated for children under 3	Hypersensitivity to fluoride or other ingredients; not indicated for children under 3	Hypersensitivity to fluoride or other ingredients
Documented Efficacy	Clinically proven to reduce caries in annual/biannual applications	Clinically proven to reduce caries	"Off-label" use since it is only approved by the FDA for treatment of hypersensitivity; however, effective for caries prevention
Flavor Analysis	Slightly tart due to low pH	No tartness or aftertaste due to neutral pH	No tartness or aftertaste due to neutral pH
Fluoride Strength	12,300 ppm	9,040 ppm	22,600 ppm
pH	3.0 to 4.0	7.0	7.0
Potential Adverse Effects	In vitro studies demonstrate aesthetic damage of porcelain, composite resin, glass ionomers, filled sealants, and titanium implants	No documented reports	No documented reports
Recommended Application Time	4 minutes	4 minutes	Apply as directed; sets on contact
Target Patients	Preferred agent for most caries-prone patients	Preferred agent for those • With aesthetic restorations • With reduced salivary flow due to chemotherapy, radiation, or medications • Who cannot tolerate acidic fluorides • With root exposure; caries • With bulimia	Preferred agent for • Children • With aesthetic restorations • With reduced salivary flow due to chemotherapy, radiation, or medications • Demineralized areas around orthodontic appliances • With root exposure; caries

This table has been adapted with permission from R. VanHorn. "A Review of Professional and Home Fluorides." *Journal of Practical Hygiene*, 9(2), 30–31, 2000.

(3) Concentration—1.23 percent fluoride; consists of 12,300 ppm of fluoride

(4) pH—3.0 to 4.0 (acidic)

(5) Application method—most generally given in a tray, but can be painted on using a cotton-tip applicator; usually applied twice annually to patients who are moderate to high risk for caries

(6) Contraindications/disadvantages—low pH level etches ceramic, porcelain, composite, or titanium restorations;[7, 8] therefore, if using APF, coat these surfaces with a petroleum jelly lubricant or cocoa butter prior to application

b. Sodium fluoride (NaF)—also known as neutral sodium fluoride

(1) Forms—foam, gel, liquid, and varnish

(2) Characteristics—absence of taste, therefore acceptable by patients; does not stain teeth, affect restorative materials, or irritate tissues

(3) Indications—can use on porcelain and composite restorations; also recommended for use by bulimic patients who cannot tolerate acidic fluorides

(4) Concentration—2 percent; ready-to-use solution or gel; liquid is prepared by dissolving 0.2 g of powder in 10 ml of distilled water; consists of 9,040 ppm fluoride

(5) pH—7.0 (basic)

(6) Application method—tray form and can also be painted on with a cotton-tip applicator

(7) Varnishes—lacquer-like solution consists of a high concentration of fluoride painted directly on the teeth

  (a) Recommendation—special needs patients because of ease of application and its ability to set rapidly in the presence of saliva, but can be used on everyone; repeat applications at four-month intervals

  (b) Concentration—5.0 percent sodium fluoride (2.26 percent [22,600 ppm] fluoride); treatment requires 0.3–0.5 ml, which contains 3–6 mg of varnish

  (c) Application method—clean teeth by toothbrushing or professional prophylaxis, dry teeth and use paint-on technique; sets promptly

  (d) Protect varnished surfaces as long as possible—instruct patient not to rinse, drink, eat, brush, or floss for at least three to four hours after application to encourage calcium fluoride formation

  (e) Retention—24 to 48 hours; provides a slow release of fluoride

  (f) Advantages—easy to apply, nonoffensive taste, sets upon contact with water or saliva, limits total amount of fluoride swallowed;[8] remains on teeth until brushing or chewing removes it

  (g) Disadvantages—some varnishes cause a temporary discoloration of the teeth on the day of application[8]

c. Stannous fluoride (SnF_2)

(1) Forms

  (a) Powder mixed with distilled water

  (b) Solution in combination with APF as a professional dual-rinse form—not accepted by the ADA

(2) Characteristics—unpleasant taste; staining of demineralized lesions and margins of composite restorations;[8] possibly causes gingival sloughing

(3) Concentration—8 percent; powder form prepared by dissolving 0.8 g of powder in 10 ml of distilled water; consists of 19,360 ppm of fluoride

(4) pH—2.4–2.8; acidic

(5) Application method

  (a) Powder/distilled water form—teeth are isolated, dried, then solution is painted on with cotton tip applicator for one minute

  (b) Solution in combination with APF as a dual-rinse form—swish half of mixture for one minute, expectorate, then swish other half of mixture for another minute and expectorate

(6) Contraindications/disadvantages

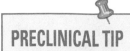

PRECLINICAL TIP

Strengthening Your Knowledge: Varnishes were introduced in 1964 under the trade name Durophat®.[10]

   (a) Powder/distilled water form—not stable, therefore must be prepared immediately before application;[8] not commonly used in dental offices today; however, stannous fluoride is an active ingredient in prescription, self-applied products

   (b) Strong, bitter, metallic taste

   (c) Produces a brownish pigmentation of carious tooth structure

   (d) Gingival irritation—burning sensation of mucosa

  d. Fluoride-containing prophylactic pastes—commonly added to commercially prepared polishing pastes used for polishing

   (1) Contain 4,000 to 20,000 ppm

   (2) Replace fluoride lost from outer layer during polishing, but do not deliver a therapeutic level of fluoride

 2. Application methods

  a. Tray technique (gel or foam)

   (1) Seat patient in an upright position—helps prevent patient from swallowing fluoride

   (2) Select appropriate size tray for patient (Figure 10–1)

    (a) Tray should cover entire dentition; avoid pinching the soft tissues

    (b) Depth of tray should cover beyond neck of teeth and contact the alveolar mucosa—ensures complete coverage of facial and lingual tooth surfaces and prevents saliva from diluting the fluoride gel; if patient has recession, a custom-made tray may be necessary to adequately cover the exposed root surfaces (Figure 10–2)

   (3) Dispense a ribbon of fluoride into the tray; avoid overfilling to prevent ingestion by patient[11]

    (a) Small children—place no more than 2 ml gel in each tray (Figure 10–3)

    (b) Patients with permanent dentition—place 2.5 ml of gel per tray—approximately 40 percent of tray capacity

   (4) Dry teeth thoroughly using compressed air—increases fluoride uptake by enamel

    (a) First dry maxillary facial surfaces

    (b) Then dry over occlusals to palatal surfaces

Figure 10–1   Large, medium and small size fluoride trays.

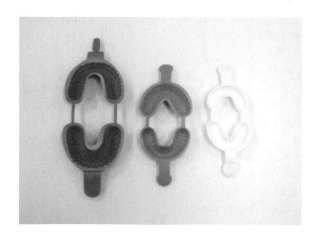

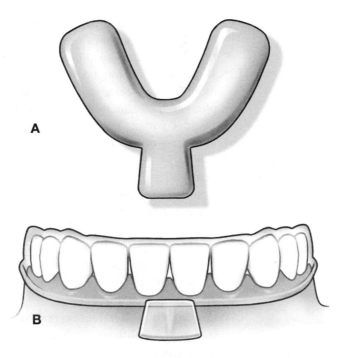

Figure 10–2   Tray Selection. A. Tray. B. A properly fitting tray should cover the entire enamel surfaces.

  (c) Proceed to mandibular linguals

  (d) Then over mandibular occlusals

  (e) Complete drying on the mandibular facial surfaces

 (5) Gently insert tray(s), mandibular portion first—maxillary teeth can maintain a drier state longer than mandibular teeth—followed by maxillary portion when using two trays

 (6) Insert saliva ejector between mandibular and maxillary arches for effective saliva removal; use during entire application—helps prevent swallowing the fluoride and causing acute toxicity (see VI. Fluoride Toxicity)

 (7) Instruct patient to tilt head forward; close teeth and gently tap together—allows excess fluoride to flow to anterior portion of mouth and forces the gel into the proximal areas respectively

 (8) *Do not* leave patient unattended

 (9) Time for four minutes—gives patient the maximum cariostatic benefit; use a timer for accurate length of time

(10) Remove tray

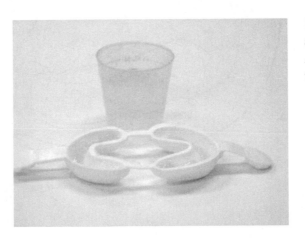

Figure 10–3   Dispense the proper amount of fluoride in the tray. Avoid overfilling to prevent ingestion by the patient.

(11) Reinsert saliva ejector and/or have patient expectorate thoroughly for 30 seconds or until all fluoride is removed from mouth—prevents swallowing remaining saliva and fluoride

(12) Wipe patient's tongue with a gauze sponge dipped in a mouth rinse—removes excess gel and eliminates any unpleasant taste remaining from the fluoride

(13) Instruct patient not to eat, drink, chew, or smoke for 30 minutes—results in increased fluoride deposition

b. Paint-on technique (solution or gel)

(1) Seat patient in an upright position—helps prevent patient from swallowing

(2) Place cotton rolls on garmers (cotton-roll holders) (Figure 10–4)

  (a) Place short cotton roll on lingual surface

  (b) Place long cotton roll on facial surface

(3) Place a Dri-angle over opening of parotid duct in cheek—helps keep area dry

(4) Insert cotton roll holder on one half of mouth—both maxillary and mandibular teeth will be isolated and treated simultaneously

(5) Insert saliva ejector on opposite side of garmers

(6) Dry teeth with compressed air—dry maxillary teeth first, since they can maintain dryness longer

  (a) First dry maxillary facial surfaces

  (b) Then dry over occlusals to palatal surfaces

  (c) Proceed to mandibular linguals

  (d) Then over mandibular occlusals

  (e) Complete drying on the mandibular facial surfaces

(7) Apply fluoride gel or solution with cotton-tip applicator

(8) Set timer for four minutes

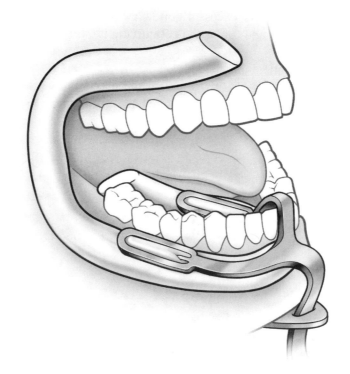

Figure 10–4 Using cotton rolls to isolate the teeth. Each half of the mouth will be treated separately. Use a long cotton roll and extend from the mandibular anterior vestibule to the maxillary anterior vestibule. A small cotton roll is placed next to the tongue over the floor of the mouth.

(9) Continue application of fluoride moistening all tooth surfaces

(10) After time is completed, remove cotton rolls

(11) Reinsert saliva ejector and/or have patient expectorate for 30 seconds or until all fluoride is removed from the mouth

(12) Continue to opposite side and repeat procedure

(13) Wipe patient's tongue with a gauze sponge dipped in a mouth rinse—removes excess and eliminates any unpleasant taste from the fluoride

(14) Instruct patient *not* to eat, drink, rinse, brush, chew, or smoke for 30 minutes

  c. Varnish

    (1) Preparation—by quadrant for ease of application

      (a) Isolate teeth with cotton rolls

      (b) Remove excess moisture from teeth with a cotton roll or a gentle stream of compressed air; however, *varnish will adhere to moist teeth*

      (c) Apply a thin covering of varnish with a swab, cotton-tipped, or disposable brush applicator

      (d) Use saliva ejector if necessary; however, sets rapidly even in the presence of saliva

    (2) Instructions to patient

      (a) After application, have patient rinse with water before leaving; helps remove any residual material from the tongue

      (b) Do *not* eat crunchy foods or brush for at least 3 to 4 hours after application—allows for maximum retention of the varnish; varnish should remain on teeth overnight

      (c) Brush and floss the following day to remove varnish—allows slow release of the fluoride onto the enamel

D. Self-applied topical fluorides (Table 10–4)[9]: Self-applied topical fluorides are available for patients with a high-caries rate, high caries risk

Table 10–4   Comparison of Home Fluoride Gels

	Stannous Fluoride (SnF$_2$) 0.4%	Neutral Sodium Fluoride (NaF) 1.1%
Application Frequency	Daily application	Daily application
Application Methods	Brush (typically at bedtime) following dentifrice or tray	Brush (typically at bedtime) following dentifrice or tray
Documented Efficacy	Clinically proven to reduce incidence of caries	Clinically proven to reduce incidence of caries
Flavor Analysis	Pleasant; slight metallic taste	Pleasant
Fluoride Strength (ppm)	1,000 ppm	5,000 ppm
pH	2.8 to 5.0	7.0
Potential Side Effects	May produce extrinsic stain; not recommended when aesthetic restorations are present; not recommended for children under 6 years of age	Keep out of reach of children; not recommended for children under 6 years of age
Target Patients	Recommended for • Patients who need both caries control and plaque reduction • Some orthodontic and periodontal patients • Patients with dentinal hypersensitivity	Recommended for • Patients with porcelain or composite restorations • Patients who cannot tolerate acidic fluorides as a result of xerostomia, bulimia, soft tissue radiation chemotherapy, or systemic disease • Orthodontic patients with decalcification • Patients using home whitening

This table has been adapted with permission from R. VanHorn. "A Review of Professional and Home Fluorides. *Journal of Practical Hygiene,* 9(2), 30–31, 2000.

(e.g., radiation/chemotherapy treatments), root caries, root sensitivity, xerostomia, and/or those in orthodontia. They include use of OTC or prescribed products, such as toothpastes, mouth rinses, and gels, and provide additional forms of frequent, low-concentration fluoride to promote remineralization (bacteriostatic effect). It is recommended patients not drink or eat after application.

1. Applied by rinsing, using trays, or toothbrushing
   a. Rinsing
      (1) Patient swishes measured amount of solution for one minute and expectorates upon completion
      (2) Contraindicated in children under 6-years-old—swallowing reflex is immature
   b. Trays
      (1) Trays can be custom-made—fabricated specifically for patient—or disposable; choose a size that properly fits the dentition
      (2) Requires good manual dexterity for placement and removal
      (3) Requires dispensing correct amount of gel per manufacturer's directions
      (4) Time correctly as recommended per manufacturer's directions
      (5) Expectorate upon completion
      (6) *Do not* eat or drink for 30 minutes
   c. Toothbrushing
      (1) Use instructed brushing techniques to apply gel or paste to dentition, usually once a day; use interproximal brush to apply fluoride to furca or accessible proximal areas
      (2) Allow gel to remain on teeth for one minute
      (3) Expectorate upon completion
      (4) *Do not* eat or drink for 30 minutes

E. Fluoride in dental products[3]—provides low concentration of fluoride on a regular basis, which is highly effective in controlling caries activity; provides bacteriostatic affect
   1. OTC products
      a. Dentifrices—contain approximately 1,000 to 1,500 ppm F (e.g. 1.0 mg F/g); sodium fluoride is the most commonly used fluoride; use at least twice daily
      b. Mouth rinses (Table 10–5)—concentrated solution intended for daily use; contain 225 ppm—0.05 percent sodium fluoride
   2. Prescription products
      a. Mouth rinses—

Table 10–5   Comparison of Fluoride Rinses[4]

	NaF (OTC) 0.05%	NaF (Rx) 0.2%	APF (Rx) 0.044%	SnF$_2$ (OTC) 0.1%
Application Frequency	Daily Application	Weekly Application	Daily Application	Daily Application
Fluoride Strength	230 ppm	900 ppm	225 ppm	244 ppm
Indications	Caries prevention; children over 6 years of age	Moderate to high-risk caries; school-based rinse programs	Moderate to high-risk caries	Moderate to high-risk caries; dentinal hypersensitivity
Other	Alcohol-free available		Can etch some restorative materials	

        (1) Neutral sodium fluoride (NaF) 0.2%—contains 900 ppm fluoride; commonly used in school-based programs; intended for weekly use

        (2) Acidulated phosphate fluoride (APF) 0.044%—contains 225 ppm fluoride; used on a daily basis

     b. Brush-on gels; intended for use on a daily basis; include

        (1) Neutral sodium fluoride (NaF)—1.1 percent (5,000 ppm) fluoride

        (2) Stannous fluoride (SnF_2)—0.4 percent (1,000 ppm) fluoride—accepted by the ADA as a desensitizing agent as well

        (3) Acidulated phosphate fluoride (APF) gel—0.5 percent (5,000 ppm) fluoride

VI. Fluoride Toxicity

Fluoride is safe when used as directed. Fluoride toxicity can occur by ingesting too much fluoride during tooth development (chronic), which can lead to fluorosis, or by ingesting fluoride, by accident, during a professional or self-applied method causing an acute toxic reaction.

A. Acute fluoride toxicity

   1. Signs and symptoms—usually begin approximately 30 minutes after exposure and can last for up to 24 hours

     a. Gastrointestinal—includes nausea, vomiting, abdominal cramping, and discomfort; caused by the formation of hydrofluoric acid in the stomach

     b. Neurological—tetany, paresthesia, and central nervous system depression

     c. Cardiovascular—weak pulse, hypotension, and cardiac irregularities

     d. Other—increased thirst and salivation

     e. Onset of three Cs—coma, convulsions, and cardiac arrhythmias

   2. Emergency treatment

     a. Initiate first aid treatment

        (1) Administer—fluoride-binding agent such as milk or other calcium or aluminum preparations (lime water, Maalox®, or condensed milk)—protects the lining of the stomach and provides the necessary calcium to which the fluoride can bind

        (2) Induce vomiting (emesis) digitally or with syrup of ipecac—often happens simultaneously and helps expel majority of fluoride

     b. Seek medical treatment—refer patient to emergency room; blood calcium levels will need to be maintained; patient may need intravenous calcium

   3. Toxicology of fluoride—determined by weight by kilogram (2.2 pounds equals one kilogram);[12] (see Table 10–6)

     a. Certainly lethal dose (CLD)—amount of drug likely to cause death if not intercepted be antidotal therapy

        (1) Adult CLD—can occur when 5 to 10 grams of sodium fluoride is taken at once

        (2) Child CLD—can occur when approximately 0.5 to 1.0 grams of sodium fluoride is taken at once (varies with size and weight of child)

     b. Safely tolerated dose (STD) = one quarter of CLD

Table 10–6   Treatment for Fluoride Ingestion

Milligram Fluoride Ion per Kilogram Body Weight	Treatment
Less than 5 mg/kg	1. Administer calcium, aluminum, or magnesium.
More than 5 mg/kg (toxic)	1. Induce vomiting. 2. Administer soluble calcium. 3. Seek medical treatment.
More than 15 mg/kg (lethal)	1. Admit to hospital immediately. 2. Monitor heart.

     (1) Adult STD—1.25 to 2.5 grams of sodium fluoride taken at one time

     (2) Child STD—0.5 grams of sodium fluoride taken at one time

  c. Prevention

     (1) In office

        (a) Seat patient in an upright position with head tilted forward

        (b) Dispense proper amount of fluoride in trays—no more than 40 percent of tray capacity

        (c) Use suction throughout procedure

        (d) After application, have patient expectorate and/or use saliva ejector for 30 seconds or until all fluoride is removed

        (e) *Never* leave patient unattended

     (2) At home

        (a) Provide thorough instructions on how to properly use product

        (b) Promote parental supervision at home with children

        (c) Keep products out of the reach of children

        (d) Limit amount of gel placed in each custom-made tray to 5 to 10 drops

        (e) Use only a pea-sized amount of toothpaste (approximately 0.25g) for children; make sure child expectorates and *does not* swallow toothpaste

        (f) *Do not* allow children less than 6 years of age to use mouth rinses—swallowing reflex is immature

B. Chronic fluoride toxicity

  1. Fluorosis (also known as "brown stain" or "mottled enamel") is a permanent hypomineralized change of the tooth enamel caused from excess ingestion of fluoridated water (more than 2 ppm) during enamel mineralization. Those at risk for enamel fluorosis are limited to children aged ≤ 8. After this age, the crowns of all the permanent teeth have already developed, except for the third molars.

    a. Forms

     (1) Very mild to mild—appears as chalk-like markings across enamel

     (2) Moderate (mottled enamel)—covers ≥ 50 percent of enamel surface as opaque white with possible brown stain

     (3) Severe (mottled enamel)—brown staining and discrete pitting; enamel may break away and is modified with elective cosmetic treatment

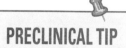

PRECLINICAL TIP

Strengthening Your Knowledge: Using a pea-sized amount of toothpaste twice a day requires two tubes of toothpaste per year.[3]

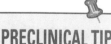

PRECLINICAL TIP

Strengthening Your Knowledge: There is an increasing prevalence of dental fluorosis among children from both fluoridated and nonfluoridated communities due to an increased intake of various fluoride sources.[13]

(4) Skeletal fluorosis—results from high level of continual intake of fluoridated water (10 to 25 ppm) over a period of years or through an industrial exposure; may include isolated instance of osteosclerosis

b. Prevention

(1) Use an optimally adjusted concentration of fluoride in community water—0.7 ppm to 1.2 ppm depending on average maximum daily air temperature

(2) Use only a pea-sized amount of toothpastes for children under 8 to help reduce incidence of fluorosis

(3) If drinking water from a private source, such as a well, have fluoride measured to determine amount; may need to consider drinking bottled water

Fluorides have been proven to greatly reduce the incidence in caries in both children and adults. However, caution must be taken when administering fluoride to prevent acute and chronic toxicity. Caution must also be taken at home when using products daily such as toothpastes and mouth rinses, especially with children. They are at risk for swallowing rinses when under the age of 6, since their swallowing reflex is immature.

QUESTIONS

1. When evaluating a patient's diet, the MOST important contributing factor in the demineralization process is the
   a. amount of fermentable carbohydrates consumed.
   b. consistency of the food.
   c. frequency of intake of fermentable carbohydrates.
   d. amount of sugar added to the food.

2. All of the following are causes of decreased salivary flow EXCEPT one. Which one is the EXCEPTION?
   a. Use of sedatives
   b. Tobacco use
   c. Drinking water low in fluoride
   d. Diabetes

3. Which of the following is a contraindication for using acidulated phosphate fluoride as a professional topical application?
   a. Etches ceramic surfaces
   b. Strong, metallic, bitter taste
   c. Produces a brownish pigmentation of carious tooth structures
   d. Burning sensation of mucosa

4. For children, which of the following is the proper amount of fluoride, in milliliters, to dispense into a tray?

   a. 1
   b. 2
   c. 2.5
   d. 4

5. Professional topical fluorides have been proven to reduce tooth decay. They should be applied on all patients at routine prophylaxis appointments, regardless of necessity, as a preventive measure.
   a. Both statements are TRUE.
   b. Both statements are FALSE.
   c. The first statement is TRUE. The second statement is FALSE.
   d. The first statement is FALSE. The second statement is TRUE.

6. Approximately what percent of communities in the United States receive optimally fluoridated water?
   a. 20
   b. 50
   c. 65
   d. 75

7. A patient comes to the dental hygiene clinic for a routine prophylaxis appointment. Upon examination, it is determined the patient has active caries and lives in an area that has < 0.7 ppm of fluoride in the community water system. Which of the following recommendations should be made regarding professional topical fluoride application?

a. No topical fluoride application is necessary.
b. Apply topical fluoride two times per year.
c. Apply topical fluoride three times per year.
d. Apply topical fluoride four times per year.

8. All of the following are recommendations to prevent a 6-year-old from swallowing fluoride at home EXCEPT one. Which one is the EXCEPTION?
   a. Have parental supervision.
   b. Use only a pea-sized amount of toothpaste.
   c. Use a saliva ejector.
   d. Do *not* use mouth rinses.

9. In parts per million (ppm), which of the following is the ideal concentration of fluoride in community drinking water systems?

a. 1
b. 2
c. 3
d. 4

10. The patient should be instructed to not eat, drink, or smoke after a professional topical fluoride application. In minutes, what is the recommended length of time?
    a. 10
    b. 20
    c. 30
    d. 40

REFERENCES

1. Featherstone, J. Elements of a Successful Adults Caries Preventive Program. *Compendium of Continuing Education in Oral Hygiene,* 8(1), 3–9, 2001.

2. VanHorn, R. Fluoride Therapy–Not Just for Kids. *Journal of Practical Hygiene,* 9(3), 51–55, 2000.

3. Centers for Disease Control and Prevention. MMWR. Recommendations for using fluoride to prevent and control caries in the United States. 50(RR-14). 2001.

4. Caries Diagnosis and Risk Assessment: A Review of Preventive Strategies and Management. *Journal of the American Dental Association,* Supplement 126 (1-S-24-S), 1995.

5. Mallott, M. E. Preventive Strategies for the Older Dental Patient. *Journal of the Indiana Dental Association,* 76(4), 44–49, 1997–98.

6. Carberry, F. J., & A. Hazelwood. A Practical Guide to Adult Caries Risk Assessment Fluoride Use. *Compendium of Continuing Education in Oral Hygiene,* 8(1), 10–17, 2001.

7. Warren, D. P., H. A. Henson, & J. T. Chan. A Survey of In-Office Use of Fluorides in the Houston Area. *Journal of Dental Hygiene,* 70(4), 166–171, 1996.

8. Newbrun, E. Evolution of Professionally Applied Topical Fluoride Therapies. *A Supplement to Compendium of Continuing Education in Dentistry,* 20(1), 5–9, 1999.

9. VanHorn, R. A Review of Professional and Home Fluorides. *Journal of Practical Hygiene,* 9(2), 30–31, 2000.

10. Warren, D. P., H. A. Henson, & J. T. Chan. Dental Hygienists and Patient Comparisons of Fluoride Varnishes to Fluoride Gels. *Journal of Dental Hygiene,* 74(2), 94–101, 2000.

11. Garcia-Godoy, F., M. J. Hicks, C. M. Flaitz, & J. H. Berg, Acidulated Phosphate Fluoride Treatment and Formation of Caries-like Lesions in Enamel: Effect of Application Time. *Journal of Clinical Pediatric Dentistry,* 19(2), 105–110, 1995.

12. Harris, N. O., & F. Garcia-Godoy. *Primary Preventive Dentistry,* 6th ed. Prentice Hall, New Jersey 2003.

13. Kleber, C. J., M. S. Putt, C. E. Smith, & C.W. Gish. Effect of Supervised Use of an Alum Mouthrinse on Dental Caries Incidence in Caries-Susceptible Children: A Pilot Study. *Journal of Dentistry for Children,* 63(6), 393–401, 1996.

APF/SODIUM FLUORIDE SKILL SHEET

Student _____

Date _____

Instructor _____

Re-evaluation
Instr: _____
Date _____

Re-evaluation
Instr: _____
Date _____

	S	U	Comments	S	U	Comments	S	U	Comments
1. Selects correct tray size.									
2. Places adequate amount of solution in tray.									
3. Seats patient in an upright position.									
4. Thoroughly dries teeth prior to application—maxillary arch first.									
5. Inserts tray in mouth–mandibular arch first.									
6. Inserts saliva ejector between arches, which remains throughout procedure.									
7. Instructs patient to tilt head forward and gently tap teeth together.									
8. Continuously monitors patient.									
9. Follows proper timing of fluoride.									
10. Removes saliva ejector and tray from mouth.									
11. Wipes excess fluoride from tongue.									
12. Reinserts saliva ejector.									
13. Gives appropriate postoperative instructions.									

Courtesy of Indiana University Purdue University Dental Hygiene Program

Index

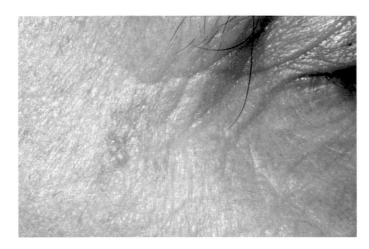

Figure 4–4   Basal cell carcinoma.

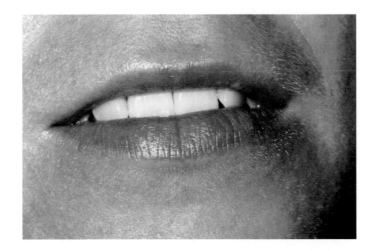

Figure 4–5   Normal lips.

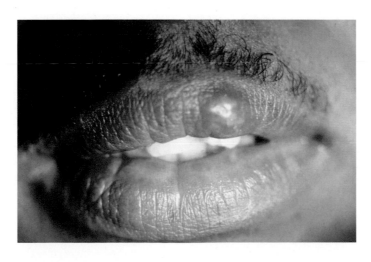

Figure 4–6   Herpes labialis.

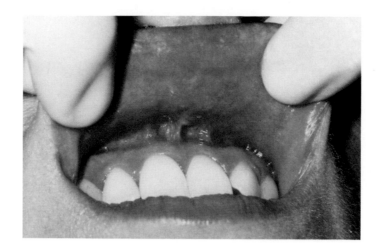

Figure 4–23   Retracting upper lip.

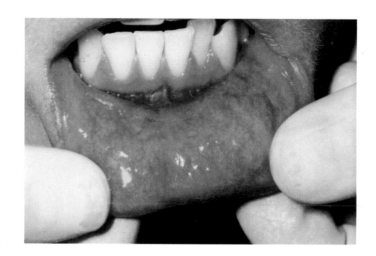

Figure 4–24   Retracting lower lip.

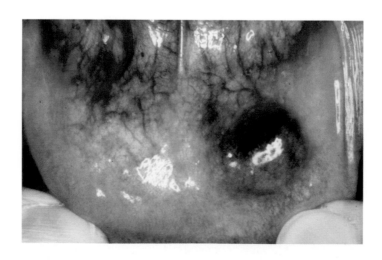

Figure 4–26   Hemangioma.

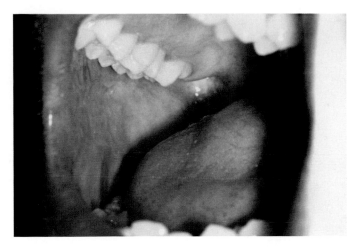

Figure 4–27   Right buccal mucosa.

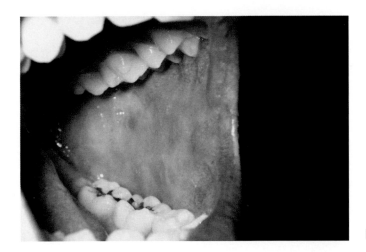

Figure 4–28   Left buccal mucosa.

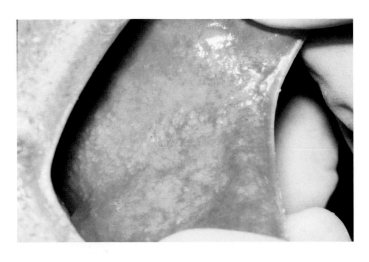

Figure 4–30   Fordyce granules.

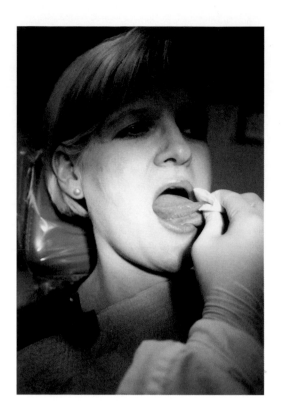

Figure 4–31   Inspecting right lateral border of tongue.

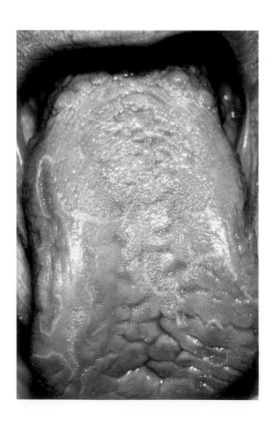

Figure 4–34   Fissured tongue.

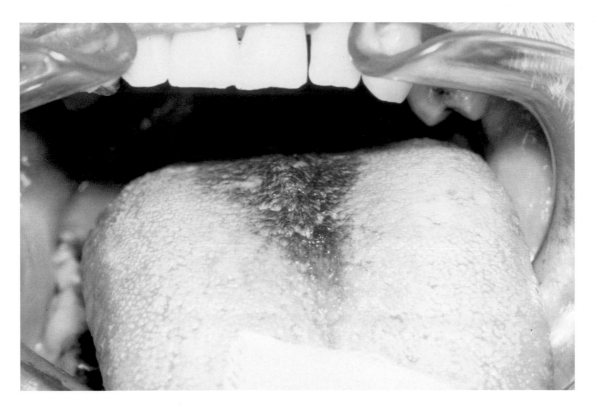

Figure 4–35   Black hairy tongue.

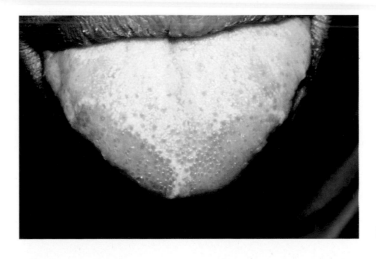

Figure 4–36   Geographic tongue.

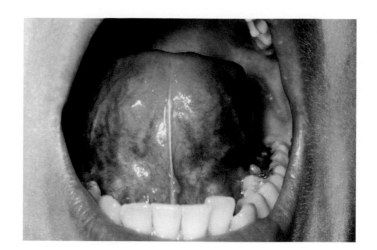

Figure 4–37   Ventral surface of tongue.

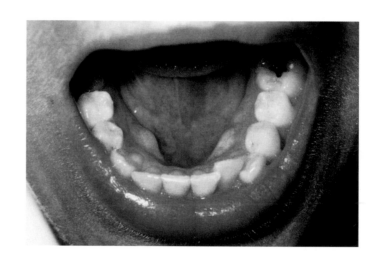

Figure 4–38   Floor of mouth.

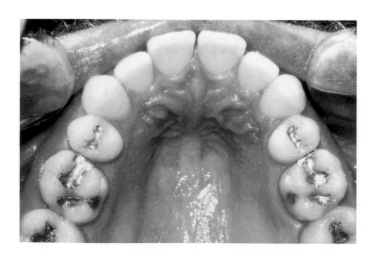

Figure 4–42   Hard palate.

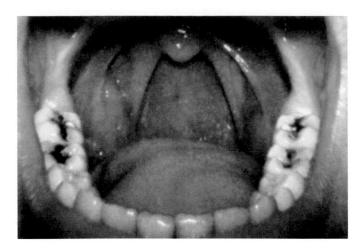

Figure 4–44   Palatine tonsils.

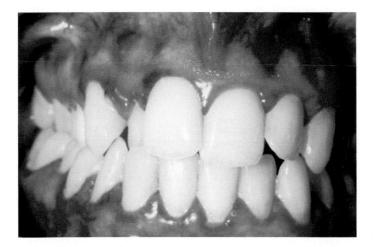

Figure 4–47   Gingivitis.

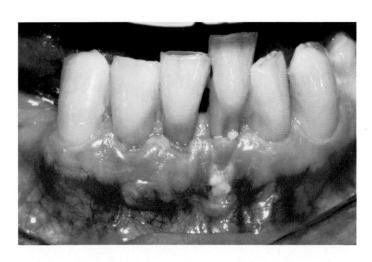

Figure 4–48   Recession, plaque, and purulis.

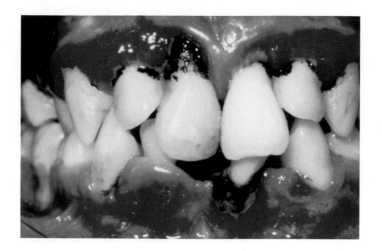

Figure 4–49 Progressed periodontitis.